BIOLOGY OF CANCER

Second Edition

Dedication

To all who nurse, take care of and
administer to patients with cancer.

BIOLOGY OF CANCER

Second Edition

Editors:

E. J. AMBROSE, D.Sc.

Chester Beatty Research Institute
Institute of Cancer Research, London

F. J. C. ROE, D.M., D.Sc., F.R.C.Path.

Member of the Institute
of Cancer Research, London

ELLIS HORWOOD LIMITED

Publisher · Chichester

Halsted Press · a division of
JOHN WILEY & SONS, Inc.
New York · London · Sydney · Toronto

First published in 1975 by
ELLIS HORWOOD LIMITED
Coll House, Westergate, Chichester, Sussex, England

Distributed in:

Australia, New Zealand, South-east Asia by
JOHN WILEY & SONS AUSTRALASIA PTY LIMITED
110 Alexander Street, Crow's Nest, N.S.W. Australia

Europe, Africa by
JOHN WILEY & SONS LIMITED
Baffins Lane, Chichester, Sussex, England

Canada by
JOHN WILEY & SONS CANADA LIMITED
22 Worcester Road, Rexdale, Ontario, Canada

United States, Mexico, South America and the rest of the world by
HALSTED PRESS a division of JOHN WILEY & SONS INC.
605 Third Avenue, New York, N.Y. 10016, U.S.A.

Library of Congress Cataloging in Publication Data

Ambrose, Edmund Jack, ed.
Biology of Cancer.

Based on Lectures given at the Chester Beatty Research Institute,
Institute of Cancer Research, Royal Cancer Hospital, London.
Includes bibliographies and index.
I. Cancer. I. Roe, Francis J. C., joint ed. II. Title.
(DNLM: 1. Neoplasms. QZ200 A496b)
RC262.A4 1975 616.9'94 74-26860
ISBN 0-470-02527-1 (Halsted Press)
ISBN 85312-016-1 (Ellis Horwood)

Printed in Great Britain by
Cox & Wyman Ltd,
London, Fakenham and Reading

CONTENTS

PREFACE TO SECOND EDITION

The First Edition of this book was based on a course of lectures held at the Institute of Cancer Research, London. The decade since its inception has witnessed an explosion in fundamental and technical knowledge and the waves caused by this explosion have transformed our understanding of the mechanisms involved in the initial development and subsequent natural history of neoplastic processes. Four new chapters have been incorporated into the text and others have been completely revised. It would have been difficult to subdivide the subject of the book into discrete topics and to have succeeded in doing so would have detracted from the value of the book. Many areas of knowledge dovetail with each other in such a way that their clean separation would have been artificial and misleading. The subject of this book could, perhaps, be thought of as a piece of sculpture, which the various authors have described from different view-points, depending on their training interests and experience. The same is there for all to see, but each author discusses different features.

We have tried to assemble a book which is a reasonably comprehensive and up-to-date survey of the principal biological mechanisms underlying cancer as a disease process. Constraints affecting the overall length of the book forced us to be selective and with regret we felt obliged to omit certain topics, notably tumour cell kinetics and the relevant biological properties of ionising radiation.

The book is intended for graduates in medicine and science, whose interests or work lead them to seek knowledge about cancer — its incidence, causation and some principles underlying its treatment. For such individuals the book provides an initial insight and references to the principal research papers.

We owe many debts of gratitude for help in preparing this Second Edition: to the Authors and their Secretaries, to Dr. Richard Carter who helped with the editing, to our own Secretaries and to Mr. Ellis Horwood, the Publisher.

E. J. Ambrose
F. J. C. Roe
January, 1975

Note

The Editorial Royalties will be given to St. Joseph's Hospice, Hackney, London—a place pre-eminently concerned with the care of terminal cancer patients.

Chapter **1**

THE NATURE AND OCCURRENCE OF NEOPLASTIC DISEASES

FRANCIS J. C. ROE, D.M., D.SC., F.R.C.Path.
Member of the Institute of Cancer Research, London

During the eight years since the first edition of this book was published, knowledge about neoplastic diseases has greatly increased. Bridges have been built between different areas of special knowledge and more scientists working in the field share a common understanding of the nature of the problems facing them. It is, therefore, no longer necessary to start the second edition with a lengthy account of the nature of neoplastic diseases. The same ground is covered in summary form only, but additional comments dealing with certain other general aspects of neoplastic diseases have been added.

The nature of neoplastic diseases

Cancer is a disease process which may affect multicellular organisms and which is characterized by the seemingly uncontrolled multiplication and spread within such organisms of abnormal forms of their own cells.

Theoretically, biological processes similar to those which are manifested as cancers in higher animals may also affect simpler forms of animal life including unicellular organisms. But if so, cancer must be defined in such a way that it may apply to both higher and lower species. The definition given above does not meet this requirement.

Theoretically, in a higher organism, a cancer could be the result of a fault at the organizational level—a defect in the way an organism maintains its structure despite various environmental assaults. We are, however, profoundly ignorant of the factors concerned in the establishment and maintenance of normal supracellular organization—the sociology of cells—and fundamental cancer research is dominated by studies directed at elucidating abnormalities in cancers at the cellular and subcellular levels. Although there is scope for debate as to whether cellular and subcellular changes are primary or secondary in relation to the disease process, most of the contents of this book are based on the assumption that they are indeed primary; this does not, however, mean that cancers are diseases *of* cells. Cancers should be regarded as diseases affecting whole animals—including human animals—and not as diseases of particular tissues or of particular cells.

In the course of unravelling the mysteries of neoplastic disease, investigators have sought and used comparatively simple model systems. In the past, confusion, misunderstanding and disappointment has resulted from the too ready assumption that the human body is an accumulation of non-interacting simple model systems.

Until about ten years ago, much cancer research, including most of the attempts to develop drugs intended for the treatment of patients with cancers, was concerned almost solely with the uncontrolled multiplication of cells. It is now widely appreciated that in many normal tissues cell replication takes place more rapidly than in most cancers; indeed, in some of the more lethal types of neoplastic disease, cell multiplication proceeds only relatively slowly. It is therefore obvious that the selective elimination of cancer cells cannot be achieved by treating a patient with a drug which indiscriminately damages all dividing cells. Accordingly, the chapter in the present edition dealing with the chemotherapy of patients with cancer is mainly concerned with the development of agents which selectively attack cancer cells, selectively being attempted by exploitation of differences between particular kinds of cancer cell and normal cells.

Immunological approaches to the treatment of patients with cancerous diseases did not, historically, arise as an extension of attempts by scientists trying to find effective drugs based on the exploitation of differences between cancer cells and normal cells. None the less, the antigenic peculiarities of cancer cells are eminently exploitable. Current attempts to exploit immunological differences in cancer treatment may well be regarded as naïve and crude, but the fund of basic knowledge in this area is accumulating rapidly (Chapter 12).

It would be wrong to omit from any general discussion of the nature of neoplastic disease a statement to the effect that cancer is not a single disease process but a galaxy of disease processes. No well-informed scientist would nowadays postulate a single all-embracing theory relevant to the occurrence of all forms of cancer; and no such scientist would expect to be able to formulate any useful general theory or hypothesis that could lead to a single new effective method of preventing all forms of the disease or of treating cancer patients irrespective of which form of cancer they had. Not only is cancer not a single disease entity but, in the case of most of the forms of the disease, multiple factors contribute to its causation and clinical course. Thus exposure to a variety of environmental agents may predispose to the same kind of cancer, and whether and when an individual develops cancer may be determined by a number of different factors or conditions acting simultaneously or sequentially, some more important and some less important. The combined effects of two or more agents may be additive or multiplicatory. Factors which delay or inhibit the appearance of cancers after exposure to carcinogens are known in experimental animals—for instance, reduced calorie intake and absence of the bacterial flora in the gut. Increasing recognition of these aspects of the problem has laid the foundations of bridges between specialized research disciplines. It is no longer questioned that a virus might be implicated in the development of a cancer in response to exposure to a chemical agent, or that an immunological disturbance might tip the balance —in favour or against—the development of cancer following exposure to a virus or to a chemical agent.

In the last analysis, it is probably true that each example of neoplastic disease is the outcome of a unique set of circumstances, including the genetically-determined uniqueness of the individual animal (human) affected, the viruses he carries and the uniqueness of the pattern of his exposure to relevant environmental factors.

The occurrence of neoplastic diseases

Unequivocal neoplastic diseases have been encountered in animal species from the lowest forms of vertebrate up to man, it is questionable, whether diseases referred to as cancers in subvertebrates and plants are truly cancerous.

In the countries of Western Europe and North America, it has been calculated that about one in four people develop one or more forms of neoplastic disease and one out of five people die from such a disease. These figures are approximately equal for both males and females although the spectra of common types of cancer affecting the two sexes are different. In males, lung cancer accounts for 40 per cent of cancer deaths, and cancers arising in the stomach, colon and rectum make up a further 30 per cent. In women the four commonest fatal forms of cancer (in descending order of frequency) are of the breast, colon and rectum, stomach and uterus; deaths from these account for about 60 per cent of all deaths from neoplastic disease.

The relative chances of dying from cancer as opposed to dying from some other kind of disease have increased during the present century because the risk of dying from infectious diseases such as tuberculosis or pneumonia have fallen greatly with the introduction of effective chemotherapeutic drugs. After correction for the beneficial effects of new drugs, the age-standardized risk of death from different forms of cancer has changed relatively little except for cancers of the lung. The age-standardized death rates from lung cancer in women aged between sixty and sixty-five and born around 1901 is more than double that for similarly aged women born thirty years later. In men the corresponding increase is more than sevenfold (See Case, 1956[1]). These increases in death rates for lung cancer have been more than offset in women by reduced death rates from cancers of the stomach, colon and rectum, breast and uterus. But in men, reduced death rates from cancers of the stomach, colon and rectum, oesophagus and oral cavity have not been sufficient to offset the dramatic rise in lung cancer death rate; the overall result is that the age-standardized risk of death from any form of malignant disease has been increasing in men. After the Second World War, there occurred in both sexes an increased risk of death from cancers of the blood forming tissues (leukaemias). This increase appears to have stopped, but it is too early to be sure whether the incidence has started to fall.

Clearly, death from one or other form of neoplastic disease is not rare. If the chances of dying from cancer were distributed randomly among the population, most families of average size would be expected to have at least one case, and multiple cancer deaths would be seen in some. If, however, the spectrum of neoplastic disease is split up into types according to the organ or tissue primarily affected, or on some other basis, the chances of two or more deaths from the same type of cancer occurring in the same family would be much smaller. Misconceptions about the familial nature of cancer have arisen through failure to distinguish between different forms of the disease and to appreciate that common events commonly occur. The fact that a family shares the same environment may mean that all its members are exposed to a particular environmental carcinogen: thus if cigarette smokers breed cigarette smokers they are at the same time breeding children with a greater than normal risk of developing lung cancer.

A combination of careful definition of types of neoplastic disease and painstaking epidemiology has begun to enable a distinction to be made between the genetic and environmental factors which contribute to the causation of specified types of cancer. One of the most exciting recent developments in this field is the accumulation of evidence that a transmissable infectious agent may be a factor in the causation of Hodgkin's disease—a form of cancer affecting lymphoreticular tissue (Vianna *et al.*, 1971, 1972[2, 3]).

Although many people develop cancers of some kind and one in five of all deaths is from the disease, it does not follow that family doctors have great experience of diagnosing or treating any particular form of the disease. A general practitioner looking after 3,500 patients will, if their distribution by age and sex conform to the national pattern, encounter some forty deaths per annum: only eight of these will be from one or other form of cancer. In addition, each year he will see for the first time two patients with cancers of which they are subsequently cured. Of the 10 patients, two would be men with primary cancers of the lung, three would be men or women with cancers of the gastrointestinal tract, and one would be a woman with breast cancer. He would see less than one case per year of any other form of cancer.

Nearly two decades ago, Logan and Cushion (1958)[4] reported that only about one per cent of patients consulting general practitioners for the first time about a particular illness or set of symptoms had cancer. On the other hand, unlike simple colds and coughs, the development of a cancer may require many visits to the doctor. Thus Logan and Cushion found that 15 per cent of actual consultations between doctors and patients involved patients suffering from one or other form of cancer.

Figures such as these help us to see the frequency of occurrence of human cancer in a broad perspective. They also explain why every general practitioner is not and cannot be expected to be a cancer specialist: although he sees many patients with cancers, he sees only very few examples of any one form of the disease. An important recent development in Britain is the decision to establish throughout the country specialist Oncological Centres for the investigation, diagnosis and treatment of patients with cancers. At such centres it should be possible for individual doctors to accumulate experience in the diagnosis and treatment of narrowly defined forms of neoplastic disease and to undertake research on them.

The history of medical research shows that detailed investigation of many examples of what appear to be the same disease often leads to the discovery that the disease in question is not a single entity; or that the cases that are seen are the tip of an iceberg made up mostly of subclinical disease. For example, although cancer of the prostate gland is responsible for the deaths of only about two in every 100 men, careful microscopic examination of the prostates of men of eighty years and older dying from causes other than cancer of the prostate, revealed the presence of 'latent' cancers of microscopic dimensions in more than half of them (Franks 1954[5]). It could well be that a high proportion of ostensibly healthy people have latent cancers in various sites or even actively, but very slowly, growing cancers. The statement made earlier that one in five humans develops cancer would be utterly wrong if one included subclinical cancers in the definition of cancer.

Even where cancers cause death, death rates for different forms of neoplastic disease are subject to wide error. Post-mortem examination is the exception rather than the rule and yet where post-mortem examination is carried out, serious differences between ante-mortem and post-mortem diagnosis are not uncommon. The best that one can hope is that misdiagnoses in the case of deaths without autopsy, will to some extent cancel each other out, and that the sources of inaccuracy are more or less the same from year to year and from place to place. If this is not the case we are in a poor position to monitor cancer incidence by collecting and analysing epidemiological data, and we cannot be sure that the apparent upward and downward trends in death rates in Britain (see above) for cancers of different sites represent real changes in incidence.

During the last decade or so, it has become customary to suspect that genetic factors are responsible for 20 per cent or less of the human cancer burden, while 80 per cent of the burden is the result of exposure to environmental carcinogens. There is little sure scientific basis for these actual figures, and even less for the assumption that exposure to chemical agents as opposed to physical or viral agents is largely responsible for the environmental contribution to the burden.

The patterns of apparent incidence of different forms of neoplastic disease vary widely from one country to another. For most undeveloped countries with poorly developed medical services the figures for cancer morbidity and cancer mortality are, unless special surveys are made, so inaccurate as to be useless for the purposes of comparisons with other countries. This is especially true in the case of cancers of the more inaccessible sites of the body. Forms of cancer of more accessible sites such as Burkitt's lymphoma affecting the jaw, cancer of the nasopharynx, cancer of the skin, or cancer of oesophagus are known to occur in widely different incidences in different countries, and these are presently the subject of intensive study. Of special interest in this connection is the fact that widely different attack rates for particular forms of cancer are sometimes seen in neighbouring localities. Thus both in Kenya (Cook and Burkitt, 1971[6]) and on the Southern shores of the Caspian Sea (Kinet and Mahboubi, 1972[7], Mahboubi *et al.*, 1973[8]) localized communities with widely differing incidences of cancer of the oesophagus have been found side by side. Comparisons between countries with well-developed medical services are clearly more meaningful, but even here differences in diagnostic methods, standards, terminology, autopsy rates etc. may superimpose variation due to observer differences on any real differences that may be present. Even after allowing for this possibility, however, there has been justifiable interest in the very wide differences in cancer incidence between certain countries, notably Japan and the U.S.A. Cancers of the stomach occur about five times more frequently in Japan than the U.S.A., but cancers of the colon and breast are far less frequent and rates for many other forms of cancer are also lower in Japan (Haenszel and Kurihara, 1968[9]). Japanese who migrate from Japan to the U.S.A.—and to an even greater extent their children and grandchildren—tend to 'adopt' the death rates for stomach and colon cancer prevalent in the U.S.A. They retain, however, the low breast cancer death rates seen in Japan. These observations are consistent with the view that environmental factors largely determine stomach and colon cancer death rates whereas genetic factors are more important determinants of breast cancer death rates. Studies on cancer incidence in migrant populations clearly have much to offer in the elucidation of factors involved in the causation of human cancer, but the contribution they can make must depend heavily on the wider use of internationally used definitions and universally applied standards of diagnosis in different countries. Declining autopsy rates in countries such as Britain are undoubtedly associated with a decreasing accuracy in the causes of death as given on death certificates. It is important that this downward trend be reversed.

On theoretical grounds, studies on monozygotic and dizygotic twins might be useful in distinguishing between genetic and environmental influences in cancer causation. In practice, the maintenance of twin registries which are large enough to throw light on factors involved in the causation of particular forms of cancer would be very expensive. Furthermore, the fact that the environment of twins is similar, especially when they are children and when they are monozygotic, means that one cannot assume that genetic factors are responsible when monozygotic twins develop similar cancers in later life.

For certain forms of human cancer, there is evidence that a sequence of changes occurs between an initial normal state and a final stage of malignancy. For some epithelial tissues such as the surface of the uterine cervix, the sequence includes hyperplasia (increased numbers of normally arranged normal cells), dysplasia (increased numbers of normal cells with some atypical cells and some abnormal arrangement of cells but with no major disturbance of tissue structure), carcinoma-in-situ (a severe form of dysplasia, with numerous atypical cells, major disturbance of tissue structure but no invasion of surrounding tissue), and invasive cancer (spread of altered cells derived from one tissue into adjacent different tissues). Some investigators regard carcinoma-in-situ as a 'pre-cancerous change but this is a misleading term. In so far as cancers may arise from normal tissues, the latter may be regarded as 'pre-cancerous'; but in so far as dysplastic lesions and carcinoma-in-situ lesions do not always progress to cancer but sometimes regress instead, they are not pre-cancerous. The concept that is needed is one of *increasing risk*: there is a greater risk of invasive cancer developing at the site of a dysplastic lesion than from normal tissue, and there is a greater risk still of invasive cancer developing from a carcinoma-in-situ lesion than from a dysplastic lesion.

Related to the development of invasive cancers through stages is the phenomenon known as 'tumour progression' (see Foulds, 1969).[10] A tumour, after it is recognizable as such, suddenly starts to grow more quickly, cell types of more abnormal kinds appear in it, and its ability to invade surrounding tissues becomes more evident. It is possible that the sequence of changes from dysplasia → carcinoma-in-situ → low-grade malignancy → cancer of higher-grade malignancy are all programmed at the time of the first essential change from normal to cancerous. Alternatively, the sequence of changes may represent responses to a sequence of stimuli or to changes in the host's reaction to the growing tumour. Examples of all these possibilities can be cited. For instance, agents (tumour promoters) are known which facilitate the development of overt tumours from pre-cancerous states. Yet another possibility is that one of the effects of the initial event in carcinogenesis is to introduce inheritable defects in the way that cells divide so that genetic material is apportioned inequitably between daughter cells. The result of this would be that in both cancerous and 'pre-cancerous' lesions there would be a mixed population of cells competing with each other for nutrients and survival. Selective survival of the most aggressive could account for the phenomenon of tumour progression. If this concept of tumour progression based on 'natural selection' among a mixed population of cells were correct, one would expect that severe changes in the environment—rendering it intolerable for the majority of cells—would, by favouring the survival of the most aggressive cells, tend to precipitate tumour progression. This is exactly what Hobbs (1971)[11] has seen when patients suffering from non-progressive or only very slowly progressive forms of a disease of the blood forming tissues known as myeloma (or immunocytoma) were inappropriately treated with cytotoxic drugs. Such treatment precipitated the onset of a more malignant form of the disease which might not otherwise have ensued for many years.

It would have been satisfying to begin this book on the biology of cancer with a clear description of the nature of cancerous disease and precise facts and figures referring to its frequency of occurrence. What is presented, however, is much more a list of difficulties and of reasons why clear statements cannot be made, and of warnings that much of the ground on which subsequent chapters are necessarily based is quicksand. On such ground it is unwise to erect tall buildings or plan permanent ones.

Still under the heading of 'occurrence of neoplastic diseases', it is perhaps necessary to give one further warning. I have already indicated some of the problems that arise in defining the nature of cancerous diseases and ascertaining the incidence of such diseases in man. The same difficulties apply equally to other animal species but, in the case of laboratory animals, the very attempts made to improve the situation may have made it worse. Inbreeding has led to the emergence of strains of mice and rats which are unduly susceptible to the development of particular forms of neoplastic diseases. In several instances, a particular form of cancer may occur in 100 per cent of the animals of a particular strain. Viruses have been shown to be causally implicated in development of some of these tumours. These same viruses, however, are found variously in outbred strains of mice and rats and in association with tumour development in those strains. Most laboratory strains of mice and rats would probably not survive for many generations outside the laboratory if for no other reason than their high tumour incidence. It is reasonable to wonder how much reliance should be put on experiments based on the use of animal strains which can to some extent be regarded as artificial products of the laboratory. Obviously, the development of inbred strains, particularly mice, has greatly aided our understanding of the roles that genetic factors, vertically transmitted viruses and immunological responses can play in the causation of neoplasms in the species studied; but part of the price paid for the use of this tool may be a change in the overall balance between the mouse and the potentially oncogenic viruses which prey on it. From this point of view, the known facts suggest the need for considerable caution in the interpretation of the results of laboratory animal experiments and in the extrapolation from these to man. This is especially true where mice are used in tests of chemical (or other) agents for putative carcinogenicity, where cancers arise that are the commonly occurring cancers of the strains of animals used, or are cancers in which viruses carried by the test animals may be or are known to be implicated.

In the long run the cancers whose biology we have to elucidate are primarily the cancers that afflict man. There is a constant danger that the very availability of convenient laboratory tools will divert the emphasis in research towards the investigation of artificially created laboratory phenomena.

References

1. Case, R. A. M., *Br.J.prev.Med.,* **10,** 172 (1956).
2. Vianna, N. J., Greenwald, P. and Davies, J. N. P. *Lancet, i,* 1209 (1971).
3. Vianna, N. J., Greenwald, P., Brady, J., Dwork, A., Polan, A., Mauro, T., and Davies, J. N. P., *Ann. Int. Med.,* **77,** 169 (1972).
4. Logan, W. P. D., and Cushion, A. A., 'Morbidity Statistics from General Practice', *Studies in Medical and Population Subjects,* General Registry Office, London (1958).
5. Franks, L. M., *Ann.R.Coll.Surg.,* **15,** 236 (1954).
6. Cook, P. J., and Burkitt, D. P., *Br.med. Bull.,* **27,** 14 (1971).
7. Kmet, J., and Mahboubi, E., *Science,* **175,** 846 (1972).
8. Mahboubi, E., Kmet, J., Cook, P. J., Day, N. E., Ghadirian, P., and Salmasizadeh, S., *Br.J.Cancer,* **28,** 197 (1973).
9. Haenszel, W., and Kurihara, M., *J.nat.Cancer Inst.,* **40,** 43 (1968).
10. Foulds, L., *Neoplastic Development,* Academic Press, London & New York (1969).
11. Hobbs, J. R., *Brit.med.J.,* **2,** 67 (1971).

Chapter **2**

CHROMOSOMES: THE GENETIC COMPONENT OF THE TUMOUR CELL

P. C. KOLLER, D.SC.

Emeritus Professor of Cytogenetics, formerly of the Chester Beatty Research Institute, Institute of Cancer Research, London.

Transformation of a normal cell into a cancer cell is a permanent alteration in cell behaviour, maintained and transmitted to descendant generations of cells through the chromosomes which represent the genetic component of the cell. In both cell multiplication and transmission of altered cell behaviour, the chromosomes play an important role. Thus it may reasonably be assumed that the chromosomes are somehow implicated in bringing about or maintaining the malignant behaviour of cancer cells.

Genetic research during the past fifty years has established that chromosomes provide the physical basis of heredity; they are the carriers of the genes which control all the characteristics of the individual. It has been demonstrated experimentally that the genes occupy definite sites in particular chromosomes and are arranged in chromosomes in linear order. During the past two decades a new branch of science, 'molecular biology' has come into being; it includes within its compass studies on the most fundamental problems of genetics such as: what is the structural organization of chromosomes by which genetic information is stored? What is the genetic code which determines specificity?; How is gene activity controlled in differentiation? It is now established that the genetic information is carried by the DNA (deoxyribosenucleic acid) of the chromosome. The DNA helix has a backbone of sugar-phosphate units that bears the four nucleic acid side chains (*Fig. 2.1*). The spatial orientation or sequence of the nucleic acid bases (cystosine—thymine—guanine—adenine) provides the 'code' by which genetic information is transmitted from cell to cell, from generation to generation. The DNA also mediates the functional activity of the cell, by transmitting its information via 'messenger' RNA (ribosenucleic acid) and 'transfer' RNA. These units pick up amino acids and line them up to form polypeptides and proteins, many of which function as cellular enzymes. It is now known that cellular activity is the result of a finely integrated genetic system (genome). Although not all genes are operating at a particular time, normal cellular activity requires an intact set of chromosomes. The furnishing of cells with a complete chromosome complement is brought about during mitosis when each daughter cell receives a replica of the chromosomes of the parent cell. When a chromosome is lost from, or added to, the genome through some error during mitosis, the delicate balance of the integrated genetic system is disrupted.

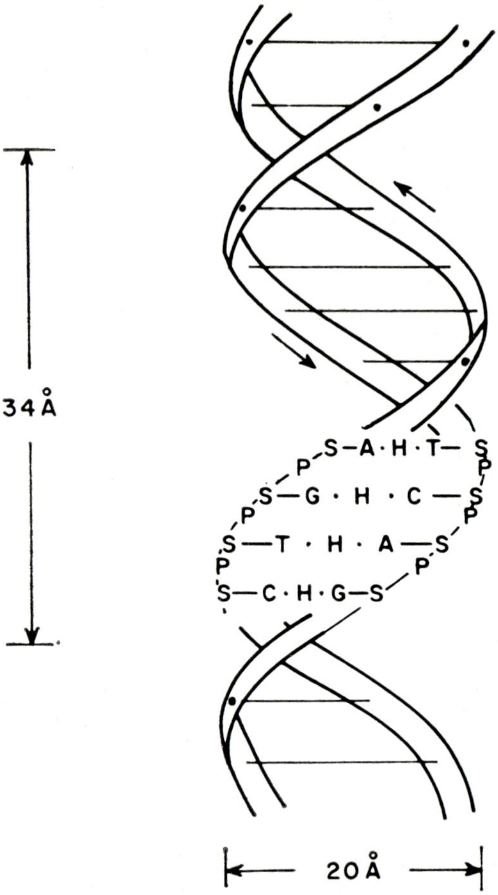

Fig. 2.1. Schematic representation of the DNA molecule, consisting of two sugar-phosphate chains (S – P – S) which form a double helix, held together by H bonds between the bases of the two chains: A: adenine; T: thymine; G: guanine; C: cystosine. (After Watson, J. D. and Crick, F. H. C., *Nature*, 171, 965 (1953).)

This may have fatal consequences, not only in the cells affected but eventually in the whole organism. Much information has now been collected by cytologists which shows that structural and numerical changes in the chromosomes of plants and animals, including man, all have genetical repercussions.

This is the basic information in the light of which the behaviour of chromosomes in tumours must be studied (Koller, 1972).[11]

Chromosomes of tumour cells

BOVERI'S THEORY

The idea that the chromosomes are involved in malignant or neoplastic growth is a very old one. The term 'chromosome' (stained body) was only two years

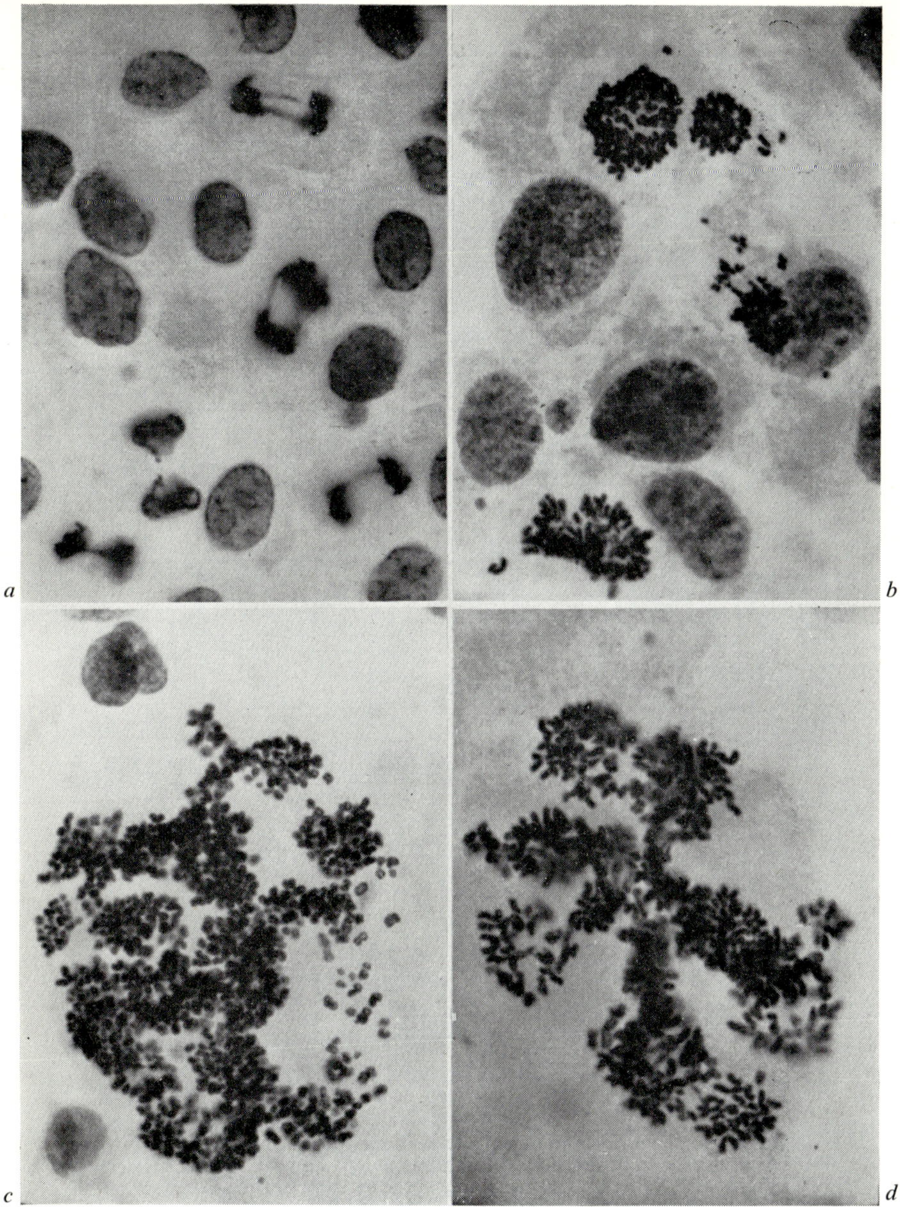

Fig. 2.2.

(*a*) Dividing tumour cells showing chromosome bridges at anaphase and telophase. The tumour was induced by an aromatic mustard in the rat.

(*b*) Four tumour cells in division, each has a different number of chromosomes. (Squamous cell carcinoma of cervix uteri.)

(*c*) Dividing cell in a malignant effusion of a patient with carcinoma of the ovary. The number of chromosomes is more than 600; the normal number in a human cell is 46.

(*d*) Dividing cell with a large number of chromosomes which are arranged on 12 incomplete equatorial plates. (Malignant effusion, carcinoma of the lung.)

old when Krebs, in 1889, reported that the numbers of chromosomes in tumour cells varied widely. Then, in a series of papers between 1890 and 1906, Hansemann described in great detail the mitotic abnormalities which occur in human tumours. He concluded that the presence of a large number of abnormally dividing cells in a tissue could be taken as a sign of its malignant nature and, in view of the seemingly universal occurrence of mitotic irregularities in tumours, he suggested that abnormal mitosis might be the cause of 'neoplasia'.

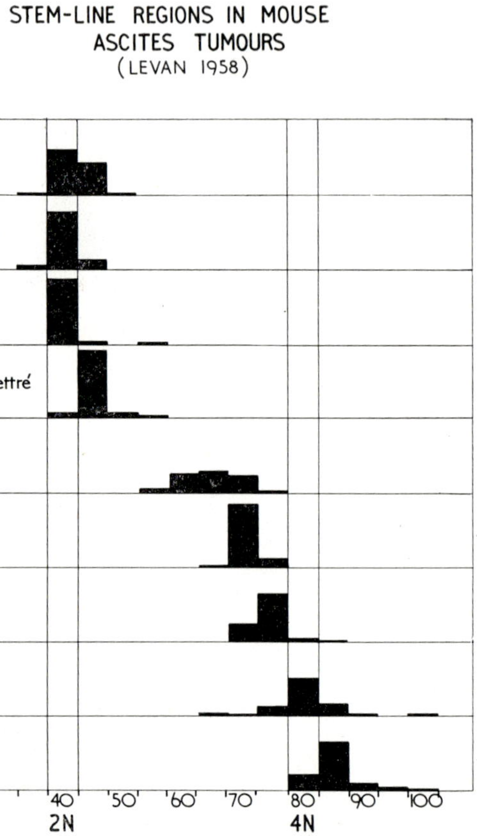

Fig. 2.3. Histograms showing the frequencies of stem cells and the range of numerical variation in different mouse ascites tumours. DBA and 6C3HED: lymphomas; TA3HA: carcinoma strain; TA3K1: a subline of the former; Ehrlich Lettré: hyperdiploid; Ehrlich: tetraploid sublines; E1 and E2: clones derived from tetraploid Ehrlich; MCIM: sarcoma strain. (After Levan, A., *Yearbook Cancer Res. Netherlands*, 8, 110 (1958).)

This proposal was put in a more definite form by Boveri (1912)[1] who postulated that malignancy was due to an abnomal chromosome content of the cell, resulting from abnormal mitosis. This is the essence of his *Chromosome Theory of Cancer*. For two decades, cytologists could not provide supporting evidence for Boveri's theory, chiefly because unsatisfactory techniques were being used for chromosome studies. But during the last twenty years new and improved methods have been introduced into cytology and much information about chromosome behaviour in normal as well as in tumour cells has emerged. Through the application of these new techniques, chromosome anomalies of various kinds have been observed in a great number of animal and human tumours, and the high incidence of such anomalies would seem to provide evidence in favour of Boveri's theory: a few examples of mitotic anomalies are illustrated in *Fig. 2.2.* Abnormal mitoses are common in tumour tissue and can be used as one of the morphological criteria for diagnosing malignancy (Koller, 1960).[10]

CELL HETEROGENEITY

Recent cytological studies have established that most experimental tumours, in terms of chromosome constitution, are composed of a heterogeneous population in which few or no normal diploid cells may be present (*Fig. 2.3*). These studies led to the 'stem-line' concept: among the chromosome variants, the stem-line is a class of cells which shares the same karyotype and forms the major numerical component of the tumour cell population.

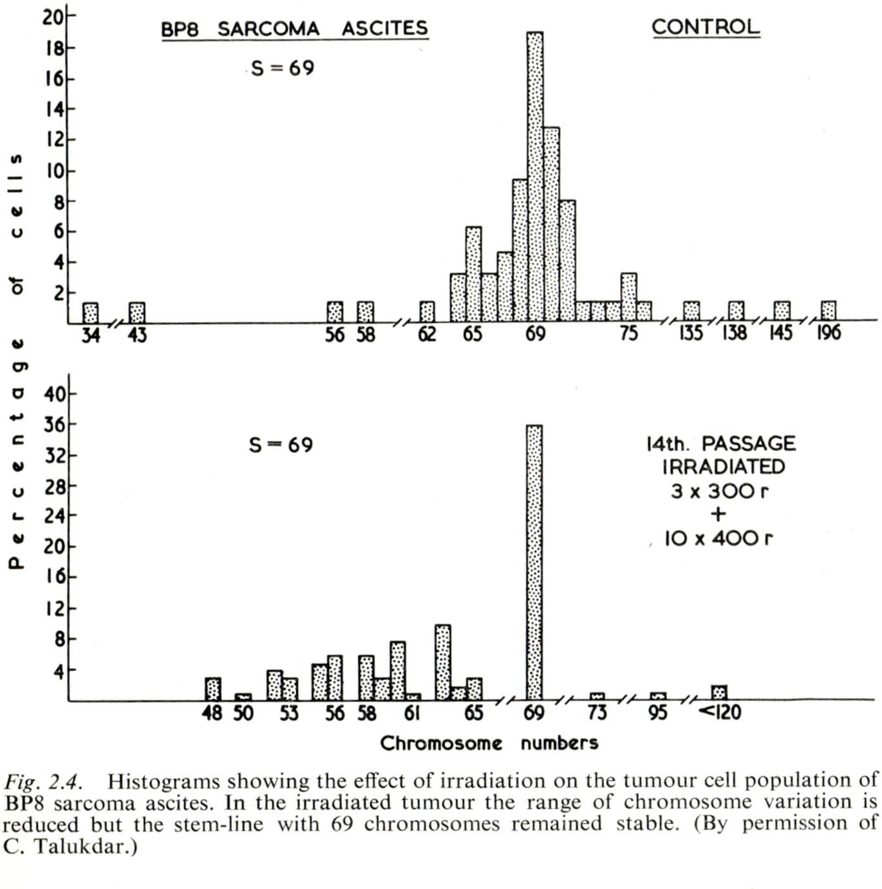

Fig. 2.4. Histograms showing the effect of irradiation on the tumour cell population of BP8 sarcoma ascites. In the irradiated tumour the range of chromosome variation is reduced but the stem-line with 69 chromosomes remained stable. (By permission of C. Talukdar.)

In experimental tumours in mice the chromosome constitution is stable in some and variable in others; transplantation or other alterations of environmental conditions can change the cell composition (*Fig. 2.4*). Structurally altered chromosomes may also appear in tumour cells and may be used as 'marker' chromosomes in cell population studies. It has been observed that the frequency of stem-line cells in clones derived from single cells can differ from that of the parent tumour.

PRIMARY TUMOURS

Studies of chromosomes in primary tumours, particularly in man, are beset by three major difficulties: (*a*) technical shortcomings; (*b*) the problem of determining whether the chromosome anomalies seen at the time of diagnosis were present *de novo* from the earliest stages of development, or whether they appeared subsequently as a secondary or epiphenomenal consequence of cancer development; and (*c*) whether such changes might in part be due to treatment, particularly with radiotherapy or chemotherapy.

Cytological studies have shown that by the time primary tumours are visible, many of them are already composed of a chromosomally heterogeneous cell population. These studies have also shown that there is no chromosome pattern which is a characteristic or exclusive feature of the malignant cell. Primary tumours of animals appear to be of two kinds: one composed mostly of cells with diploid (normal) chromosome constitution, the other characterized by a cell population which contains a great number of chromosome variants deviating from the diploid condition. The deviation may be small (as in X-ray-induced leukaemias) or large (as in chemically-induced sarcomas). The chromosome pattern in early primary tumours, particularly those with a diploid modal number, frequently undergo progressive alteration in chromosome constitution during the later stages of tumour development. Cytological studies have shown that primary tumours are individual in respect of chromosome number, spectrum of chromosome variants, frequency of cells with different chromosome numbers, and marker chromosomes. Tumours induced by the same carcinogenic agent may vary in their cytology. Cellular instability, indicated by mitotic aberrations, can persist for long periods and result in a wide spectrum of chromosome variants in the developing tumour. So far, very few tumours have been found in which every malignant cell contains the same chromosome anomaly. Amongst such neoplasms chronic myeloid leukaemia in man is the most important.

Nowell and Hungerford (1960)[14] observed that in chronic myeloid leukaemia the chromosome number is 46 (i.e. the normal diploid number) but that one chromosome is abnormal (*Fig. 2.5*). This abnormal chromosome has now been identified as chromosome 22 of the G group. It is found in blood and bone marrow cells and has been designated as the 'Philadelphia' chromosome (Ph′). The identification of this chromosome was made possible by the technique of Caspersson and his associates (1970*a*, *b*)[2, 3] who found that quinacrine mustard, an alkylating agent, produced sharply defined fluorescent bands in metaphase chromosomes. The Ph′ chromosome is identified by its highly characteristic banding pattern. The close association between the Ph′ chromosome and chronic myeloid leukaemia suggests that the anomaly might be associated with the cause of the disease, or that it predisposes to malignant change in cells carrying it. So far, chronic myeloid leukaemia represents a unique situation because particular chromosome anomalies have not been seen consistently in association with any other form of malignant disease.

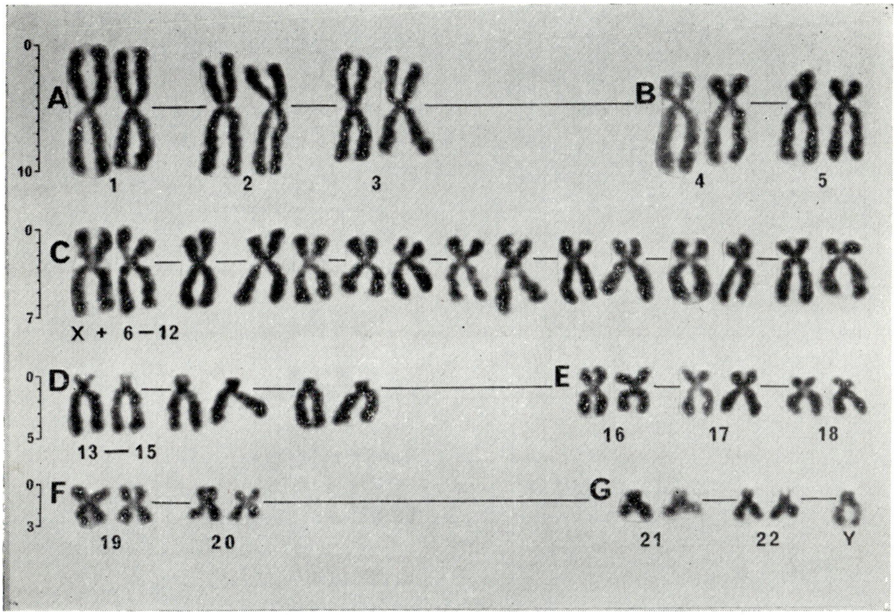

Fig. 2.5. Normal male karyotype of man showing the 46 chromosomes arranged according to size. In patients with chronic myeloid leukaemia one chromosome-21 is abnormal. (By permission of D. T. Hughes.)

There is no doubt that tumour cells can differ from normal cells in respect of chromosome constitution; but the question as to whether a chromosome anomaly, when present, is directly related to the primary event of malignant transformation is still unanswered.

Heteroploid transformation of cells *in vitro**

Most cell populations grown *in vitro* for a long time have properties very similar to those of cell populations of tumour tissue: they contain cell variants which differ in their chromosome constitution, not only from the normal diploid cells (from which the population was derived) but also from each other. Analysis of a large number of cell lines seems to indicate that 'heteroploid transformation' is common when cells are grown in an artificial environment outside the body.

*A heteroploid population of cells is one predominantly composed of cells with anomalous chromosome numbers and (possibly) anomalous structure.

Several experiments have shown that certain cell lines, which have grown *in vitro* for a long time and undergone such a heteroploid transformation, produce tumours when grafted into suitable animal hosts. A classic example was provided by Levan and Biesele (1958)[12] who cultured cells of embryonic mouse skin *in vitro* and analysed the chromosome behaviour of the cell population at successive passages (*Fig. 2.6*). They found that the proportion of

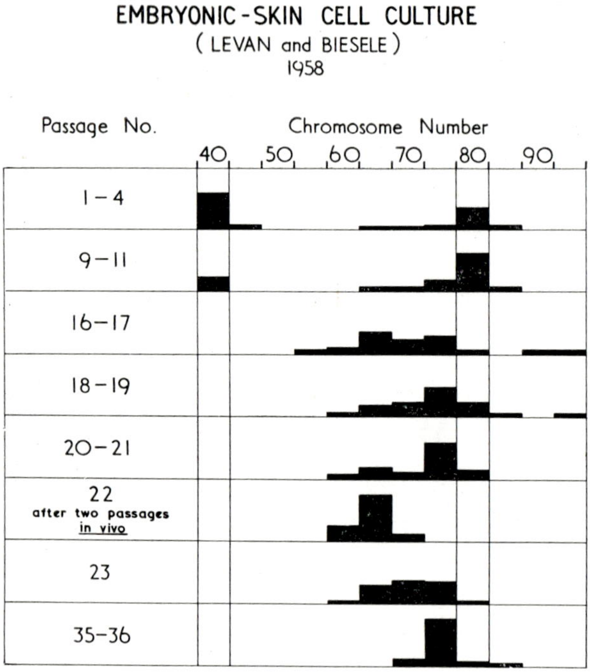

Fig. 2.6. Histograms showing the changes in chromosome constitution in an embryonic mouse skin cell culture which showed malignancy when tested *in vivo* at the 22nd passage. (After Levan, A. and Biesele, J. J. *Ann. N.Y. Acad. Sci. 71*, 1022 (1958).)

cells with the normal diploid chromosome number gradually decreased and that, after the sixteenth passage, the 'normal' class had entirely disappeared from the culture. After the twenty-first passage, the chromosomally altered cell population was implanted into mice and local subcutaneous tumours developed at the injection site. This finding has been corroborated by many similar observations of other investigators.

It seems that when cells adapt to autonomous existence *in vitro*, they also undergo changes in chromosome constitution. But it should be stressed that cytological changes in a cell line are not always associated with malignant behaviour. Many chromosomally-aberrant cell lines do not give rise to tumours on implantation into animals. Heteroploid transformation *per se*, which accompanies the adaptation of cell lines to *in vitro* existence and growth, is not equivalent to real cancerization; some other additional characteristics are also required by these cells to turn them into 'cancer' cells (Hsu, 1961).[7]

Chromosome anomalies in precancerous states

Although chromosome changes in a cell population grown *in vitro* do not necessarily confer malignant behaviour, it has been found that such alterations in chromosome behaviour and constitution commonly precede malignant change.

In the liver of rats fed on a diet containing dimethylaminoazobenzene for several months, progressive alterations occur, culminating in the development of malignant tumours. One of the changes concerns the number of chromosomes; it has been observed that hepatic cells with a normal diploid chromosome number are gradually replaced by cells with abnormal chromosome constitution (*Fig. 2.7*). However, the transplantation of such hepatic tissue,

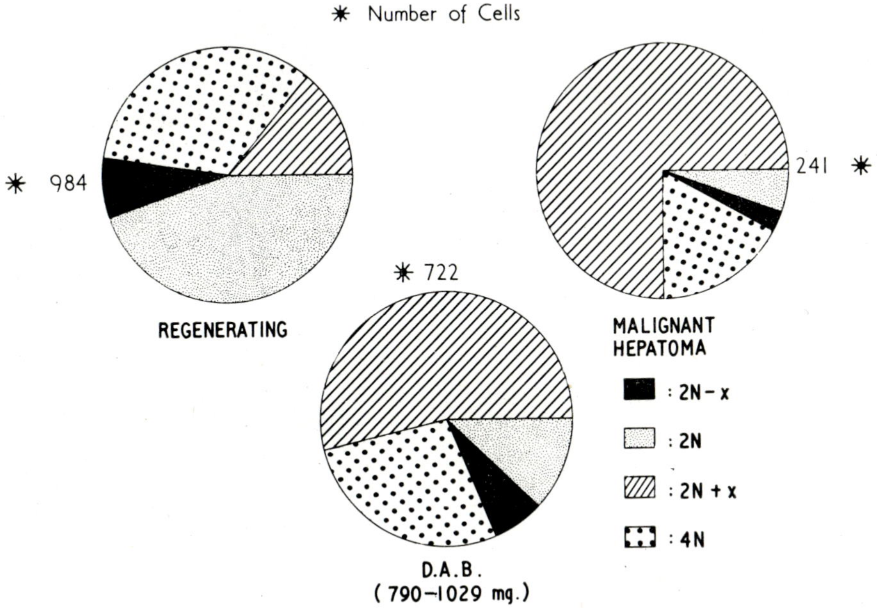

Fig. 2.7. Diagram illustrating the frequency of cell types with different chromosome constitutin in regenerating liver, in liver of rat fed on *p*-dimethyl-aminoazo-benzene (D.A.B.) and in malignant hepatoma. (After Glass, E., *Krebsforsch. 60*, 362 (1960).)

containing chromosomally-altered cells, does not always result in tumour growth. A similar observation was made in relation to the enlarged thymus of irradiated C57BL mice, which eventually developed into malignant thymoma with subsequent leukaemic spread. It has been found that the enlarged thymus contains many chromosomally-anomalous cells; yet when transplanted into other C57BL mice it fails to produce leukaemia. Studies on a preinvasive carcinoma of the cervix (carcinoma *in situ*) revealed that cells with an abnormal chromosome number were already present. These observations show that chromosome changes in cells may occur during the early stages of carcinogenesis; and it is conceivable that such changes predispose the cells to malignant transformation (Spriggs, 1963).[15]

The type of mitotic anomalies and their origin

It was mentioned earlier that the chromosome constitution of the cell populations in both transplanted and autochthonous tumours often differs from the normal diploid chromosome complement of the species because of mitotic irregularities, e.g. abnormal spindle formation resulting in non-disjunction of chromosomes. The frequency of mitotic anomalies increases during the growth of the tumour and there is much evidence that this increase is attributable to abnormal environmental conditions prevailing in tumour tissue (*Fig. 2.8*)—

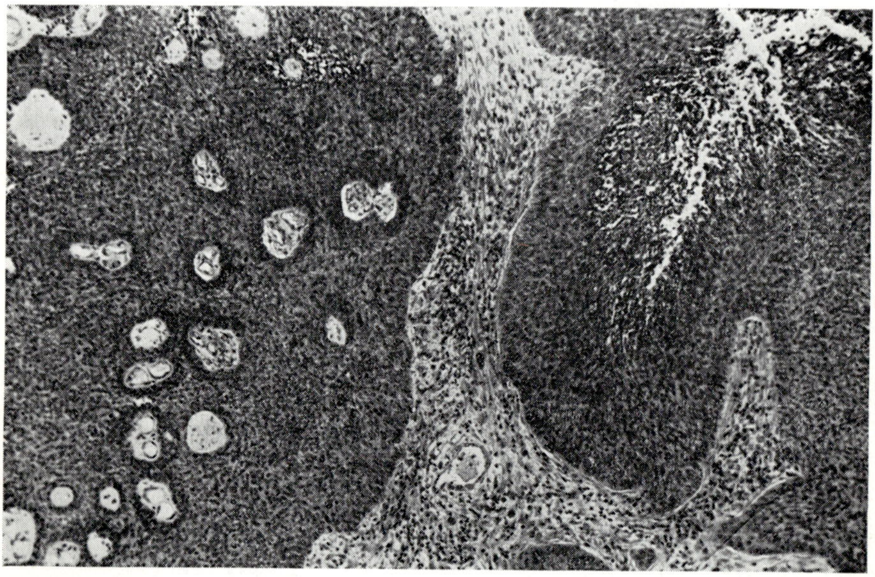

Fig. 2.8. Photomicrograph showing the histological structure of two tumour-cords of carcinoma cervix uteri. The deficient blood supply of one (on the right) results in cellular necrosis.

e.g. necrosis due to an inadequate blood supply. The most common types of mitotic anomalies are stickiness of chromosomes at metaphase, lagging of chromosomes and the formation of chromosome bridges at anaphase. All these irregularities can result in an abnormal distribution of chromosomes to the daughter cells. Abnormal mitosis is an exception in normal tissues and chromosome anomalies are correspondingly rare.

On the other hand, cells with gross deviation from normal chromosome constitution can, under certain circumstances at least, exist and proliferate; it seems that their viability is not impaired. Such is the case when cells are cultured *in vitro*. The chief function of these cells is replication, and for this purpose their metabolism is channelled into a simple pattern, requiring less integration of intracellular genic control than does the pattern in cells which are differentiated for other functions. These cells are adapted to existence outside the body, and they may achieve autonomy. Similarly, neoplastic transformation of cells involves functional simplification, and adaptation to an autonomous existence. In these cells, heteroploidy can apparently be tolerated as long as the genetic mechanism (chromosomes and genes) controlling basic cell metabolism is retained. Thus tumour cells can exist with grossly altered chromosome constitution because they are malignant.

Significance of heteroploidy

During the early stages of tumour development, tumour cells retain many of the morphological and metabolic features characteristic of the tissue of origin. At this stage, cells with chromosome anomalies are rare or may be entirely absent. This is well illustrated by the 'minimum deviation' hepatomas. In these tumours, deviation of cells from the morphological and metabolic characteristics of the normal hepatic cell is 'minimal', and their chromosome constitution has revealed none of the gross alterations which, nevertheless, became apparent when they were successively transplanted several times. It seems that, during the growth of such tumours, 'de-differentiation' of cellular metabolism takes place and that this tends to be associated with the appearance of various chromosome anomalies in the cells. Some of the cell variants are better adapted to the new environment and will have a reproductive advantage over other cells; consequently they will replace the cells that are less adapted.

It has been found that tumours can change during growth and development. Thus, as their growth-rate increases, they attain greater autonomy and become independent of hormonal influences. This process is described as *tumour progression* and it is made possible by the heterogenerous cell composition of the tumour tissues. The mixed population represents a great advantage to the tumour tissue because the different cell types may have different survival values under adverse conditions. The cells of which a tumour is predominantly composed can be altered experimentally by exposure to environmental influences, which are more favourable to the survival of some types of cells than to that of other types. Thus, the conversion of solid tumours in mice into an ascites form (i.e. cells proliferating while suspended in fluid) is attributed to the selective over-growth of a very small number of cells, which differed from the majority of the original population in their capacity to multiply in the environment of the peritoneal cavity. Similarly, the development of drug-resistant sublines of L1210 mouse leukaemia was found to be due to the selective pressure provided by prolonged exposure to folic acid antagonists. It is now evident that the cell population of malignant tissue is composed of variants, some of which (under the forces of selection) can become the source of a new population of cells, better adapted to autonomy.

Many studies have been carried out to see if there is an association between a particular chromosome constitution and certain forms of neoplastic behaviour. As an illustration, the difference in radiosensitivity of tumours may be considered in relation to their chromosome constitution. On theoretical grounds, it might be expected that differences in chromosome number would be reflected in corresponding differences in the radiosensitivity of cells. The possibility of such correlation has been tested by comparing the radiosensitivity of neoplastic cell populations which differ in chromosome number although they have been derived from a common parental tumour. Ehrlich ascites tumour cells were irradiated with 200 rad of X-rays before intraperitoneal transplantation, and the process was repeated for twenty-three transfers. By this procedure, several radioresistant sublines were obtained. Cytological studies, however, revealed that the model chromosome number (stemline) of radioresistant clones was identical with that of sensitive ones, and the clones with the same degree of radiosensitivity had different modal chromosome numbers. Thus, in this particular study, no consistent relationship between chromosome number and radiosensitivity was found. Similarly, it was observed that by exposing a neoplastic cell population to a particular drug, resistance to the drug was obtained without any detectable change in chromosome constitution. On the other hand, some correlation between the chromosome constitution and types of serum protein has been observed in four plasma cell leukaemias of mice. While there are some tumours in which alteration in chromosome constitution is followed by a change in certain properties of tumour cells, in the great majority of tumours no such correlation has been found (Hauschka, 1958).[6]

Predisposition or susceptibility to cancer

CHROMOSOMAL

For years, geneticists had suspected that chromosomal anomalies lay behind the various aberrations in human sex differentiation and mongolism. It is now well established that certain pathological conditions in man have a chromosomal basis. Thus Down's syndrome (mongolism) and Klinefelter's syndrome are due to the presence of an extra chromosome, while in Turner's syndrome (ovarian agenesis) one sex chromosome is missing from the genome. The numerical chromosome changes originate during gametogenesis or very early foetal life. Consequently, every cell in the body of the affected individual has the abnormal chromosome constitution.

It has been found that, in mongols, the incidence of leukaemia is about eighteen times higher than in the general population. Similarly, ovarian carcinoma seems to be more common in patients with Turner's syndrome than in normal persons. One possible explanation of these associations is that chromosomal anomaly produces metabolic instability in cells, which predisposes the cell to malignant transformation.

One of the most interesting examples of what seems to be a chromosomally-determined predisposition to leukaemia has been reported from New Zealand. Fitzgerald and Hamer (1969)[4] found a family afflicted with an abnormal chromosome which is designated as Ch′. When the family was first investigated (*Fig. 2.9*), two members (No. 4 and 6) had the Ch′ chromosome and lymphocytic leukaemia. More recently it was reported that leukaemia developed in a

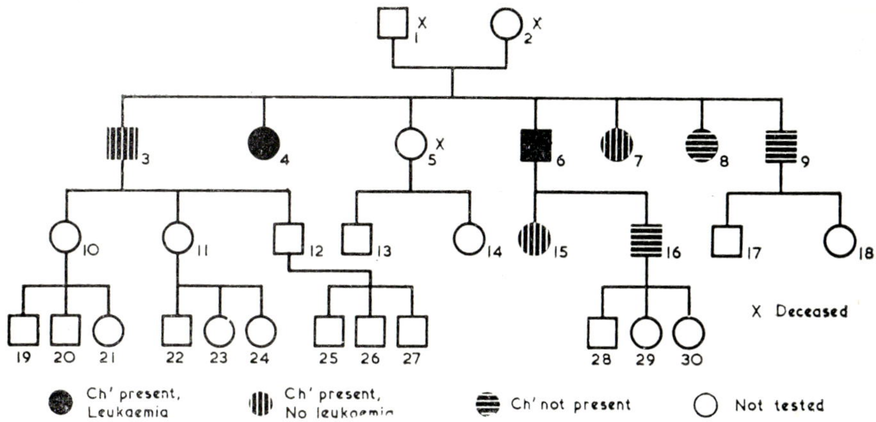

Fig. 2.9. The pedigree of the 'C' family in which the presence of the abnormal chromosome 21 (Ch') has been observed, (Gunz, F. W., Fitzgerald, P. H., and Adams, A., *Br. med. J. 2*, 1097 (1962).)

third sibling (No. 3) who was a carrier of the Ch′ chromosome. The authors suggest that this particular chromosome anomaly confers a predisposition to the development of leukaemia on those carrying it.

GENE-DEPENDENT

Experimental demonstration of gene-determined susceptibility to cancer is provided by inbred strains of mice in which the individual members have, through prolonged selective mating, identical genetical constitutions. *Table 2.1*

Table 2.1. Tumour incidence in various strains of mice

Tumour	*Strain*	*Tumour incidence in percentage*	*Average age of mice in months when tumour appears*
Mammary gland	C_3H	95	·9
	RIII	90	16
	A	80	12
	DBA	65	12
	CBA	15	20
	Balb/C	1	24
	C57BL	0·5	22
Lung	A	85	14
	C57BL	0·5	18
Leukaemia	AKR	95	10
	C58	90	10
	DBA/2	40	12
	C57BL	20	18
	Stoli	1	16

shows the incidence of particular types of cancer in some strains of mice. The incidence is never 100 per cent; there is always a certain proportion of the animals which do not develop a tumour, in spite of having an inherited susceptibility from their parents. When, however, such mice are exposed to potent carcinogens (benzpyrene, 20-methylcholanthrene, etc.) the incidence of cancer is increased; in some instances it may rise to 100 per cent and the time required to develop tumours is unusally short. There is much evidence that a general predisposition to cancer is a feature of certain strains of mice, but it has been also found that other, non-genetic, factors are necessary for the development of a particular type of cancer (Koller, 1957)[9].

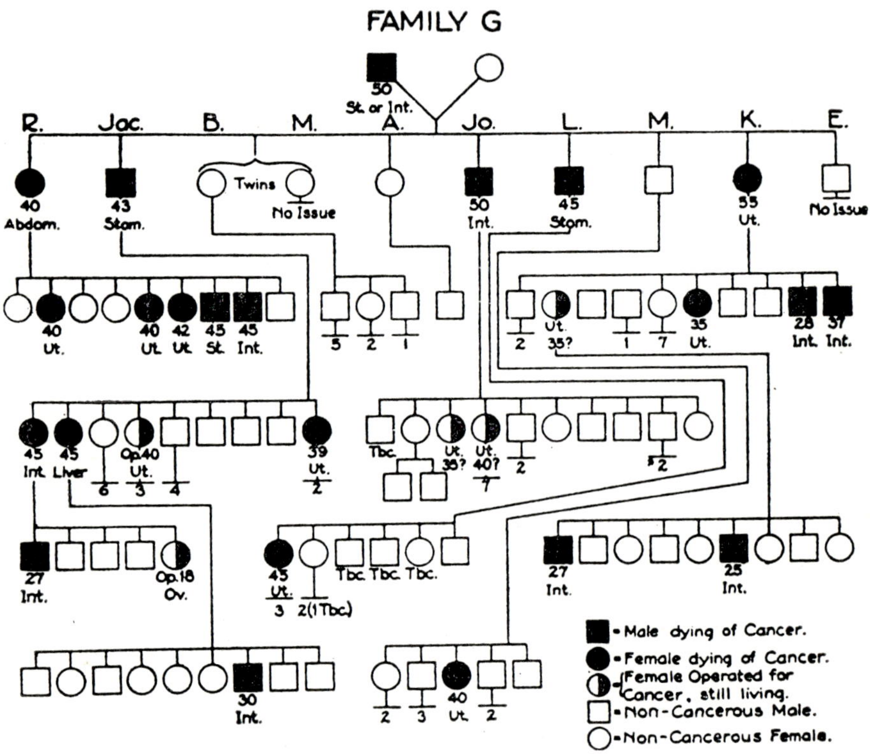

Fig. 2.10. The pedigree of 'G' family showing an extremely high incidence of cancer amongst the relations. (Warthin, A. S., *J. Cancer Res. 9*, 279 (1925).)

Studies of human families in which an excessive number of close relatives had developed cancers revealed a situation similar to that in certain mouse strains and suggested that the high incidence might be due to inherited susceptibility. One of the most famous pedigrees is provided by family 'G' in which the incidence of cancer among close relations who reached the 'cancer' age was 31·8 per cent (*Fig. 2.10*). Before accepting the assumption that susceptibility to cancer may be inherited, it should be stressed that cancer is a common disease in the human populations and the presence of several cases in one family might be due to chance alone. However, by the introduction of special statistical methods and a more critical selection of control groups, in recent studies of family pedigrees geneticists have obtained data which indicate that in *some families* there is an inherited predisposition to cancer of the stomach, of the breast and perhaps of the cervix and uterus (Lynch, 1967)[13]: the risk of contracting cancer of the stomach and breast is two to three times higher for members of such families than for members of the general public.

It is necessary to emphasize that, as yet, no general predisposition to cancer has been revealed by the surveys which have been carried out on human populations. Nor do these surveys show a simple pattern of inheritance of susceptibility. It seems that the genetic basis of predisposition to cancer is complex, and that several genes may be involved. Pedigree analysis of human material has revealed only few examples of simple Mendelian inheritance of high susceptibility to a particular type of tumour. Thus, *retinoblastoma* is determined by one gene; and *neurofibromatosis* is controlled by a single gene which behaves as a dominant gene in the affected children. Two pre-cancerous conditions, multiple *polyposis* of the large intestine (*polyposis coli*) and *xeroderma pigmentosa* are determined by single genes. But all these conditions are very rare and are not representative of the more common types of cancers, e.g. of breast or lung. Pedigree analysis suggests that susceptibility to these latter cancers is determined by many genes, probably of varying potency.

While it is an accepted fact that genetically-determined predisposition to a particular cancer exists in certain human families, such a predisposition cannot be considered as the sole aetiological factor in the origin of cancer in these cases. Studies of cancer incidence in *identical twins* show the great and decisive importance of environmental influences on the development of cancer. Such twins have identical genetic constitutions, yet the same cancer very rarely occurs in both members. The information obtained from studies of family pedigrees is, however, valuable: it enables an estimate to be made of the risks for members of a particular family in which cancer has appeared in certain forms, and it may assist the physician in his diagnosis and in his advice on preventive measures.

In particular instances genetically determined susceptibility to malignant disease can be investigated on a cellular basis by the technique of Todaro *et al.* (1966)[16]. These investigators found that the Simian virus, SV40, transforms cells grown *in vitro* and confers on them the following malignant properties: (i) loss of contact inhibition (the cells grow in multilayer clumps instead of in monolayers); (ii) the acquisition of T-antigen; and (iii) the ability to produce tumours (tested by inoculation of the transformed cells into appropriate host animals). The proportion of cells transformed can be used to measure the sensitivity of cells to transformation. Through this method it has been demonstrated that skin fibroblasts of patients with Down's syndrome and Fanconi's aplastic anaemia exhibit increased sensitivity to transformation by SV40; both conditions are known to be associated with chromosomal anomalies and to predispose to leukaemia and other malignancies. Fanconi's anaemia is an inherited disorder conditioned by an autosomal recessive gene.

Table 2.2 shows the frequency of cell transformation of skin fibroblasts in four members of a family with the syndrome of Fanconi's anaemia: two were homozygotes having inherited from both parents the genes predisposing to the disease, and two were heterozygotes having received the predisposing gene from one parent only. In the former the numbers of transformed colonies was found to be fifty times higher than in normal persons; in the heterozygotes the

Table 2.2. Frequency of cell transformation *in vitro* by SV40

Source of skin fibroblasts	*Number of transformed colonies per 10,000 cells*
Fanconi's anaemia	
Homozygotes:	
AM	79·7 ± 18·1
JV	41·4 ± 12·1
Heterozygotes:	
TM	20·1 ± 3·2
CV	28·2 ± 8·7
Normal controls:	1·6 ± 5·1

incidence was also higher than normal but much less so than in the homozygotes. The heightened incidence shown by the heterozygotes may be used to detect the carriers of the gene predisposing to the Fanconi's disease and malignancy. In this syndrome chromosomal anomaly is the 'secondary' consequence of cellular instability which is gene-determined. (German 1972)[5].

Viral carcinogenesis

Predisposition to cancer in relation to the genetic mechanism has so far been discussed at two levels. Evidence has been presented that, although anomalous chromosome constitution may not be the primary cause of malignancy, it sometimes associates with enhanced susceptibility to neoplastic transformation. Furthermore, studies of certain strains of mice and human family pedigrees suggest that genetic factors do play a role in determining susceptibility to certain forms of cancer. Thus, it is obvious that the genetic apparatus of the cell can become involved either directly or indirectly in the process of malignant transformation.

One mechanism by which the genetic apparatus of cells is involved in neoplastic transformation is indicated by studies of virus-induced neoplasia—see Chapter 11. It has been found that 'oncogenic viruses' (e.g. polyoma, SV40) transform cells not only *in vivo* but also *in vitro* making it possible to follow the various changes occurring in the cells which are infected with the virus. It has been observed that within a few hours after infection, a new antigen appears and the DNA synthesis is stimulated in the cell. Though the transformed cells do not yield infectious virus particles, the viral genome is present in them and, according to various evidence, it is integrated into the chromosomal DNA of the host cell. The strongest evidence of viral integration into the chromosomes was provided by cell hybridization; a method which consists of fusing two cells of different origin, e.g. mouse with hamster, mouse with human. This method is intensively employed in the study of inborn errors of metabolism in man. The discovery of rapid elimination of human chromosomes from mouse + human hybrid cells made the method applicable for testing the 'integration hypothesis' (Weiss, 1970)[17]. By using the specific new antigen as indicator of the presence of the virus in the cell, it was observed that when human cells transformed *in vitro* by SV40 were fused with non-transformed mouse cells, the virus specific antigen disappeared with the loss of human chromosomes from the hybrid cell. The number of viral genomes present in the cell is estimated to be between five and sixty which seem to be randomly scattered amongst the chromosomes of the host cell.

Recent investigation threw light on the mechanism by which oncogenic viruses may be integrated into the host cell's DNA and opened up a new approach in the search for the presence of potential oncogenic viruses in man (Huebner and Todaro, 1969)[8].

Conclusion

Cytological studies of the chromosome constitution of cells in tumours of varying kinds have revealed that abnormalities, both in number and structure of chromosomes, are of common occurrence. But these studies failed to demonstrate, except in chronic myeloid leukaemia, the existence of a stable chromosome pattern which would be characteristic of, and exclusive to, the malignant cell. Furthermore, it has been found that, in respect of chromosome constitution, tumour tissue is composed of a heterogeneous cell population, the structure of which can change under environmental influences. Cytological investigations have provided some evidence that predisposition of cells to malignant transformation may be facilitated by chromosomal anomalies. Though it is at present very unlikely that abnormal chromosome constitution can be considered the primary cause of malignant change, yet it seems that the genetic component of the cell plays a certain role during the process of carcinogenesis.

References

1. Boveri, T. 'Beitrag zum Studium des Chromatin in den Epithelzellen der Carcinome', *Beitr.Z.Path.Anat.und Z.allg.Path.* **14,** 249 (1912).
2. Caspersson, T., Zech, L., Johansson, C. and Modest E. J. 'Identification of Human Chromosomes by DNA-binding Fluorescent Agents', *Chromosoma,* **30,** 215–227 (1970).
3. Caspersson, T., Gahrton, G., Lindsten, J. and Zech, L. 'Identification of the Philadelphia chromosome as a number 22 by quinacrine mustard fluorescence analysis' *Exptl. Cell Res.* **63,** 238–239 (1970b).
4. Fitzgerald, P. H. and Hamer, J. W. 'Third case of chronic lymphocytic leukaemia in carrier of the inherited Ch' chromosome' *Brit. Med. J.* **3,** 752 (1969).
5. German, J. 'Genes which increase chromosomal instability in somatic cells and predispose to Cancer' *Progress in med. Genetics,* **8,** 61–101 (1972).

6. Hauschka, T. S. 'Correlation of chromosomal and physiological changes in tumours', *J. cell comp. Physiol.,* **52,** Suppl. I, 197–223 (1958).
7. Hsu, M. S. (Chromosomal evolution in cell populations', *Int. Rev. Cytol.,* **12** 69–161 (1961).
8. Huebner, R. J. and Todaro, G. J. 'Oncogenes of RNA tumour viruses as determinants of cancer' *Proc. Nat. Acad. Sci.,* **64,** 1087–1096 (1969).
9. Koller, P. C. 'The genetic component of cancer' in *Cancer,* vol. 1 (edited by R. W. Raven), 335–403, Butterworth, London (1957).
10. Koller, P. C. 'Chromosome behaviour in tumours: Readjustment to Boveri's theory, *Cell Physiology and Neoplasia,* 9–37, University of Texas Press, Austin (1960).
11. Koller, P. C. 'The Role of Chromosomes in Cancer Biology' in *Recent Results in Cancer Research,* vol. **38.** Springer-Verlag, Berlin (1972).
12. Levan, A. and Biesele, J. J. 'Role of chromosomes in cancerogenesis as studied in serial tissue culture of mammalian cells', *Ann. N.Y. Acad. Sci.,* **71,** 1022–1053 (1958).
13. Lynch, H. T. 'Hereditary factors in carcinoma' in *Recent Results in Cancer Research,* vol. **12,** Springer-Verlag, Berlin (1967).
14. Nowell, P. C. and Hungerford, D. A. 'Chromosome studies on normal and leukemic human leukocytes', *J. natn. Cancer. Inst.* **25,** 85–109 (1960).
15. Spriggs, A. I. 'Karyotype changes in human tumour cells', *Br. J. Radiol.,* **37,** 210–212 (1963).
16. Todaro, G. J. and Martin, G. M. 'Increased susceptibility of Down's syndrome Fibroblasts to transformation by SV40.' *Proc. Soc. Exp. Biol. Med.,* **124,** 1232–1238 (1967).
17. Weiss, M. C. 'Properties of somatic hybrid cell lines between mouse cells and SV40-transformed human cells' in *Genetic Concept and Neoplasia,* The Williams and Wilkins Comp. Baltimore, (1970).

Chapter 3

THE SURFACE PROPERTIES OF TUMOUR CELLS

E. J. AMBROSE, D.SC.

Professor of Cell Biology, Chester Beatty Research Institute, Institute of Cancer Research, London

Introduction

The first clear demonstration that changes in cell surface properties might be of importance in malignancy was made by Dale Coman when, in 1944[1], he carried out micromanipulation studies of squamous cell carcinoma of the skin and normal epidermis. Coman found that the tumour cells were more readily separated from each other than normal epidermal cells, suggesting that the surfaces of the tumour cells were less adhesive. More exact work in this field became possible with the introduction of suitable tissue culture methods in which the dynamic behaviour of contacts in living cells could be investigated. Abercrombie, Heaysman and Karthauser (1957)[2] carried out comparative studies of normal fibroblasts and sarcoma cells in explant culture and found that the locomotion of normal fibroblasts was controlled by cell-cell interactions (contact inhibition) whereas the movements of the sarcoma cells investigated were not regulated by contact inhibition. Later studies of the interactions between the membranes using time-lapse filming with the interference microscope (Abercrombie, Ambrose, D. Easty and Heaysman, 1958[3]; Abercrombie and Ambrose, 1958[4]) indicated that changes in cell-cell adhesion at the points of contact and arrest of the active membrane movements (undulations) were involved in contact inhibition. Efforts were then concentrated on applying physicochemical and biochemical methods to the surface structure of tumour cells (Ambrose, James and Lowick, 1956[5]; G. Easty, D. Easty and Ambrose, 1960[6]).

Studies of cell surfaces and cell membranes have expanded greatly in recent years, both as basic investigations and in the more specific context of cancer research: a world-wide effort somewhat comparable to that directed earlier to the study of DNA is now being made in this field. It has become clear that the major factors concerned with biological control in metazoa either involve the cell surface directly or must enter the cell through the surface, and that disturbance of such control mechanisms are likely to be of fundamental importance in the development of neoplasia. The problem of the cell surface in cancer can be broken down into the following major fields of investigation: (*a*) surface adhesive forces (*b*) cell surface shape and movements (*c*) biochemical constitution of the surface (*d*) immunology of cell surfaces (*e*) cell junctions and intercellular communications.

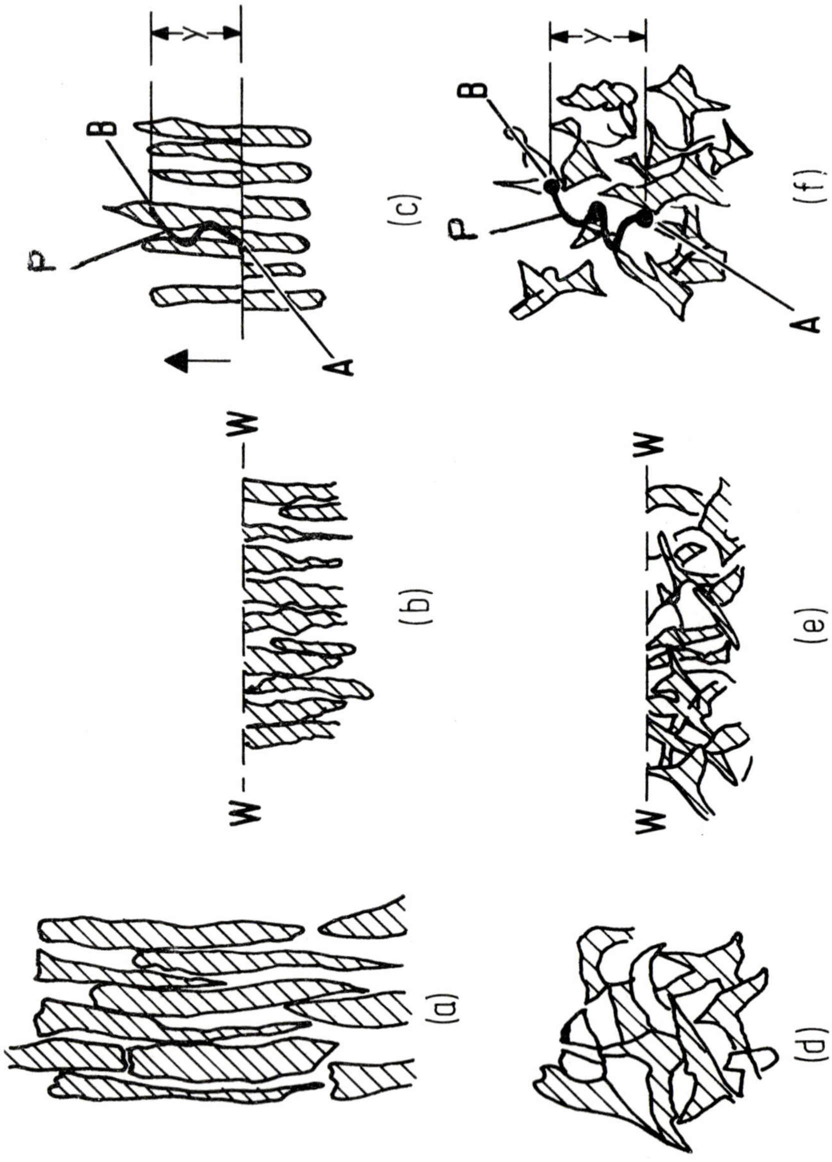
(a)
(b)
(c)
(d)
(e)
(f)
W
W
W
W
P
A
B
y
P
A
B
y

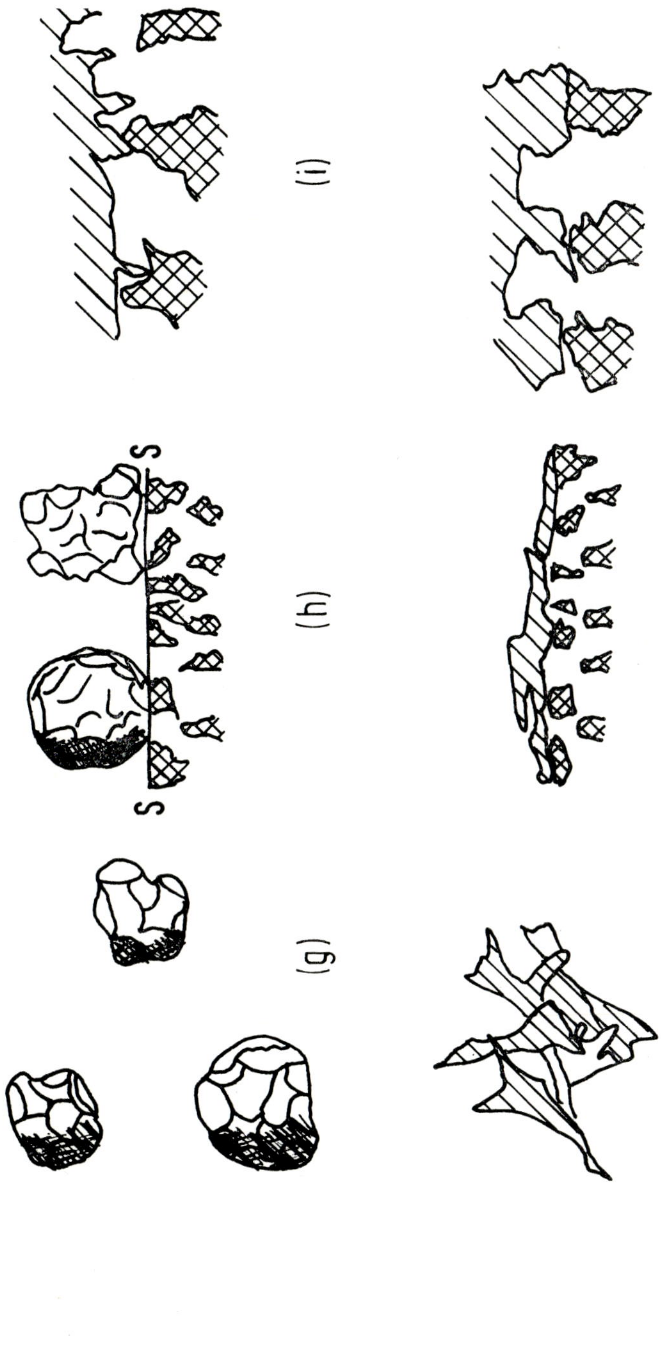

Fig. 3.1. Legend overleaf on page 30.

Recent developments in these various fields are reviewed below, while the relevance of this work to the problems of local invasiveness of tumours and metastasis is described in Chapters 4 and 5; immunological aspects are considered in Chapter 12.

Biological investigations of tumour surface properties

The availability of a range of non-malignant cells and the corresponding virally-transformed cells in culture has made possible a systematic study of changes in cell surface structure in malignancy. Cloned BHK21 (baby hamster kidney fibroblasts) and the corresponding cloned cells after transformation by polyoma virus (Macpherson and Stoker, 1962[7]) have been widely used for this work. The growth pattern in confluent culture is shown diagrammatically in *Fig. 3.1a* and *d.* A simple method for demonstrating changes in contact inhibition arising from such transformation has been the wounding procedure as described by Todaro, Lazar and Green (1965)[8] and by Vasiliev, Gelfand, Domina and Rappaport (1969)[9]. A confluent monolayer of cells is incised to produce a sharply defined edge (*Fig. 3.1b*). Polarized and well orientated groups of fibroblasts grow out from such an edge as shown in *Fig. 3.1c.* Contacts between cells (contact inhibition) operate so that the cells do not migrate appreciably in the x direction; they move perpendicularly to the wounded edge. Polyoma virus-transformed cells (which produce tumours *in vivo*) migrate in a random fashion with much cell overlap as shown in *Fig. 3.1–d–f.* Contact inhibition should not be looked upon as an all-or-none phenomenon. Phillips and Ambrose (1772)[10] used the method shown in *Fig. 3.1a–f* for the study of hybrid cells formed from malignant and non-malignant parents. Contact inhibition was measured as the mean ratio of movement in the y direction to total path length (p)—see *Fig. 3.1c.* For perfect contact inhibition $\frac{y}{p} = 1$; for completely random movement $\frac{y}{p} = 0$. Various clones derived from the hybrid populations showed a range of intermediate values for contact inhibition of movement. Contact inhibition has also been studied recently by Middleton (1973)[11] in primary cultures of pigmented

Fig. 3.1. (See pp. 28–9) Cell contacts in non-malignant and malignant fibroblasts.
(*a*) Confluent monolayer of untransformed fibroblasts showing polarized and aligned cells due to contact inhibition of movement.
(*b*) As above after wounding. W—W: wounded edge.
(*c*) As above showing migration from wounded edge. y—distance migrated perpendicular to edge. From A to B, total path length—p.
(*d*) Confluent layer of polyoma virus-transformed fibroblasts showing random appearance and overlap of cells.
(*e*) As above after wounding. W—W: wounded edge.
(*f*) As above after random migration. y—vertical distance. From A to B, total path length—p.
(*g*) Untransformed fibroblasts growing as compact colonies on G S millipore (plan).
(*h*) As above in section.
(*i*) Enlarged view of incomplete contacts between fibroblast microvilli and millipore.
(*j*) Polyoma-transformed cells on GS millipore (plan).
(*k*) As above in section.
(*l*) Enlarged view showing close contacts due to irregular polypodia of transformed cells.

retinal epithelial cells from chick embryos. The cells initially moved freely; collision between cells halted them and cell-cell contacts, once formed, were stable. The cells were strongly monolayered and freshly dissociated cells failed to spread on the surface of a pre-existing monolayer of cells. This phenomenon of contact inhibition as observed in both fibroblast and epithelial cultures can be investigated in terms of cellular adhesiveness, cell shape (topology) and cell surface dynamics; and these aspects are considered below.

CELL SURFACE ADHESIVENESS

Adhesiveness between surfaces is a complicated physico-chemical problem which will not be discussed in detail here; the subject has been reviewed by Curtis (1967)[12] and by L. Weiss (1972)[13]. Cell surfaces carry a net negative charge due to ionised acidic groups. This leads to the so-called coulomb force of *repulsion* between surfaces which falls off rather slowly with distance. The other attractive forces, which are short range in character, include electrostatic bonds between positively and negatively charged groups at the surface, covalent bonds, weak hydrogen bonds such as those found between amide $\left(> N{-}H \ldots O{=}C<\right)$ and hydroxyl $\left(O{-}H \ldots O\langle^{H}\right)$ groups also the more general van der Waals' forces. The net effect of such interactions at cell surfaces is to give rise to two positions of equilibrium between surfaces as shown in *Fig. 3.2a.* In living cells the net adhesive force between a cell and the substratum or between cell and cell is also governed by the total areas in contact. Cell surfaces are often irregular in shape and therefore only a small fraction of the surfaces may be in direct contact. Vasiliev and Gelfand (1973)[14] have therefore distinguished between *adhesiveness*, which is the true force per unit area in the regions of contact (*c*) as indicated in *Fig. 3.2a*, and *attachment* which depends on the areas of attachment of the cells to the substratum. This latter property may be measured by centrifugation methods (Easty *et al.*, 1960)[6] or by an air blast technique (Gail and Boone, 1972[15]). Ability of cells to attach to each other need not run parallel with their ability to attach to the substratum; thus, Ambrose and Ellison (1968)[16] compared the growth pattern of BHK21 fibroblasts and polyoma transformed cells (PyY) on smooth glass, rough glass, smooth plastic and millipore surfaces. In *Fig. 3.1* (*g, h, i*) is shown in plan the appearance of a culture of BHK fibroblasts grown on GS millipore on roughened glass. The cells do not adhere appreciably to the substratum but form massive spherical colonies of cells which may reach as much as 1mm in diameter. Somewhat similar growth patterns have been seen by Friedenstein, Rappaport and Murian (1967)[17] with human diploid cell lines on filter material. By contrast, the polyoma transformed cells spread as well on millipore or on roughened glass as they do on smooth glass or plastic (*Fig. 3.1 j, k, l*) despite the fact that transformed cells do not have such a strong net attachment to smooth glass or plastic (Gail and Boone, 1972[15]; Vasiliev and Gelfand, 1973[14]). Steroscan electron microscope studies suggest that this difference between relative cell-cell and cell-substrate adhesiveness shown by the two cell types on millipore may depend on differences in the cell surface shape (topology) to be discussed below.

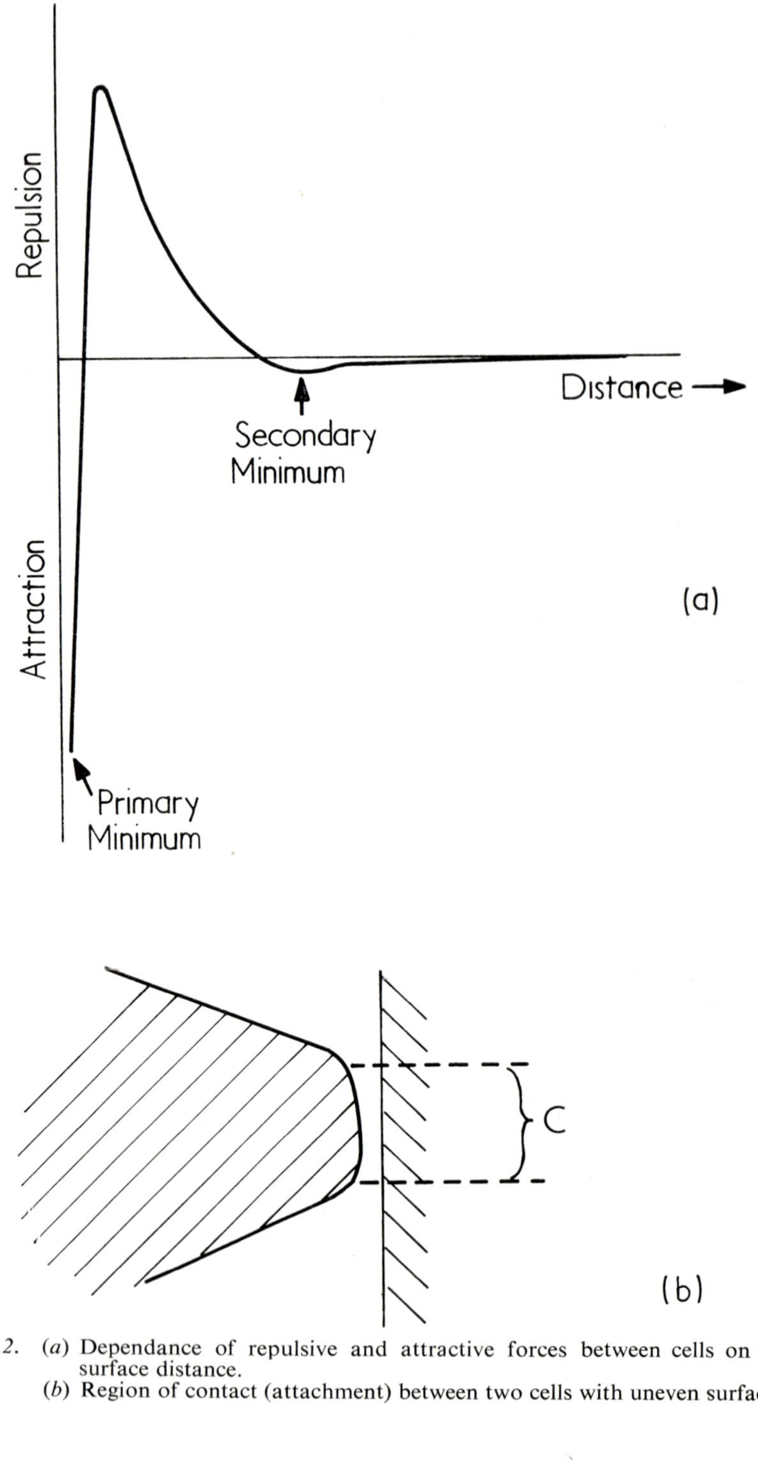

Fig. 3.2. (*a*) Dependance of repulsive and attractive forces between cells on inter-surface distance.
(*b*) Region of contact (attachment) between two cells with uneven surfaces.

CELL SURFACE SHAPE

The surfaces of cells as observed in time lapse films are seen to be in a state of flux, with constant changes of topology. Such systems have proved extremely difficult to classify and analyse, but a recent mathematical theory of transient disturbances at interfaces and other inhomogeneities of strucure has been developed by René Thom (1968)[18]. This theory has been applied to a study of cell surface topology by Ambrose (1971)[19] and the reader is referred to this paper for full details. The main types of transient disturbances observed at cell surfaces are illustrated in *Fig. 3.3.* In *Fig. 3.3 (a–d)* is shown the expansion of a

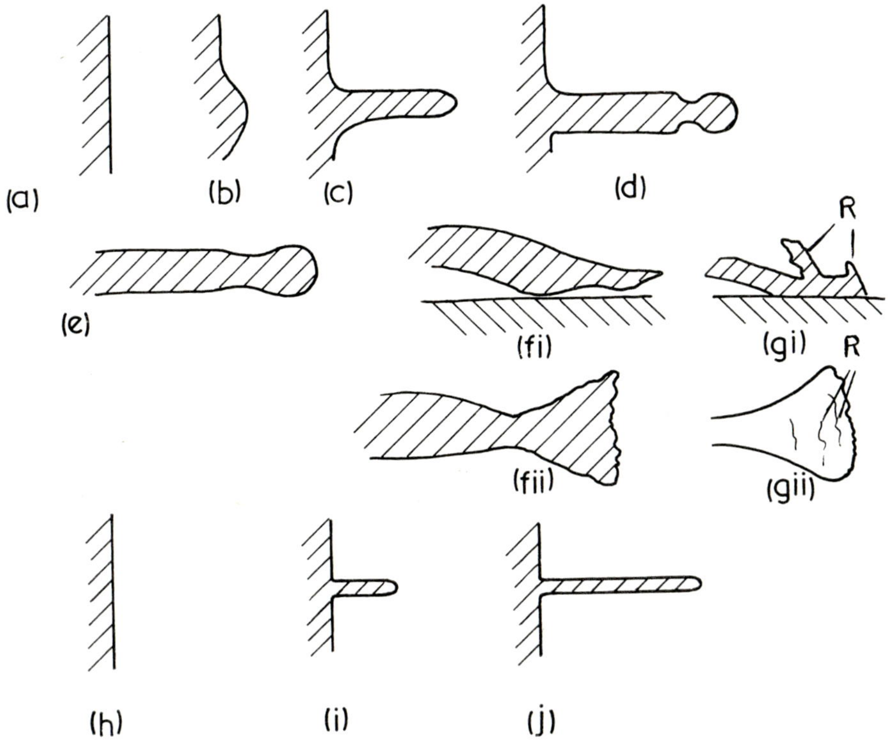

Fig. 3.3. Formation of pseudopodia by non-malignant cells. (a), (*b*), (*c*), (*d*). Stages on the evolution of a large pseudopodium. (*e*), (*f*), (*g*). Manner in which a pseudopodium attaches to a substrate. (*fi*). section (*fii*). Plan: R. ruffled membranes (*h*), (*i*), (*j*) stages on the evolution of a microvillus.

pseudopodium (*a*), (b), (*c*) which may later develop into a lobopodium (*d*). If such a lobopodium makes contact with a substrate, adhesive forces may operate and it will expand into a fan-like cone (*Fig. 3.3 ef,*). This cone may later form a sheet or lamellipodium (*Fig. 3.3g*). Once a lamellipodium has been generated the second type of major disturbances is initiated; these are *ruffled* (*undulating*) membranes and are shown in *Fig. 3.3g*. Movements of this

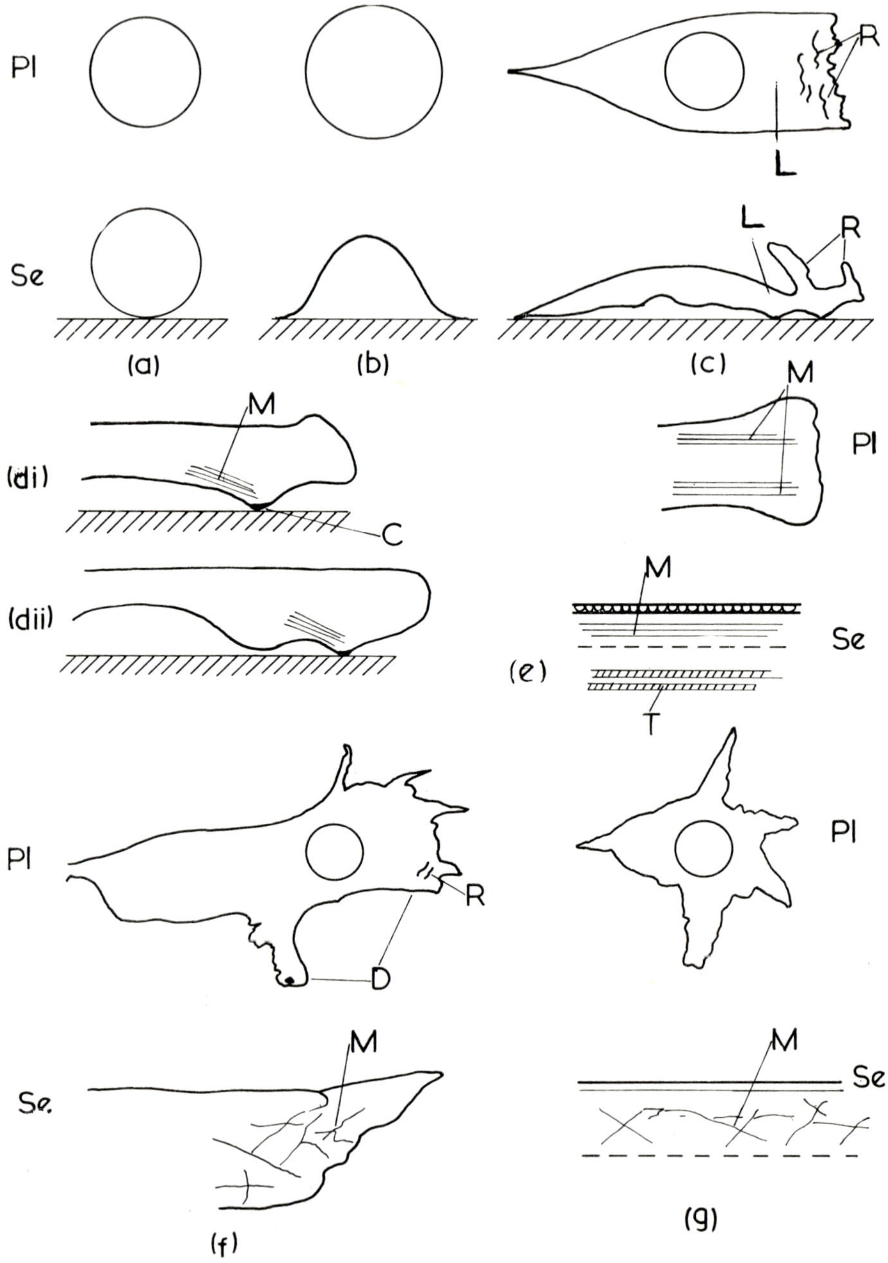
Pl
R
L
Se
L
R
(a)
(b)
(c)
M
M
(di)
Pl
C
(dii)
M
Se
(e)
T
Pl
Pl
R
D
M
Se.
M
Se
(f)
(g)

kind, on the *lower* surface of the cell, provide the locomotory mechanism. The third type of disturbance commonly seen is the formation of fine hair-like processes or microvilli of about 2000 Å in diameter. These microvilli extend from the surface, remain stable for a time and are then withdrawn (*Fig. 3.3* (*h, i, j*).

CELL SURFACE DYNAMICS

The simplest way to study the relationship between surface adhesiveness, surface topology and surface movements in non-malignant and malignant cells is to examine their behaviour while settling on to a flat surface from a suspension. The spherical form, being the shape with the least surface energy, is generally assumed by cells in suspension (*Fig. 3.4a*). When contact is made with the substratum, the cell spreads due to adhesive forces in the way that a drop of water spreads on a slightly greasy surface (*Fig. 3.4b*). Undulating membranes begin to form at the cell boundary, lamellipodia are produced and the cell becomes elongated (*polarized*). The cell soon begins to move (*Fig 3.4c*) by advancing the leading lamellipodium. Cellular locomotion takes place by the generation of intermittent contacts of small areas of the lower surface of the cell with the substrate as was first demonstrated by surface contact microscopy (Ambrose, 1961[20]). This has since been confirmed by direct observation from the side of fibroblasts moving on glass fibres (Korohoda, 1971[21]). Using the interference reflection microscope, Harberey (1971)[22] has seen similar intermittent contacts on the lower surface of *Amoeba proteus* when migrating on a glass surface. It now appears from the work of Abercrombie, Heaysman and Pegrum (1971)[23] that the formation of ruffled membranes is associated with local surface flow, as indicated by the movement of particles, and that the main locomotory force is generated in regions of strong cell-substrate contact near the front of the cell. Intermittent contacts are also observed further back from the leading edge (Ambrose, 1961[20]; Vasiliev and Gelfand, 1973[14]) but these contacts appear to prevent the uniform close approach of the cell surface to the substrate, a situation which would lead to enormous viscous resistance to cell locomotion. The cells move like front-drive motor cars, the motive force and the transmission being located at the front of the cell, the trailing intermittent contacts behaving somewhat like bogey wheels. Cytoplasmic microfilaments are also seen near the regions of contact at the leading edge which may provide a tensile force (Heaysman, 1973[24]).

Fig. 3.4. Attachment of untransformed and transformed cells to smooth glass (pl-plan se-section).
(*a*) Rounded fibroblast from suspension settling on glass.
(*b*) Uniform spreading stage.
(*c*) Extension to polarized form. L—Lamellar cytoplasm: R—Ruffled membranes.
(*d*) Intermittent cell-substrate contacts on leading edge. (i) 1st stage: (ii) 2nd stage. M—microfilaments; C—region of thickening.
(*e*) Arrangement of sub-surface microfilaments in region of lamellar cytoplasm. M—microfilaments: T—microtubules.
(*f*) Transformed cell of low malignancy. D—polypodia: R—ruffled membranes. M—Disorientated microfibrils.
(*g*) Highly malignant cell showing irregular pseudopodia.

The subject of cell locomotion has been described in detail in an excellent Ciba Foundation Symposium (Ed. Abercrombie, 1973[14]). There is now fairly general agreement that the locomotion of fibroblasts, epithelial cells and probably macrophages is mainly a cell surface phenomenon, the active movements of the cell surface required to generate the motive force being found in sub-surface microfilaments (Ishikawa, Bischoff and Holtzer, 1969[25]; Spooner, Yamada and Wessels, 1971[26]) of 60 Å diameter and similar in constitution to the actin of smooth muscle (*Fig. 3.4e*). Myosin-like ATPase activity is also found in this region (Bryn Jones, Kemp and Groschel Stewart, 1970[27]). Vasiliev and Gelfand (1973)[14] note that the spreading of fibroblasts and the development of polar form is accompanied by the formation of a region in the leading part of the cell called *lamellar* cytoplasm. This region contains plasma gel 0·1–1μ thick on its inner surface, also microfilaments which can be seen in the stereoscan electron microscope to be arranged in bundles as shown in *Fig. 3.4e*. Vasiliev and Gelfand (1973)[14] have made a careful comparative study of the spreading of non-malignant fibroblasts (one passage after preparation of primary culture), a line of L strain fibroblasts of low malignancy, and the highly malignant CIM and S40 lines; the results were obtained by time-lapse filming and by transmission and stereoscan electron microscopy. The conclusions reached are summarized in Fig. *3.4* (*f* and *g*). The L cells spread somewhat similarly to the normal fibroblasts but with *numerous microvilli* at the borders (*Fig. 3.4f*). The periphery of the cell was also thicker than the normal cell. The areas of *lamellar cytoplasm* were found to be much reduced or separated into discrete areas. Fibrillar bundles were *reduced in number*, or *absent*. The CIM and S40 cells showed similar characteristics but to a more pronounced degree. Cells with 1–3 long processes were often seen (*Fig. 3.4g*). The less ordered regions of microfilaments on the periphery of neoplastic cells had previously been noted by Ambrose, Batzdorf, Osborn and Stuart (1970)[28], and Ambrose, D. Easty and Batzdorf (1972)[29] in cultures of human glial cells before and after removal of the outer coat and plasma membrane by ion etching.

McNutt, Culp and Black (1973)[30] have demonstrated comparable changes using replica and thin section methods. When epithelial cells spread in culture the chief difference in properties as compared with fibroblasts lies in the high cell-substrate adhesiveness which causes them to form an extremely thin disc; also, the sub-surface filaments do not play such an important role in morphology. Membrane undulations at the borders and locomotion occur as with fibroblasts except that the cells lack the polarized form of fibroblasts and myoblasts. Examples of the type of morphological change observed in carcinoma transformation are illustrated in Plate 3.1.

CELL CONTACTS

Once cells in a monolayer have spread and grown to produce a confluent sheet, many cell junctions are formed. Studies by Trinkhaus, Betcheku and Krurkowski (1971)[31] have shown that direct contact between cell membranes is involved in the arrest of movement by contact inhibition and that signalling molecules are not required. The stages have been described by Abercrombie

(1970)[32] as inhibition of formation of lamellipodia, retraction of the leading edge and sometimes cell-cell adhesion. Depending on the degree of attachment of adjacent cells to the substratum, some degree of *underlap* may occur leading to penetration of one cell beneath another before movement is finally arrested. The initial formation of junctions has been carefully investigated by Heaysman (1973)[24] using electron microscopy. A typical cell-cell junction is shown in *Fig. 3.5a.* Some overlap of the edges of the two cells may take place and there is adhesion over a limited area characterized by a zone of intracytoplasmic secretion just below the membrane surface. The detailed structure of the types of junction which later develop between various cell types on contact have been extensively studied both in cultures and whole tissues using thin sectioning electron microscopy and freeze etching procedures. In early work, the most striking feature of cell-cell contacts was their uniformity of appearance with an apparent gap of ~ 100 Å between the adjacent plasma membranes. Curtis (1960)[33] proposed that this gap was a real gap, the distance between the cells being stabilized by a balance between attractive and repulsive forces. The mathematical theory of Derjaguin and Landau (1941)[34] and of Vermey and Overbeek (1968)[35] would explain how such conditions could be satisfied at the secondary minimum shown in *Fig. 3.2a.* Later work has indicated that a glycoprotein gel of low density may fill the gap. Nevertheless, the surprising uniformity of the gap suggests some underlying physical basis. In addition to this general lining up of cells in contact, special types of junction at limited areas occur. They are shown diagrammatically in *Fig. 3.5* (*b, c* and *d*), and are described below:

The *macula adhesions* or desmosome junctions (*Fig. 3.5b*) are regions where plaques are secreted between the cells; fibrous plaques also form in the adjacent cytoplasm within the two cells. Fine tonofilaments (100 Å in diameter) become attached to the internal plaques. The gap between the membranes is ~ 350 Å. These junctions are thought to play an important role in maintaining cell adhesion and tension; in tissues subject to mechanical stress the tonofibrils probably provide additional strength. They are, for example, particularly conspicuous in the squamous epithelium of the skin. Somewhat similar but less differentiated junctions with gaps of about 200 Å occur over larger areas; such a junction is known as a zonula or fascia adherens.

Small gap junctions (*nexus junctions*) are small areas of adjacent cells which come into much closer contact, the distance between the two trilaminar membranes as seen in electron microscope sections being only 20–30 Å (Revel and Karnovsky, 1967[36]; McNutt (1972)[37]. These junctions play a role in adhesion and communication between cells. Muir (1967)[38] incubated cardiac muscle in a calcium-free medium and found that after a short time all junctions except the nexus gap junctions were broken. Hyperosmotic Krebs–Henseleit solution (2·5 mM calcium, Barr, 1965[39], 1968[40]) will, however, separate the nexus junctions at the mid-plane if the cells are slightly stretched. An important feature of these junctions is that they are packed with subunits 70–80 Å in diameter (Benedetti and Emmelot, 1965[41]; Revel and Karnovsky, 1967[36]). There is evidence to suggest that these subunits are embedded in their respective plasma membranes but meet at their apices to provide an

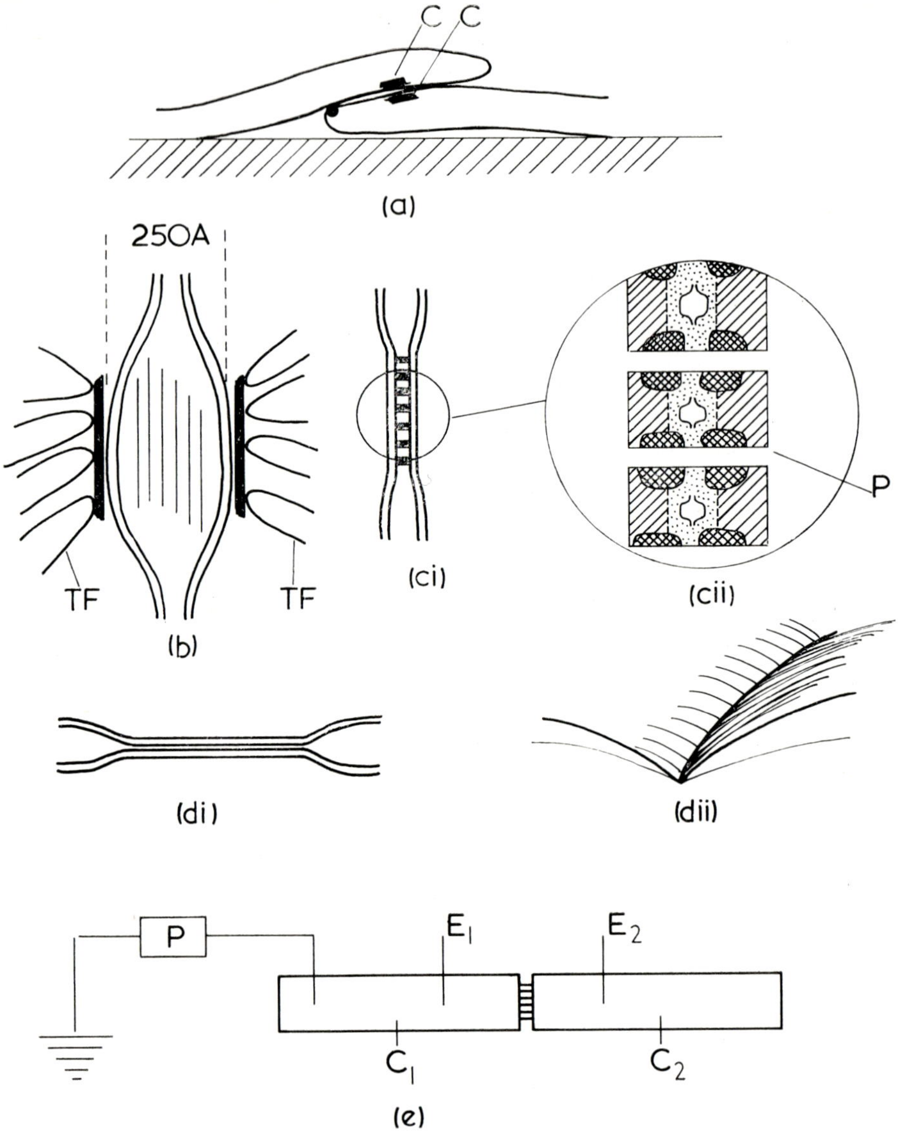

Fig. 3.5. Cell junctions.
(*a*) Initial stage in junction formation seen in fibroblasts in monolayer culture C—region of cytoplasmic thickening.
(*b*) Desmosome junction. TF—tonofibrils.
(*c*) (i) nexus junction
(ii) enlargement of same showing pores (P).
(*d*) (i) tight junction.
(ii) The same showing its banded form in perspective.
(*e*) Arrangement for testing intercellular coupling. P—pulse generator. E_1, E_2—electrodes C_1, C_2—cells.

ion-permeable channel from cell to cell as indicated in *Fig. 3.5c*. For this reason the nexus junctions provide small areas of electrical communication between cells. These junctions have proved to be of importance in malignant transformation following the work of Lowenstein *et al.* (1967)[42]. A clear-cut picture has been obtained by comparing non-malignant hepatocyte cell lines with hepatomas. Electrical communication is demonstrated by means of the electrode assembly shown in *Fig. 3.5e*. A measurement of the resistance between the electrode E_1 in the medium and E_2 indicates a high or low ion permeability (10^{-4}mho/cm^2) being a measure of the membrane resistance of Cell C. If the resistance between E_2 and E_3 is measured, a high value is again obtained if the cells C_1 and C_2 are not in communication. If low resistance junctions (nexus gap junctions) exist between C_1 and C_2 the resistance is low (150Ω/cm^2) being about the same as that of cellular cytoplasm. Azaria and Lowenstein (1973)[43] have also studied non-malignant rat cell lines of epithelial origin and fibroblasts and an A strain rat tumour. They have found that malignancy *in vivo* is suppressed in hybrid lines formed from malignant and non-malignant lines and contact inhibition as indicated by ability to form a stable monolayer is restored. In addition, the non-malignant lines show electrical communication whereas the malignant lines do not (Borek, 1972[44]).

Unfortunately the situation is not so clearcut with fibroblasts and sarcoma cells. The junctions in polyoma-transformed cells do in fact appear to have considerable coherence as observed in time-lapse films. It is partly the topological factor, i.e. production of irregular pseudopodia and hence of reduced *areas* of adhesion (attachment) which also play an important role in the surface changes in malignant fibroblasts. The disadvantage of the technique for measuring electrical communication is essentially that it measures an all-or-none effect. If the number of nexus junctions is reduced but a few remain after transformation, the cells will still show electrical communication and this may happen during transformation of fibroblasts to sarcoma cells. The nexus junctions also allow the passage, for example, of the dye Procion yellow (mol. wt. 500) from cell to cell (Payton, Bennett and Pappas, 1969[45]). They may play a role in permitting ions and moderately large metabolites to pass from cell to cell in living tissues.

Zonula Occludens (*Tight Junctions*) are continuous belt-like regions of intimate contact between adjacent cells where no actual separation of the cells can be observed (*Fig. 3.5e*). They were first described by Farquhar and Palade (1963)[46] in the terminal bar region of columnar epithelia; they are also seen linking hepatocytes at the bile canaliculus (Matter, Orci and Rouiller (1969)[47]. Freeze cleavage reveals that they are formed by ridges on one cell surface which fit into grooves on the other surface, so that a continuous band is formed to provide a barrier. The function of these junctions is to provide a complete barrier to the passage of fluids along cell surfaces. McNutt and Weinsten (1969)[48] observed that nexus junctions were abundant in normal cervical epithelium while they were deficient in squamous carcinoma. Martinez–Palomo (1970)[49] studied pre-lactating and lactating mouse mammary glands and mouse mammary carcinoma. Tight junctions were absent in many tumours and the apical junctions became permeable to lanthenum.

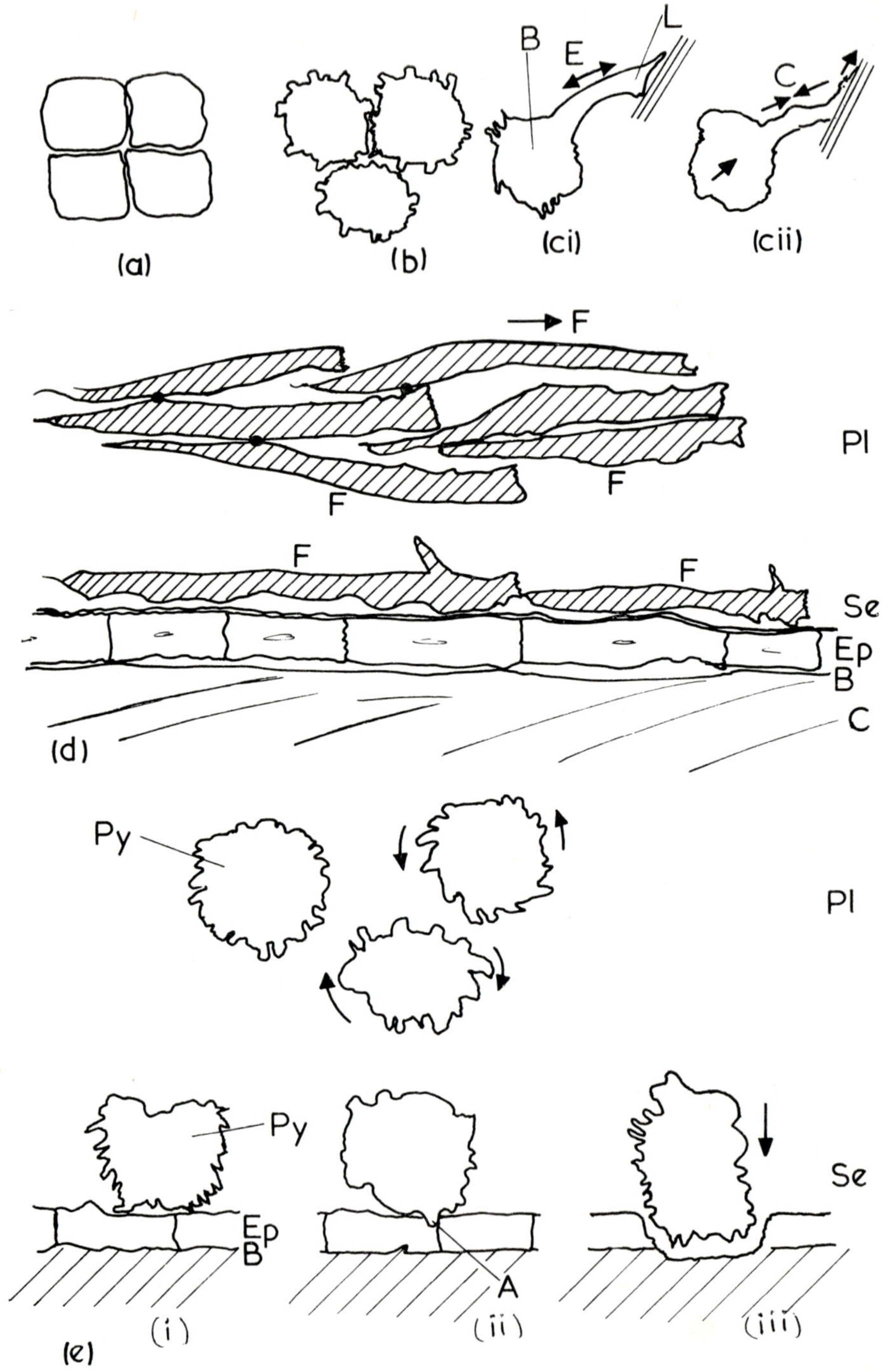
B
L
E
C
(a)
(b)
(ci)
(cii)
F
Pl
F
F
F
F
Se
Ep
B
C
(d)
Py
Pl
Py
Se
Ep
B
A
(i)
(ii)
(iii)
(e)

Gap junctions (nexus junctions) were also scarce. Sirsat *et al.* (1970)[50] have observed a decrease in the number of desmosome junctions in malignant transformation of buccal mucosa to oral cancers in man.

There is little to suggest that any basic structural changes take place in these three types of cell junctions during malignant change, though various workers have found some reduction in the number of cell-cell junctions in certain tumours.

Cell surface movements and contacts in whole tissues

The extensive investigations made in the cell surface dynamics of non-malignant and malignant cells in monolayer tissue culture as described above have not been matched by corresponding studies of cells in whole tissues. This is partly because a problem in two dimensions is easier to analyse than the corresponding problem in three dimensions. In addition, optical conditions are most unfavourable for the direct observation of the behaviour of living cells in whole tissues. The most suitable tissues for such studies are transparent embryos, and Gustafson and Wolpert (1961)[53] have studied the movements of mesenchymal cells during morphogenesis in the gastrulation of developing sea urchins.

In monolayer culture, the cells have every opportunity to attach to the flat surface of plastic or glass, whereas *in vivo* the substrata are more variable in morphology and may consist of other cells in the form of strands or sheets, collagen fibres, linings of vessels, cavities etc. Trinkaus (1973)[52] has made a detailed study of the movements of deep cells during the early embryonic development of the fish Fundulus. During the blastula stage the cells are comparatively non-adhesive and can be readily broken up into separate cells in culture. In the embryo they grow and divide up to the 128-cell stage but without showing detectable membrane movements (*Fig. 3.6a*). After this, blebbing of the surface begins to occur (*Fig. 3.6b*). This is followed by the formation of lobopodia. These lobopodia (*Fig. 3.6c* (i) and *Fig. 3.6c* (ii) may adhere by their ends to other cell surfaces, and may spread to form lamellipodia where they can find attachment. Cell migration then begins. A somewhat similar sequence of events was observed by Wolpert and Gustafson (1961)[51] in the mesodermal cells during gastrulation in the sea urchin. The lobopodia

Fig. 3.6. Movements of cells in whole tissues.
(*a*) Group of growing and dividing cells in early blastula stage.
(*b*) The same at a later stage showing irregular blebbing of the surface.
(*c*) (i) Development of pseudopodium during gastrulation with lamellipodium attaching to filaments or other surface. E—Extending pseudopodium. B—Cell body.
(ii) The same later showing cell body being pulled up by contraction (C) of pseudopodium.
(*d*) Behaviour of non-malignant fibroblasts when placed on the surface of the chick chorioallantoic membrane or rat omentum. P—plan: S—section: F—fibroblast: Ep—Epithelium: B—Basement membrane: C—connective tissue.
(*e*) Behaviour of polyoma transformed fibroblasts (Py) under similar conditions. P—plan: S—section.
(i) Rounded cell with irregular polypodia not yet attached.
(ii) Cell forming cavity and
(iii) invading the normal tissue. A—point of anchorage.

extended into the cavity of the blastula, attached to a surface and then retracted, possibly due to their elasticity, so drawing the cell body with them. Korohoda has described similar behaviour in fibroblasts growing on glass fibres. A lobopodium may be generated on the upper surface of a cell when it attaches to a neighbouring fibre and later draws up the body of the cell. With non-malignant cells, the key to locomotion appears to lie in the formation of the lamellipodia. Ambrose and D. Easty (1973)[54] studied the spreading of non-malignant BHK21 fibroblasts and macrophages on a surface of normal epithelial or mesothelial cells using a new time-lapse filming technique for organ cultures. In spite of the somewhat irregular topology of the surface of the normal tissues, the fibroblasts and macrophages migrated smoothly over these normal cells, apparently as a consequence of intermittent contacts generated by undulating motion of the cell membranes (*Fig. 3.6d*) The fibroblasts formed polarized groups of cells similar to those found when fibroblasts are growing on glass (*Fig. 3.6e*). Fibroblasts which had been transformed by polyoma or SV40 virus behaved quite differently. The malignant cells did not spread well on the normal tissues but showed continuous production of polypodia over their entire surface. *Fig. 3.6e* (i)). After a short time most of the cells became anchored at one place on the normal epithelium (*Fig. 3.6e* (ii). From then on no further translational movement parallel to the normal tissue surface occurred. The polypodial activity remained just as intense throughout the observations and the cells eventually drove a passage down between the normal tissues (*Fig. 3.6e* (iii)). Under these circumstances the difference between the surface dynamics of the tumour and non-malignant cell surface was considerably more striking than that seen in monolayer culture for these cells. Other factors are involved in the local invasion of normal tissues by tumour cells (see Chapter 4) such as a release of enzymes which break down the intercellular cement in the normal tissues (Sylvén, 1962[54a]). But the rather special type of cell surface dynamics and adhesiveness observed in films of organ cultures also play a key role, e.g. non-motile cells show little tendency to invade the normal tissues.

Surface dynamics of human tumours

Although it would clearly be desirable to examine the surface dynamics of living human tumours in an organ culture system or *in vivo*, this is not at present a feasible routine procedure. Useful information can, however, be obtained from studies made in monolayer culture based on the experimental work described above, namely:

(1) Cell-substrate adhesion (2) Cell-cell adhesion
(3) Cell polarity (4) Pseudopodial morphology
(5) Cell overlap and piling up in confluent layers.

This is illustrated in a group of renal carcinomas cultured by a new technique which give small discrete explants, often homogenous in cell type (Ambrose, G. Easty and Tchao, 1974[55]).

Epithelium from the normal human kidney (Plate 3.1.I) shows the characteristic close contacts at the cell borders which give rise to a continuous sheet

Plate 3.1. Microexplant cultures of human carcinomas of the kidney.

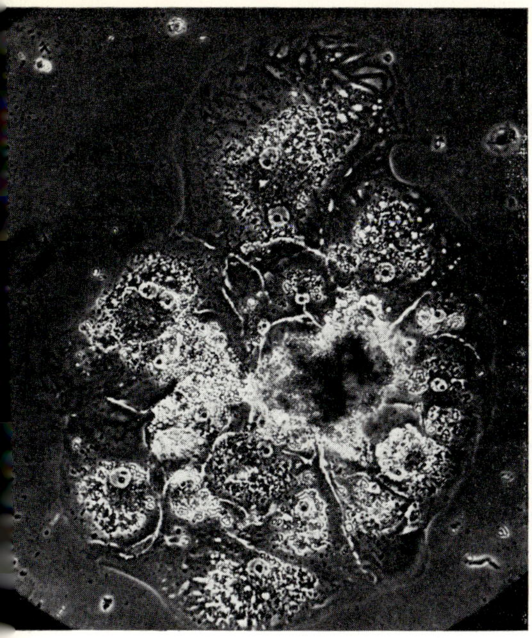

Plate 3.1.I. (*Left*) Cell group showing normal contacts and morphology of cortical epithelium.

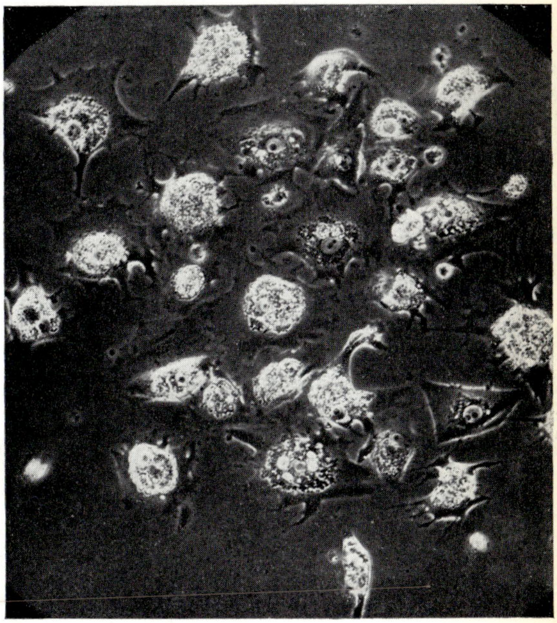

Plate 3.1.II. (*Right*) Group showing monolayer but with irregular (polypodial) contacts.

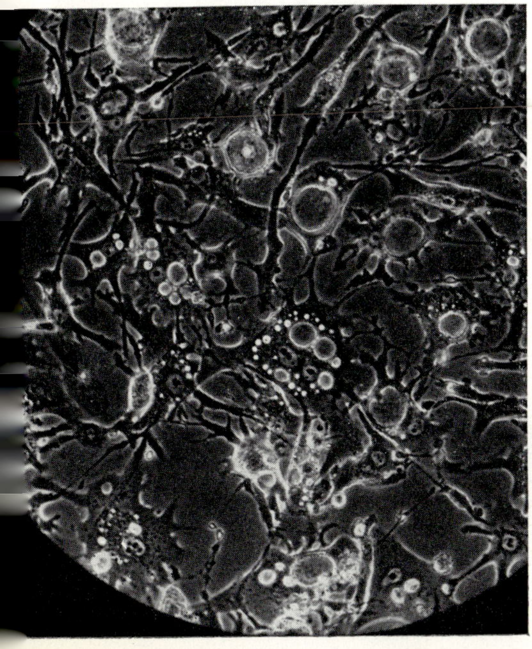

Plate 3.1.III. (*Left*) Bizarre cells, high lipid contact.

Plate 3.1. Microexplant cultures of human carcinomas of the kidney (*cont.*)

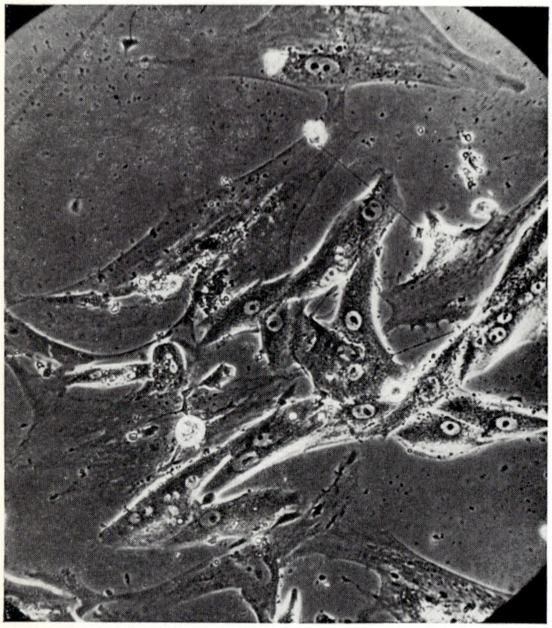

Plate 3.1.IV. (*Left*) Cells showing piling up, loss of contact inhibition.

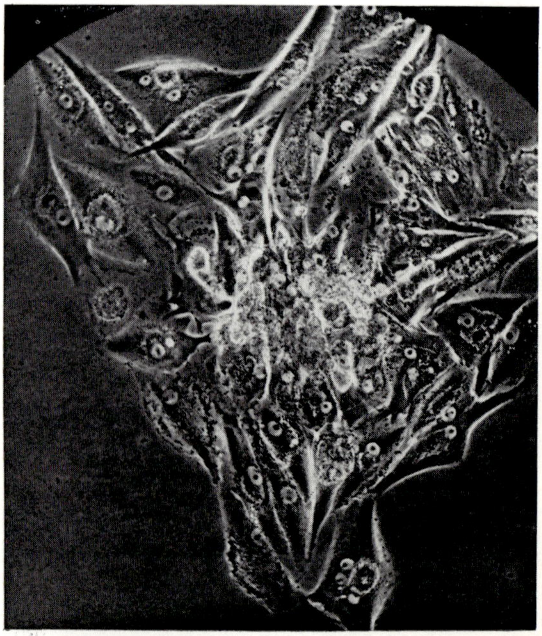

Plate 3.1.V. (*Right*) Microcolony from a pulmonary metastasis similar in morphology to d.

of cells. These are similar in appearance to renal cortical epithelial cells of normal rat and hamster, growing in culture. The three renal carcinomas show an interesting progressive alteration in surface properties. The first of these (Plate 3.1.II) shows little deviation from normal morphology, with polypodia at the cell borders of the type already described; cell-substrate adhesion, as judged by spreading, is still good. In the second tumour (Plate 3.1.III) there are bizarre forms with cell overlap and high lipid production, also considerable cell overlap. The third tumour (Plate 3.1.IV) shows marked piling up and loss of contact inhibition. Plate 3.1.V shows a culture obtained from a needle biopsy of a lung metastasis from a renal carcinoma. There is a remarkable resemblance between these cells and the tumour of Plate 3.I, suggesting that this cell type may be one of those capable of forming metastases.

Cell contacts and the control of growth

The accounts given above have shown the importance of cell surface phenomena in the dynamics of cell movements and in the escape from control of locomotion in malignancy. Another important aspect of escape from control relates to the failure of growth regulation in malignancy. Abercrombie and Ambrose (1962)[56] suggested that surface changes might also lead to loss of control of mitosis in addition to affecting cell movements in malignant cells. Experimental work in this field has been carried out by Todaro, Lazar and Green (1965)[57], Levene, Becher, Boone and Eagle (1965)[58], Dulbecco and Stoker (1970)[59] and others. When non-malignant fibroblasts grow in culture they generally proliferate until a confluent sheet of cells is produced; then the rate of DNA synthesis and of mitosis falls to a low level. This phenomenon has been variously named 'contact inhibition of cell division' (Levene, 1965[58]), 'density dependent inhibition' (Stoker and Rubin, 1967[60]), and 'post confluent inhibition of cell division' (Steinberg, 1972); 3T3 cells show the effect particularly clearly. Cell-cell contacts play an important role in this phenomenon, but not in quite the same sense as in contact inhibition of cell movements. Steinberg (1972)[61] has shown that one further mitosis can occur after cells have become completely surrounded by other cells. In addition, a serum factor plays an important role; this factor is found in the γ globulin fraction and does not appear to be species-specific (Temin, 1967[62]). Untransformed cells cannot begin to synthesise DNA in the absence of serum factor (Clarke, Stoker, Ludlow and Thornton, 1970[63]). But the capacity of the untransformed cells to respond to this serum factor depends on their relationship to other cells; cells in a confluent layer are much less responsive than migrating cells. By contrast, polyoma-transformed BHK 21 cells continue to grow after reaching confluence and produce multilayers. Transformed cells do not require a serum factor to initiate DNA synthesis; but both cell types require an additional serum factor to initiate mitosis (Clarke, Stoker, Ludlow and Thornton, 1970[63]). Nevertheless, the clear involvement of direct cell contacts in growth control can be illustrated with the help of wounded edge cultures of the type shown in *Fig. 3.1a, b, c.* If such a wound is formed in a confluent non-growing culture of non-malignant cells, migration is initiated (*Fig. 3.1c, d*), DNA synthesis begins and mitoses occur. This is in the identical culture medium containing the same serum factors as the confluent layer which does not grow.

Korohoda has studied the role of cell contacts on cellular metabolism in cultured chick embryo fibroblasts using a microrespirometer (Zurcycki and Starzecki, 1970[65]). The mean respiration rate in μl 0_2/million cells was as follows—in suspension: 4·07 ± 0·66; confluent layer: 2·35 ± 0·85; locomoting: 18·87. He concludes that an important property of metazoan cells is the control of growth, and that growth is a *permissive phenomenon.* It is the failure of the cell-cell interactions leading to growth regulation which is deficient in malignancy and the cell surface is clearly involved. A somewhat similar view has been expressed by Holly (1972)[66].

Another important development relating to the role of the cell surface in growth control relates to the discovery that cyclic AMP (adenosine 3′5′ monophosphate) is involved as a regulator of cytoplasmic activity. The cyclei form is produced by enzymes, adenylate cyclases, which are located on the cell surface. These enzymes can act as specific receptors for hormones which appear to induce some kind of allosteric change in the molecule that is transmitted across the membrane resulting in the generation of cyclic AMP within the cytoplasm. Cyclic AMP also plays a role in the control of cell growth. High levels of cyclic AMP are associated in some studies with reduced growth rate for cells in monolayer culture; thus, Shepperd (1972)[67] investigated the effect of cyclic AMP levels on polyoma-transformed 3T3 cells and found that the cells grow to a lower saturation density if theophylline and dibutyryl cyclic AMP was added to the medium. Smets (1972)[68] has proposed that this effect is not due to a phenotypic reversion to normal cell surface behaviour but to the effects of cyclic AMP on later stages of the cell cycle. However, the level of cyclic AMP rises when non-malignant cells reach a confluent layer and the growth rate falls, suggesting that cell-cell contacts may also play a role in the activation of adenylate cyclases and hence to the regulation of growth by the second messenger molecules of cyclic AMP. It has also been found that non-malignant cells in the rapid growth phase contain a higher cyclic AMP level than malignant cells in the growth phase. The work of Teel and Hall (1973)[69] using KB cells indicated that the plating density was reduced by a factor of 3 on addition of 10^{-4}M dibutyryl cyclic AMP. They ascribed the effect to an inhibition during the G_1 phase of the cell cycle. Burger *et al.* (1972)[70] found that pronase treatment of untransformed cells leads to overgrowth; pronase also exposes receptor sites for concanavalin A. Dibutyryl cyclic AMP will block this increased growth after pronase treatment.

Molecular structure of the cell surface

The cell surface complex, as defined by Ambrose and D. Easty (1971)[71], is illustrated diagrammatically in *Fig. 3.7a.* Three distinct regions can be recognized—the outer coat, the plasma membrane, and the sub-surface plasma gel containing microfilaments. Changes in all three of these structures may occur to varying extents during malignant change, depending on the cell concerned and on the type of malignant transformation.

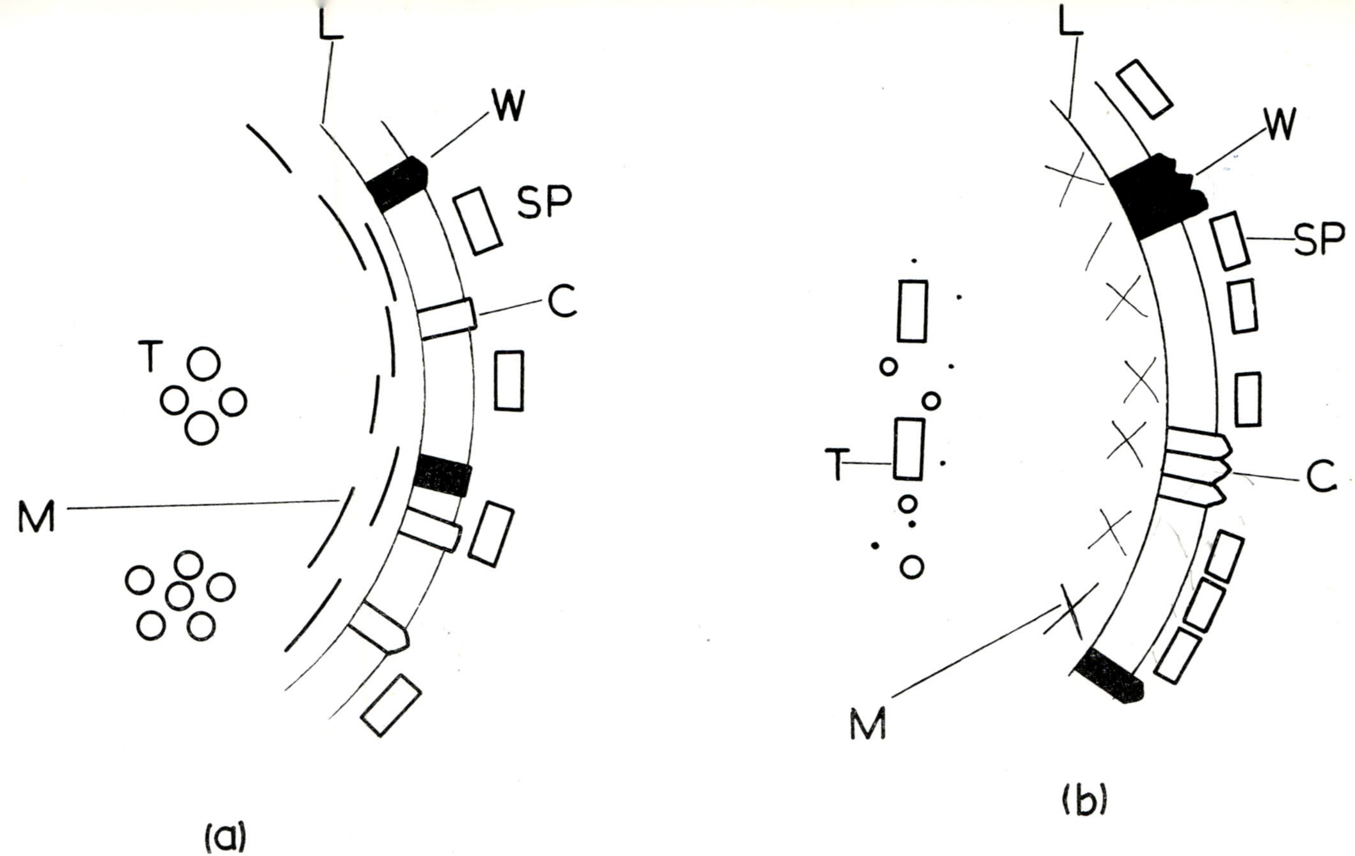

Fig. 3.7. Generalized model for the cell surface in normal and malignant cells.

(*a*) *Normal cell:* L—Lipid bilayer; SP—outer coating of sialo-mucoproteins; W—receptors for wheat germ agglutinin; C—receptors for concanavalin A; M—sub-surface microfilaments, well orientated; T—microtubules packed in regular arrays.

(*b*) *Malignant cell:* L Lipid bilayer, increased cholesterol; SP—more sialo-mucro proteins available at the cell surface; W—aggregated wheat germ receptors.;C—aggregated concanavalin A receptors; M—disorientated microfilaments; T—disaggregated microtubules.

OUTER COAT

Glycoproteins constitute a major component of the outer coat material and are involved in many biological phenomena concerned with specificity at the molecular level—for instance, in the form of blood group substances and transplantation antigens. The sugar residues mainly found in the carbohydrate portion of glycoproteins are D-galactose, D-mannose, D-glucose (rarely), L-fucose, N-acetyl glucosamine, N-acetyl galactosamine and sialic acids. The sialic acids are five carbon sugars based on D. mannosamine with various portions substituted with acyl groups. They carry acidic carboxyl groups which can be detected at cell surfaces. The carbohydrate chains may be straight or branched, ranging in length from two to thirty sugar residues. The glycoproteins also contain polypeptide chains. The carbohydrate chains are linked through the C_1 position of the reducing terminal sugar residues to the side chains of amino acid residues in the polypeptide chain. These may be amide groups of asparagine residues, hydroxyl groups of serine, threonine, hydroxylysine or hydroxyproline. The enzyme neuraminidase cleaves the linkage between the terminal sialic acid residues of glycoproteins and the adjacent sugar residue. Cell electrophoresis before and after treatment with neuraminidase can therefore be used as an indicator for the presence of sialic acid residues at the cell surface. The first evidence that changes in acidic groups at the cell surface might be involved in the malignant change was obtained by Ambrose, James and Lowick (1956)[5]. An almost two-fold increase in mobility was observed in a stilboestrol-induced renal tumour in the hamster as compared with the normal epithelial cells from which the tumour cells were derived (*Fig. 3.8*). Increases were also observed when hepatoma cells were compared with normal liver parenchymal cells.

Earlier studies of the cell surface change in malignancy had suggested that surface charge might play a significant role in preventing close approach of cell surfaces and thus lead to the failure of the contacts that form in normal tissues. This simple explanation has to be modified in the light of the more recent work described in this chapter. Nevertheless, a number of biological systems have been studied in which a correlation between rate of growth and surface charge density has been obtained. Hughes, Sandford and Jeanlos (1972)[72] found that ascites tumour cells from a strain mice showed decreased tumour-forming ability in allogeneic mice after treatment with neuraminidase which reduced their surface charge density. Yamada (1972)[73] found a reasonably good correlation between electrophoretic mobility and growth rate (measured at the maximum rate) for a number of cell types *in vivo*. There is, in fact, an increase in surface charge density during mitosis (Brent and Forrester, 1970[75]) but recent work by Shank and Barski (1972)[76] suggests that this is due in the case of cells growing on a solid substrate, to changes in shape (cells round up during mitosis). No such changes in mobility and mitosis were observed with mouse lymphoblasts growing in suspension. The increased surface charge on rapidly growing cells seen throughout the cell cycle may well be conducive to growth. Hagmar (1972)[77] has studied the growth of the MCG–SS tumour in CBA mice. Dextran and dextra–

sulphate gave rise to increased surface charge and to increased growth rate, the polycation DEAD-dextran reduced surface charge and blocked tumour transplantation. (This latter was not a toxic effect because it could be reversed by the polyanion dextran sulphate.)

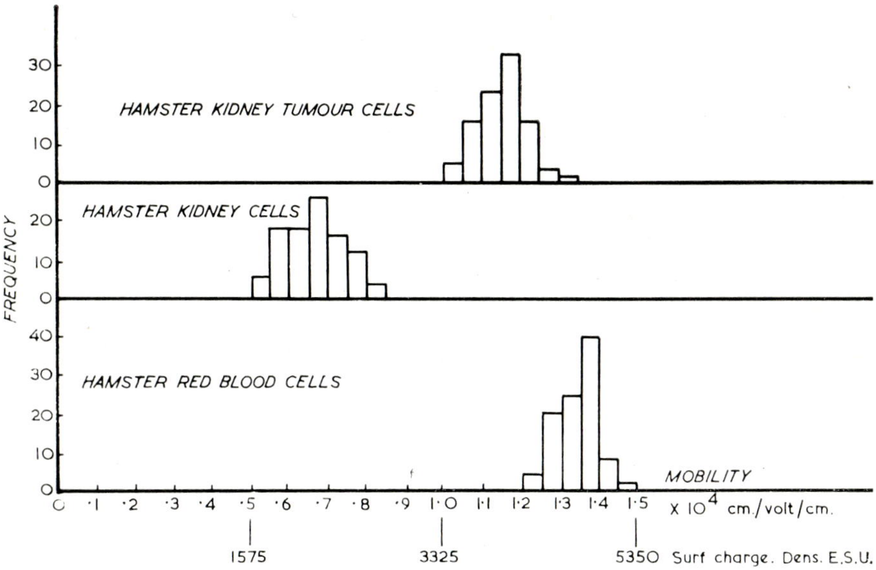

Fig. 3.8. Electrophoretic Mobility of normal hamster kidney cortical epithelium and of stilboestrol-induced renal tumour cells.

The changes in cell-cell interactions cannot, however, be understood only in terms of an increased amount of acidic glycoprotein in the outer layers of the cell surface. Conformational changes may also be important: acidic glycoproteins may be drawn to the outer surface by the attraction of the counter ions in the electrical double layer in preference to other materials. Cell electrophoresis only registers groups lying within 10Å of the outer surface. A net increase in the total amount of sialic acid within the membrane as detected in biochemical extracts may not be necessary—Meezan, Wu, Black and Robbins (1969)[78] studied normal and virus-transformed mouse fibroblasts and found no increase in the total content of sialic acid in the virus-transformed cells. Another type of conformational change which can occur at surfaces is an alteration in the distribution in the plane of the surface, i.e., in the mosaic pattern of the numerous components in the plane of the surface. The importance of this aspect has been discussed by Weiss (1972)[13] and by Steinberg (1962)[79]. The important role of bivalent cations should also be mentioned. Calcium ions play a major role in the reaggregation of suspensions of sponge cells and of amphibian embryo cells, and they are important in mammalian cell aggregation which is affected by chelating agents: the key factor in determining adsorption of calcium ions lies in the position of adjacent charged groups either on the surface of one cell or of neighbouring cells so that the calcium ions are able to form a bridge (chelation) $-COO^{-}-Ca^{++}-{}^{-}OOC-$.

Sialic acid and fucose provide the common terminal groups of the polysaccharide side chains in glycoproteins of the plasma membrane. The structure of these cell surface glycoproteins has been studied by three methods; biochemical analysis of the isolated plasma membranes, separation of glycoprotein fragments directly from the cell surface by mild treatment with trypsin or other proteolytic enzymes, and by cell electrophoresis.

The structure of the glycoproteins located at the surface of the erythrocyte membrane was investigated extensively by Cook, Seaman and Heard (1962)[80] using both cell electrophoresis and biochemical isolation of the coat material (see review by Cook, 1968[81]). Comparable studies were made on tumour cell surfaces by Forrester, Ambrose and Stoker (1964[82]). Both sialic acid and phosphate groups of phospholipid were found to contribute to the surface charge (Forrester, 1964[82]); also, in certain instances, ribosenucleic acid (Mayhew and Weiss 1968[86]). But the main interest has centred on the glycoproteins with terminal sialic acid residues. Treatment with neuraminidase, which removes terminal sialic acid residues, reduces the charge on both untransformed and transformed BHK21 fibroblasts (Forrester *et al.*, 1962[87]); it also reduces the difference in electrophoretic mobility of the untransformed and transformed fibroblasts. These findings suggest that the main factor affecting a change in surface charge here is an alteration in the sialomucoproteins. More general evidence in support of this view has been provided by the work of Emmelot (1973)[88] who finds that all neoplastic cells so far investigated in his laboratory (virus transformed fibroblasts, lymphosarcoma, hepatoma grown *in vitro*, etc.) show increased sialic acid density of a fucose-containing glycoprotein fraction as compared with non-malignant counterparts (this does not necessitate an overall net increase in all sialomucoproteins). At present, this is the most universal change in the surface of neoplastic cells, regardless of cell type and mode of transformation. Detailed biochemical investigations of surface glycoproteins in tumours cells were made by Langley and Ambrose (1964–67)[83, 84] who isolated a peptide fragment from Ehrlich ascites tumour cells, containing equal proportions of sialic acid and N-acetyl galactosamine.

Extensive biochemical work on membrane glycoproteins from normal mouse and rat liver cells has been carried out by Emmelot and Benedetti (1968)[89]. Membranes from rat liver contain 33 μ moles N-acetylneuraminic acid, 65 μ moles of neutral hexose and 61 μ moles of hexosamine per mg of proline. At least 70 per cent of the sialic acid, predominantly N-acetylneuraminic acid, was released by neuraminidase. Later work by Evans and Gurd (1971)[90] showed that galactosamine was in fact largely confined to the glycolipids in these membranes.

Buck, Glick and Warner (1970)[91] compared the glycoproteins in untransformed and virally transformed cells. They demonstrated a fucose-containing glycoprotein on the surface of the transformed cells which was also present in much smaller amounts on normal cells. An ascitic mammary carcinoma of A strain mice was shown by Gasic and Gasic (1962)[92] and Gasic and Berwick

(1963)[97] to have a coat of sialic acid containing glycoproteins which were important in metastasis. Codington, Sandford and Jeanlos (1971)[94] isolated a glycoprotein from the surface of these cells. Homogeneity was not established. The composition was galactose (26%), N-acetylgalactosamine (19%), N-acetylglucosamine (9%), N-acetylneuraminic acid (13%), threonin (12%) and serine (8%) with a total of about 10 per cent of eight other amino acids. N-acetylgalactosamine provided the main links to polypeptide by P-glycosidic linkages to threonine.

An alternative approach to the problem of cell surface biochemistry has developed from the use of plant lectins which attach to the surface of tumour cells. During a study of enzyme preparations which might be expected to combine with cell surfaces (G. Easty, D. Easty and Ambrose, 1960[6]), it was found that a wheat germ lipase preparation caused agglutination of ascites cells in suspension. When later tested on primary cultures of normal hamster kidney cells and corresponding renal tumour cells, the wheat germ lipase preparation was found to inhibit the growth of the tumour cells selectively (Ambrose, D. Easty, G. Easty and Dudgeon, 1961[95]). Fluorescent labelling of fractions of the preparation showed a combination with the cell surface which did not run parallel with lipase activity (Cormack and Ambrose, 1962[96]). Aub *et al.* [97,98] isolated agglutinin for tumour cells from wheat germ. Burger and Goldberg (1967)[99] purified a glycoprotein from wheat germ lipase preparation which was found to be a specific inhibitor for the reaction. The reaction is not an all-or-none process; either a quantitative difference exists between the number of chitobiose groups on malignant cells or some changes in surface conformation takes place so that these groups become exposed at the surface, a possibility that has been discussed by Burger (1969)[100]. Gentle treatment of normal cells with trypsin under strictly controlled conditions caused the normal cells to agglutinate in a similar manner to malignant cells and, indeed, the total amount of wheat germ agglutinin bound to the cell surface of normal and malignant cells is not strikingly different (Malluci, 1971[101]). The increased agglutinability of the malignant cells could therefore be explained in terms of a rearrangement of the groups in a plane perpendicular to the membrane. Another possibility has been discussed by Singer and Nicholson (1972)[102], who propose that a rearrangement of the binding sites takes place within the plane of the membrane so that those groups which are dispersed in a monomolecular pattern in the non-malignant cells become aggregated in clusters on the surface in transformed cells (*Fig. 3.7b*). Whatever the explanation may be for the change in the malignant cell surface, it seems more likely to be conformational than chemical. The receptor sites for the wheat germ agglutinin can be detached from the cell surface of L1210 leukaemic cells by hypotonic shock, a procedure commonly used for releasing transplanation antigens (Burger, 1968[105]). Using gel filtration, and ion exchange chromatography, Smith, Neri and Walborg (1973)[106] have isolated and partially characterized the cell surface glycopeptides which possess binding sites for wheat germ agglutinin and concanavalin A. They were partially purified and showed specific reactions with wheat germ agglutinin and with concanavalin A; they also selectively inhibited the agglutination of tumour cells by the two lectins. Other plant agglutinins have been studied including concanavalin A (Inbar and Sachs, 1969[107]) isolated from the jack bean, soya bean agglutinin etc. A comparison of agglutinin of 3T3 cells, before and after transformation, by wheat germ agglutinin and soya bean agglutinin indicated a highly specific agglutination of the transformed cells with concanavalin A; specific agglutination was not observed in one-day old cultures but only after four days in culture (Inbar and Sachs, 1972[108]). The plant lectins have therefore proved to be useful tools for the investigation of cell surface conformations and have demonstrated a surprising degree of specificity in malignant cell surfaces.

Some of the highly specific surface glycoproteins are antigens. Of particular interest is the glycoprotein found in the circulation of patients with colonic and other tumours. This is an antigen which cross reacts with an antigen found in foetal gut (Gold and Freedman, 1965[109]; Gold, Gold and Freedman, 1968[110]; Laurence and Neville, 1972—see also Chapter 7). This carcinoembryonic antigen can be shown by immunofluorescence to be associated with the tumour cell surface. It is a glycoprotein containing sucrose, galactose, fucose, glucosamine and sialic acid, (Krupey, Gold and Freedman, 1967[111], 1968[110]). Tumour specific antigens, present on the surface of cells in tumours induced by chemical carcinogens, oncogenic viruses and radiation (see Chapter 12), may also be glycoproteins. So too, are the transplantation antigens of the H2 and HL-A loci (Davies, 1969; Natherson, 1960). It should, however, be noted that the 'strong' histocompatibility antigens described by these investigators do not seem to be disturbed in malignant transformation; and the possibility arises that new antigenic determinants may arise in tumours by slight modification of pre-existing histocompatability antigens, eg. by acquisition or loss of one or more monosaccharides in the carbohydrate units of these membrane glycoproteins (Hughes, 1973[114]).

The neurominidase-sensitive glycoproteins on the outer layers of the cell surface may plan an important role in interfering with the immunological response of the host in malignancy, in that they may mask the specific recognition sites remaining on malignant cells. The immune response of the host can be enhanced if innoculated with tumour cells which have previously been treated with neuronimidase (Bagshawe, 1970). The extent to which surface charges in glycoproteins affect metastases is discussed in Chapter 4. The problem is complicated because metastasis involves several stages—local invasion, penetration of blood vessels and renewed adhesion in the new site of (potential) metastatic growth in which surface charge may well be implicated.

In view of the increasing interest in glycoproteins as biological markers for malignancy—notably the carcinoembryonic antigens (Gold and Freedman, 1968[110]) and the α–foetoprotein (Abelev)—the study of the synthesis of surface glycoproteins and of their release into the general circulation of patients has become important. Using an optical ellipsometric method to measure the synthesis of coat material after deposition from suspension, Malluci, Poste and Wells (1972) found that polyoma-transformed cells had a thicker coat than untransformed cells; the difference was, however, only marginal in chemically induced tumours. Hughes, Sandford and Jeanlos (1972)[119] found that the rate of regeneration of surface coat by strain A mouse ascites cells treated with neuraminidase was similar to that of untreated cells, suggested a continuous production of surface coat by cells, at least by cells capable of mitosis; this may be important for future developments in the use of glycoproteins as biological markers in malignancy.

PLASMA MEMBRANE

The detailed molecular structure of the lipid component of the cell surface complex has been the subject of study by electron microscopists in recent years. Several techniques have been used, particularly the freeze cleavage method (Moor, 1966[120]; Benedetti and Emmelot, 1968[89]). On the basis of these investigations and other data, Singer and Nicholson (1972)[102] have proposed a fluid mosaic model for the plasma membrane—see *Fig. 3.9.* The model

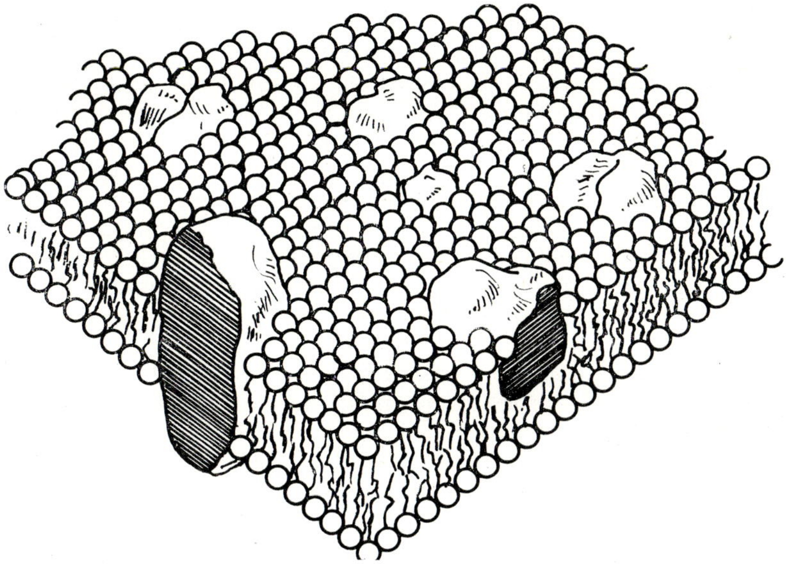

Fig. 3.9. Fluid mozaic model for the plasma membrane as proposed by Singer and Nicholson (1972).[102] Corpuscular protein molecules lie within a liquid crystal of a lipid bilayer.

consists basically of a phospholipid bilayer as originally proposed by Danielli (1958)[121] with the polar groups of phospholipid orientated towards the aqueous plane. This layer is a liquid (or, rather, a liquid crystal) in which the order is maintained under conditions in which molecules can readily interchange with one another within the surface layer. Embedded in this liquid crystal lie compact globular proteins and glycoproteins which sometimes extend completely across the membrane from one side to the other; such proteins may provide membrane pores involved in active transport etc. Mention has already been made of the evidence, that association of these penetrating molecules on adjacent cells in contact may provide a channel for ionic penetration, as observed in electrical coupling described by Lowenstein (1970). Evidence for fluidity of the lipid matrix has been obtained by de Petris and Roff (1973)[122]. Mouse spleen cells were labelled with fluorescent antibody raised against cell surface immunoglobulins. Univalent antibody was first spread uniformly over the cell surface. When labelled with bivalent antibody, clusters were formed due to linkage by antibody which gradually migrated to form a mass at the tail region of the cell. This 'capping' phenomenon is also observed with concanavalin A receptors, H2 and HL-A antigens. According to Singer and Nicholson, the change from non-malignant to malignant cells is associated with an aggregation phenomenon of this sort by the wheat germ or concanavalin A receptors as shown in *Fig. 3.8*. Such clusters could have an increased probability of linking via plant lectin with neighbouring cells.

The biochemistry of the lipid phase of the cell surface complex has been intensively investigated (Emmelot 1967). The most interesting components of the membrane from the point of view of malignant change have proved to be the glycolipids. These components represent a small fraction (about 1 %) of the major lipid constituents which consist of phospholipids such as lecithin, phosphatidyl, ethanolamine and sphingomyelin, and also cholesterol. The (glycolipid) blood group antigens of the Lewis and H type (Hakomori, 197)[126] were isolated from a human gastric carcinoma whereas the red cells from the same patient carried A group activity. This field has been extensively studied by Hakomori, and Siddiqui (1971)[124]. Robbins and Macpherson (1971)[126] compared untransformed and transformed cells from the NIL2 hamster line and found that three glycolipids were suppressed in the transformed cells. These glycolipids were also found to be present at lower concentration in growing untransformed NIL2 cells than in the same cells after forming a contact inhibited monolayer. Hakomori *et al.* (1971)[124] have shown that glycolipids with longer carbohydrate chains were generally deleted in transformed cells, suggesting incomplete synthesis of carbohydrate chains; some-times this led to the accumulation of a glycolipid having a precursor residue.

THE SUB-SURFACE STRUCTURE

The region of the cytoplasm lying immediately below the plasma membrane is the plasma gel. Many microns thick in *Amoeba proteus*, the plasma gel in mammalian cells is generally 0·1–0·2μ (Vasiliev and Gelfand 1973[14]). This gel region is free from cytoplasmic organelles such as ribosomes and mitochondria and has considerable tensile strength; according to Goldacre (1968)[127], this region provides the strength of the cell surface region, it was noted earlier that the sub-surface region contains the actin-like microfilaments which may be arranged in well orientated sheets or bundles, or in a looser network. The importance of these structures in the maintenance of cell polarity and morphology has already been mentioned, also the decreased organization of these elements in malignant cells (Ambrose, Batzdorf, Osborn and Stuart, 1970[28]; Vasiliev and Gelfand, 1973[14]). The biochemical basis for changes in the organization of these elements is at present unknown.

General conclusions

Dr. John Paul summarized the problem of malignancy at the end of a Conference on 'in vitro' carcinogens (Patterson Symposium, 1972) in the following terms:

'Although malignancy is manifestly a complex phenomenon in which many properties both of the tumour and the host need to be investigated, it can be said in general terms that some relaxation of the factors regulating growth and some relaxation of the control of motility are essential for malignancy.' The work described in this chapter has shown that cell surface properties play a major role in regulatory mechanisms of this type. For this reason, cell surface studies in cell biology, immunology and biochemistry have done much to provide a unified concept of the nature of cancer, perhaps more so than any other single field of investigation.

In conclusion, when considering the various stages of deviation from normal behaviour by malignant cells either in the case of a group of tumours or during progression within the same tumour, the following factors are important.

(1) Escape from growth control is the first step in deviation from normal behaviour; the specific receptors associated with cell-cell contact may be rearranged so that adenylate cyclases do not respond and cyclic AMP levels are kept low.
(2) Production of fucose-containing glycoprotein with increased sialic acid content takes place. This protein tends to increase the net surface charge on the cells, and reduces further the cell-cell interactions; cells become motile and may commence local invasion. Nexus junctions and electrical cell-cell communications break down.
(3) Constitutive synthesis of surface coats takes place so that outer coat glycoproteins are secreted into the intercellular spaces and eventually reach the circulation. These include the carcinoembryonic antigens, and probably tumour specific antigens. At this stage the serum glycoproteins may provide useful indicators for the presence of viable tumour cells.
(4) Failures of the organization of sub-surface microfilaments and cytoplasmic microtubules occur. The cells become polypodial in form and exhibit pronounced membrane activity at their contact with normal tissues. Invasiveness becomes pronounced.
(5) Lysosomes and plasma membranes produce enzymes and toxic factors. Normal tissue destruction ensues; metastases are formed.

This sequence of events does not necessarily take place in the same order in different tumour types, nor even in the same types of tumour. The normal cells from which tumours arise themselves differ in surface properties so that changes arising in the course of neoplastic development are likely to be different, epithelial tissues are highly adhesive but are not generally polarized and molecular changes in the surface—increased surface charge, loss of nexus junctions—are likely to be critical. Fibroblasts, on the other hand, are polarized cells and loss of microfilament organization may be more important than molecular changes at the surface. Surface charge may show only marginal differences.

References

1. Coman, D. R. *Cancer Research*, **4,** 625–629 (1944).
2. Abercrombie, M., Heaysman, J. E. M. and Karthauser, H. M. *Exp. Cell Res.,* **13,** 276–292 (1957).
3. Abercrombie, M., Ambrose, E. J., Easty, D. M. and Heaysman, J. E. M. Time Lapse Ciné Film. VIIth International Cancer Congress, London (1958).
4. Abercrombie, M. and Ambrose, *E. J. Exp. Cell Res.,* **15,** 332–345 (1958).
5. Ambrose, E. J., James, A. M. and Lowick, J. H. B. *Nature, Lond.,* **177,** 576–577 (1956).
6. Easty, G. C., Easty, D. M. and Ambrose, E. J. *Exp. Cell Res.,* **19,** 539–547 (1960).
7. Macpherson, I. and Stoker, M. *Virology,* **16,** 147 (1962).
8. Todaro, G. J., Lazar, G. K. and Green, H. *J. Cell comp. Physiol.*, **66,** 325 (1965).
9. Vasiliev, Ju. M., Gelfand, I., Domina, L. V. and Rappaport, R. I. *Exp. Cell Res.,* **54,** 83–93 (1969).
10. Phillips, B. J. and Ambrose, E. J. Ph.D. Thesis. University of London (1972).
11. Middleton, C. A. *Locomotion of Tissue Cells.* Ciba Foundation Symp. (ed. Abercrombie, M.) pp. 251–262 (1973).
12. Curtis, A. S. G. *The Cell Surface.,* Logos Press, Academic Press (1957).
13. Weiss, L. *The Chemistry of Biosurfaces*, (ed. Hair, M. L.) Marcel Dekker Inc. 377–438 (1972).
14. Vasiliev, Ju. M. and Gelfand, I. *Locomotion of Tissue Cells*, Ciba Foundation Symp. (ed. Abercrombie, M.) pp. 311–329 (1973).
15. Gail, M. H. and Boone, C. W. *Exp. Cell Res.,* **70,** 33–40 (1972).
16. Ambrose, E. J. and Ellison, M. *Europ. J. Cancer,* **4,** 459 (1968).
17. Friedenstein, A. Y., Rappaport, R. I. and Luria, E. A. *Exp. Cell Res.,* **49,** 488–494 (1967).
18. Thom, René. Towards a Theoretical Biology. I.U.B.S. Symp. ed. C. H. Waddington (Edinburgh Univ. Press) p. 152 (1968).
19. Ambrose, E. J. *Symp. Faraday Soc.,* No. 5, 175–186 (1971).
20. Ambrose, E. J. *Exp. Cell Res. Suppl.,* **8,** 54–73 (1961).
21. Korohoda, W. *Folia Biologica,* **19,** 191–199 (1971).
22. Harberey, M. *Mikroscopie,* **27,** 226–234 (1971).
23. Abercrombie, M., Heaysman, J. E. M. and Pegrum, S. M. *Exp. Cell Res.,* **62,** 389–398 (1971).
24. Heaysman, J. E. M. and Pegrum, S. M. *Exp. Cell Res.,* **78,** 71–78 (1973).

24a. Harris, A. K. *Locomotion of Tissue Cells.* CIBA Found. Symp., (ed. Abercrombie, M.' pp. 3–20 (1973).

25. Ishikawa, H., Bischoff, R. and Holtzer, H. *J. Cell Biol.,* **43,** 312–327 (1969).
26. Spooner, B. S., Yamada, K. M. and Wessells, H. *J. Cell Biol.,* **49,** 595–613 (1971).
27. Jones, B. M., Kemp, R. B. and Gröschel Stewart, U. *Nature,* Lond., **226,** 261–262 (1970).
28. Ambrose, E. J., Batzdorf, U., Osborn, J. M. and Stuart, P. R. *Nature,* Lond., **227,** 397 (1970).

29. Ambrose, E. J., Batzdorf, U. and Easty, D. M. *J. Neuropath. and Exp. Neurology*, **31**, 596–610 (1972).
30. McNutt, N. S., Culp, L. A. and Black, P. H. *J. Cell Biol.*, **50**, 691–708 (1971).
31. Trinkhaus, J. P., Betcheku, T. and Krurkowski, L. S. *Exp. Cell Res.*, **64**, 291–300 (1971).
32. Abercrombie, M. *In vitro*, **6**, 128–142 (1970).
33. Curtis, A. S. G. *Amer. Naturalist*, **94**, 37–56 (1960).
34. Derjaguin, B. V. and Landau, L. D. *Acta Physiochimica URSS*, **14**, 633–662 (1941).
35. Vermey, E. J. W. and Overbeek, J. Th. G. Theory of Stability of Lysophylic Colloids. Elsevier Amsterdam (1948).
36. Revel, J. P. and Karnovsky, M. J. *J. Cell. Biol.*, **33**, C.7 (1967).
37. McNutt, N. S. and Weinstein, R. S. *J. Cell. Biol.*, **47**, 666–688 (1970).
38. Muir, A. R. *J. Anat.* (*Lond.*), **101**, 239 (1967).
39. Barr, L., Dewey, M. M. and Berger, W. *J. Gen. Physiol.*, **48**, 797 (1965).
40. Barr, L., Berger, W. and Dewey, M. M. *J. Gen. Physiol.*, **51**, 347 (1968).
41. Benedetti, E. L. and Emmelot, P. *J. Cell. Biol.*, **26**, 299 (1965).
42. Lowenstein, W. R. and Kanno, Y. *J. Cell Biol.*, **33**, 225 (1967).
43. Azaria, A. and Lowenstein, W. R. *Nature, Lond.*, **241**, 455–457 (1973).
44. Borek, C. *Proc. Nat. Acad. Sci.*, **69**, 956–959 (1972).
45. Payton, B. W., Bennett, M. V. L. and Pappas, G. D. *Science*, **166**, 1641 (1969).
46. Farquhar, M. G. and Palade, G. E. *J. Cell. Biol.*, **17**, 375 (1963).
47. Matter, A., Orci, L. and Rouiller, C. *J. Ultrastruct. Res.* (*Suppl.*), **11**, 1 (1969).
48. McNutt, N. S. and Weinstein, R. S. *Science*, **165**, 597 (1969).
49. Martinez–Palomo, A. *Lab. Investigation*, **22**, 605 (1970).
50. Sirsat, S. M. and Pinday, J. J. *Indian J. Cancer*, **5**, 301–308 (1967).
51. Wolpert, L. and Gustafson, T. *Biol. Rev.* (Camb.), **42**, 442–498 (1967).
52. Trinkhaus, J. P. Locomotion of Tissue Cells, Ciba Foundation Symp. (ed. Abercrombie, M.) pp. 233–243 (1973).
53. Gustafson, T. and Wolpert, L. *Exp. Cell Res.*, **24**, 64–79 (1961).
54. Ambrose, E. J. and Easty, D. M. *Differentiation*, **I**, 39–50 (1973).
54a. Sylvén, B. E. G. V. Biological Interactions in Normal and Neoplastic Growth. Henry Ford Symp. (ed. Brennan, M. J. and Simpson, W. L.), Little, Brown & Co. Boston. 635–670 (1962).
55. Ambrose, E. J., Easty, G. C. and Tchao, R. In Course of Publication (1974).
56. Abercrombie, M. and Ambrose, E. J. *Cancer Research*, **22**, 525–548 (1962).
57. Todaro, G. J., Lazar, G. K. and Green, H. J. Cell comp. *Physiol.*, **66**, 325 (1965).
58. Levene, E. M., Bocher, Y., Boone, C. W. and Eagle, H. *Proc. Nat. Acad. Sci. U.S.*, **53**, 350–356 (1965).
59. Dulbecco, R. and Stoker, M. G. P. *Proc. Nat. Acad. Sci. US.*, **66**, 204–210 (1970).
60. Stoker, M. G. P. and Rubin, H. *Nature, London.*, **215**, 171–172 (1967).
61. Martz, E. and Steinberg, M. S. *J. Cell Physiol.*, **79**, 189–210 (1972).
62. Temin, H. M. Growth Regulating Substances for Animal Cells in Culture. (Ed. Defendi, V. and Stoker, M.) Wistar Inst. Press, Philadelphia, 103–116 (1967).
63. Clarke, G. D., Stoker, M. G. P., Ludlow, A. and Thornton, M. Nature, **227**, 798–801 (1970).
64. Korohoda, W. *Acta Protozoologica*, **11**, 161–172 (1972).

65. Zurzycki, J. and Starzechi, W. Volumetric methods: Plant Photosynthesis Production (eds. Z. Sestak, J. Catskyard, P. G. Jarvis). W. Junk, The Hague, 257–275 (1971).
66. Holly, R. W. *Proc. Nat. Acad. Sci. U.S.*, **69**, 2840–2841 (1972).
67. Sheppard, J. R. *Nature New Biol.*, **236**, 14 (1972).
68. Smets, L. A. *Nature New Biol.*, **239**, 123–124 (1972).
69. Teel R. W. and Hall, R. G. *Exp. Cell Research*, **76**, 390–394 (1973).
70. Burger, M. M. *J. Dermatology*, **59**, 24–26 (1972).
71. Ambrose, E. J. and Easty, D. M. *Cell Biology. Nelsons,* London (1971).
72. Hughes, R. C., Sandford, B. and Jeanlos, R. W. *Proc. Nat., Acad. Sci. U.S.* **69**, 942–945 (1972).
73. Yamada, T. *Acta. Path.*, Japan, **22**, 1–10 (1972).
74. Yamada, T., Takaoka, T., Katsuta, H., Namba, M. and Sato, *J. Jap. J. Exp. Med.*, **42**, 377–388 (1972).
75. Brent, T. P. and Forrester, J. A. *Nature,* Lond., **215**, 92–95 (1967).
76. Shank, B. and Beurki, H. J. *J. Cell. Physiol.*, **78**, 243–250 (1972).
77. Hagmar, B. *Acta. Path. microbiol. Scand., A*.**80**, 357–366 (1972).
78. Meezan, E., Wu, H. C., Black, P. H. and Robbins, P. W. *Biochem.*, **8**, 2518–2524 (1969).
79. Steinberg, M. S. *Science,* **137**, 762 (1972).
80. Cook, G. M. W., Heard, D. H. and Seaman, G. V. F. *Exp. Cell Research,* **28**, 27–39 (1962).
81. Cook, G. M. W. *Biol. Revs.*, **43**, 363–391 (1968).
82. Forrester, J. A., Ambrose, E. J. and Stoker, M. G. P., *Nature,* Lond., **201**, 945–946 (1964).
83. Langley, O. K. and Ambrose, E. J. *Nature,* Lond., **204**, 53–54 (1964).
84. Langley, O. K. and Ambrose, E. J. *Biochem. J.*, **102**, 367–372 (1967).
85. Forrester, J. A. Ph. D. Thesis, University of London (1965).
86. Mayhew, E. and Weiss, L. *Exp. Cell Research*, **50**, 461 (1968).
87. Forrester, J. A., Ambrose, E. J. and Macpherson, I. A. *Nature*, Lond., **196**, 1068–1072 (1962).
88. Emmelot, P. *5th Int. Symp. on Biological Characterization of Human Tumours*, Bologna. Abstract 1 (1973).
89. Benedetti, E. L. and Emmelot, P. *The Membranes,* ed. Dalton, A. J. and Haguenau, F. Academic Press, pp. 33–120 (1968).
90. Evans, W. H. and Gurd, J. W. *Biochem. J.*, **125**, 615–624 (1971).
91. Buck, C. A., Glick, M. C. and Warner, L. *Biochem. J.*, **9**, 4567–4576 (1970).
92. Gasic, G. and Gasic, T. *Proc. Nat. Acad. Sci.*, **48**, 1172–1177 (1962).
93. Gasic, G. and Berwick, L. *J. Cell Biol.*, **19**, 223–228 (1972).
94. Codington, J. F., Sandford, B. H. and Jeanlos, R. W. *Fed. Proc.*, **30**, 1280 (1971).
95. Ambrose, E. J., Dudgeon, J. A., Easty, D. M. and Easty, G. C. *Exp. Cell Research,* **24**, 220–227 (1961).
96. Cormack, D. H. and Ambrose, E. J. *J. Roy. Microscop. Soc.*, **81**, 11–18 (1962).
97. Aub, J. C., Tieslau, C. and Lancaster, A. *Proc. Nat. Acad. Sci.*, **50**, 613–619 (1963).
98. Aub, J. C., Sandford, B. H. and Wang, L. *Proc. Nat. Acad. Sci.*, **54**, 400–402 (1965).
99. Burger, M. M. and Goldberg, A. R. *Proc. Nat. Acad. Sci.*, **57**, 359–366 (1967).
100. Burger, M. M. *Proc. Nat. Acad. Sci.*, **62**, 994–1001 (1969).

101. Malluci, L. Nature, New Biol. **233,** 241–244 (1971).
102. Singer, S. I. and Nicholson, G. L. *Science,* **175,** 720–731 (1972).
103. Eridani, S. and Smith, W. *Blut,* **26,** 69–73 (1973).
104. Ambrose, E. J., Smith, W. and Forrester, J. A. Cytology Automation. 2nd Tenovus Symp. Cardiff (ed. Evans, D. M. D.) Livingstone, Edinburgh, pp. 100–107 (1970).
105. Burger, M. M. *Nature,* Lond., **219,** 499–500 (1968).
106. Smith, D. F., Neri, G. and Walborg, E. F. Biochemistry **12,** 2111–2118 (1973).
197. Inbar, M. and Sachs, L. *Nature,* Lond., **223,** 710–712 (1969).
108. Inbar, M., Ben-Bassat, H. and Sachs, L. *Nature, New Biol.,* **236,** 14–16 (1972).
109. Gold, P. and Freedman, S. O. *J. Exp. Med.* **122,** 467–481 (1965).
110. Gold, P., Gold M. and Freedman, S. O. *Cancer Res.,* **28,** 1331–1334 (1968).
111. Krupey, J., Gold, P. and Freedman, S. O. *Nature,* Lond., **215,** 67–68 (1967).
112. Davies, D. A. L. Transplantation **8,** 51–70 (1969).
113. Nathenson, S. G. *Am. Rev. Genetics,* **4,** 69–90 (1970).
114. Hughes, R. C. *Progress in Biophys. and Mol. Biol.,* **26,** 189–268 (1973).
115. Currie, S. A. and Bagshawe, K. D., *Lancet,* **1,** 708 (1967).
116. Hagmar, B. *Acta Path. Microbiol.,* Scand., **A.80,** 357–366 (1972).
117. Abelev, G. I., *Adv. Cancer Research,* **14,** 295–358 (1971).
118. Malluci, L., Poste, G. and Wells, V. *Nature, New Biol.,* **235,** 222 (1972).
119. Hughes, R. C., Sandford, B. and Jeanlog, R. W. *Proc. Nat. Acad. Sci.,* U.S., **69,** 942–945 (1972).
120. Moor. H. *Int. Rev. Exp. Pathol.,* **5,** 179 (1966).
121. Danielli, J. F. Cold Spring Harbor Symp., **6,** 190–195 (1938).
122. de Petris, S. and Raff, M. C. Locomotion of Tissue Cells. CIBA Symp. (ed. Abercrombie, M.) 27–41 (1973).
123. van Deenen, L. L. M. and de Haas, G. H. Advances in Lipid Research (ed. Padetti, R. and Kritchensky, D.) *Acad. Press.,* N.Y., 167 (1964).
124. Hakomori, S. *Proc. Nat. Acad. Sci.,* **67,** 1741 (1970).
125. Hakamori, S., Kijimoto, S. and Siddique, B. Biological Membranes, 253–277 (1973).
126. Robbins, P. W. and Macpherson, I. *Nature,* Lond., **229,** 569 (1971).
127. Goldacre, R. J. *Laboratory Practice,* **15,** 53–59 (1966).

Chapter **4**

INVASION BY CANCER CELLS

G. C. EASTY, Ph.D.

Senior Lecturer in Cell Pathology, Chester Beatty Research Institute, Institute of Cancer Research, London

---

In addition to a capacity for relatively uncontrolled growth, many malignant tumours show other properties not usually possessed or expressed by the cells of the normal tissue from which they arise. One of the most sinister of these properties is the ability to spread from their site of origin. Cords of tumour cells may extend for considerable distances into apparently normal tissue and, becoming disengaged from the primary tumour, disseminate and subsequently develop into discrete secondary or metastatic tumours, quite separate from the primary lesion (see Chapter 5).

This process of dissemination may involve active migration and growth of tumour cells over free surfaces, or passive transport in the vascular or lymphatic systems. When the disseminated cells finally become lodged in a distant organ which provides a suitable environment, invasion may again take place. There are thus two phases of tumour dissemination where invasion occurs: the first consists of infiltration of surrounding normal tissue by neoplastic cells from the primary tumour, and the second involves invasion of a distant organ following dissemination. Many factors have been considered to be responsible for tumour invasion but it is probable that most (if not all) of them are involved to extents varying with the type of tumour, its site and stage of development.

Mechanical pressure

If a primary tumour arises in a tissue which does not present uniform structural and mechanical properties, it is likely that pressure developing within the tumour as a result of cellular proliferation and oedema favours extension of the growing neoplasm growing along paths of least mechanical resistance, such as in fascial planes of loose connective tissue. There is evidence that tumour cells may separate from each other more readily than cells in many normal tissues, and this property would facilitate distortion of the tumour mass and extrusion of cells. Young (1959)[1] has constructed a model invasion system in which jelly spherules representing tumour cells were discharged under pressure into gels which represented surrounding normal tissues. He found that the spherules moved freely down a pressure gradient, infiltrated the surrounding gel, and 'invaded' the walls of 'vascular elastic-jelly tubes' [sic] forming emboli.

Linear extension of tumour from the primary focus can be demonstrated by serial sections and by xeroradiography; invasion resulting from pressure within the tumour is probably an important factor in local invasion, particularly where the advancing tumour cells are still in partial or continuous contact with the central tumour mass.

Infiltration of tumours by components of normal tissue

Growing tumours are themselves infiltrated by certain components of the normal surrounding tissues. Time-lapse cinemicrography of tiny tumour implants in the hamster cheek pouch (Warren and Shubik, 1966)[2] and rabbit each chamber (Wood, 1958)[3] has demonstrated the rapid formation of new capillaries forming from proliferating endothelium in nearby vessels. Within a few days the new capillaries penetrate the tumour implant and establish the flow of blood essential for continuous tumour growth. Folkman (1971)[4] and his colleagues (Folkman *et al.*, 1971)[5] have extracted a 'tumour angiogenesis factor' from animal and human tumours, which stimulates the infiltration of tumours by normal blood capillaries.

Tumour cell migration

The development of pressure within a tumour and the local infiltration of normal capillaries are not the only mechanisms involved in the spread of tumours. Waldeyer[6] in 1872 was one of the first to suggest that invasion might be the result of migration of tumour cells through normal tissues. The demonstration of isolated tumour cells at considerable distances from the main tumour mass, and the recognition that some slow-growing tumours may invade and metastasize more readily than many fast-growing tumours (Willis, 1967)[7], support the view that tumour cells may be motile *in vivo*. Direct experimental confirmation of the motility of tumour cells *in vivo* has been provided by Wood and his colleagues (Wood *et al.*, 1967)[8] in the rabbit ear chamber. They recorded that V2 carcinoma cells migrated at a rate of 6–7 microns per minute: if the cells moved continuously in one direction they would travel 1 cm. in one day. Murine tumour cells which must have migrated several hundred microns per day through normal tissues were observed by Easty and Easty (1963)[9] in an *in vitro* system where fragments of normal and tumour tissue were cultured in contact with each other. The culture conditions were such that proliferation of the tissues was minimal and pressure could not have been responsible for tumour infiltration. Wolff and Schneider (1956)[10] have extensively studied the capacity of several tumours of animal and human origin to invade chick mesonephros in culture, and their results support the role of direct tumour cell migration in invasion. Destruction of normal cells in the region of invasion was observed. Mutual infiltration of normal cells (particularly if they are embryonic) can occur in this system, as Wolff and Weniger (1954)[11] observed using combinations of duck and mouse embryo gonads; but the rates of infiltration of the normal cells appeared to be much lower than those of tumour cells and cell destruction was not observed.

Reduced adhesiveness of tumour cells

CALCIUM IONS

Coman (1944)[12] suggested from measurements of the forces required to separate pairs of comparable normal and malignant cells that the malignant cells showed less mutual adhesiveness than normal cells, and that their greater ease of separation would facilitate invasion and metastasis. Using more reproducible techniques involving standardized conditions of agitation or aspiration, McCutcheon *et al.* (1948)[13] and Tjernberg and Zajicek (1965)[14] confirmed Coman's original observations.

The demonstration by Carruthers and Suntzeff (1944)[15] of a decrease in the calcium content of normal epithelium after an initial application of 3-methylcholanthrene, followed by a further decrease when tumours developed, led Coman (1944)[12] to suggest that the lower calcium content of tumours was responsible for the decreased mutual adhesiveness of tumours which, he proposed, had a reduced capacity to bind calcium at the cell surface. Although calcium ions are known to be involved in the establishment and maintenance of adhesions between the cells of many tissues—either by forming direct or indirect linkages between adjacent cells, or by reducing electrostatic repulsion, or by influencing the function of cytoplasmic contractile elements involved in cell motility and detachment—more recent work has complicated Coman's original hypothesis. Hickie and Kalant (1967)[16], for example, found that the calcium content of Morris hepatomas in rats was twice as high as that of normal liver though this may have been a consequence of high extracellular binding of calcium in regions of necrosis. The calcium content of the whole tissue is not, however, necessarily relevant to cell adhesion: tumour cells may possess a decreased concentration of calcium binding groups at their surfaces which are not detectable in measurements of the total calcium content in a tissue (Coman, 1961)[17]. Measurements of the calcium binding capacity of cell surfaces have not revealed any significant differences between comparable normal and tumour cells (Bangham and Pethica, 1960[18]; Patinkin *et al.*, 1970a[19]). These measurements provide only an average for the whole cell surface: some calcium binding sites may be involved in cell-cell adhesion while others are not. Weiss *et al.* (1972)[20] have published some preliminary evidence suggesting that the anionic charges on the Ehrlich ascites tumour cell surface are not evenly distributed; cells of similar surface charge density may possess very different adhesive properties which in turn may be related to differences in the pattern of distribution of surface charges. Thus, although there is a conviction that calcium associated with the cell surface and subsurface cytoplasmic structures plays an important role in the adhesive properties of cells, the relationship between calcium ions and the reduced adhesiveness of tumour cells for each other is obscure.

CELL SURFACE CHARGE

Similar ambiguities have arisen concerning the relationship between cell surface charge and invasiveness. Much work was stimulated by the important observations of Ambrose *et al.* (1956)[21] and Purdom *et al.* (1958)[22] of the increased surface charge density of tumour cells compared with their normal counterparts; also the increased charge density was associated with the increased capacity of one group of murine tumours to grow in the ascitic state and to metastasize (Purdom *et al.*, 1958[22]; Sakai, 1967)[23]. Many subsequent investigators have found no significant differences between the surface charge densities or sialic acid content of several comparable normal and malignant cells (Ohta *et al.*, 1968[24]; Wu *et al.*, 1969[25]; Vassar, 1963[26]; Weiss and Sinks, 1970[27]; Cook and Jacobson, 1968[28]; Patinkin *et al.*, 1970b)[29]. If surface charge is connected with the adhesion and invasiveness of cells, it is probably related to specific patterns of distribution and function of ionogenic groups at the cell surface rather than with the average cell surface content of such groups. There is evidence from the rapid mixing of species antigens during the formation of heterokaryons (Frye and Edidin, 1970)[30] that some of these surface components are present on the membrane in a highly mobile and even fluid state; it is thus probable that many functional groups on the cell surface involved in adhesion and motility are arranged in specific patterns which can only be detected when the cells are examined while they are performing specific functions. Observations on cells which are spherical as a result of being brought into suspension may not be relevant to their properties when they are attached to other cells or substrates and their surfaces are anisotropic.

Electron microscopy has provided considerable, albeit circumstantial, evidence of a morphological and structural basis for the reduced mutual adhesiveness of tumour cells. Easty and Mercer (1960)[31] examined surface replicas of monolayer cultures of normal hamster kidney epithelial cells and cells from an oestrogen-induced renal carcinoma; they found that while normal cells were closely apposed with a gap of ~200Å between them the tumour cells formed far fewer contacts of this type. Similar results were obtained by Martinez-Palomo *et al.* (1969)[72] from sections of cultures. They observed frequent regions of fusion between normal cell surfaces in contrast with their absence in cultured tumour cells. Martinez–Palomo (1970)[33] also found that tight junctions, which are regions of strong attachment between cells, were completely absent in the three tumours he examined, and gap junctions were much reduced in number compared with the normal tissues. Similar observations have been made by McNutt and Weinstein (1969)[34] and McNutt *et al.* (1971)[35] in a comparison of ‘benign and malignant’ cervical epithelium. McNutt and his colleagues found a decrease in the frequency of occurrence of these junctions well before stromal invasion was apparent, and they suggested that this deficiency may be an important factor permitting the eventual diffuse local invasion characteristic of squamous carcinomas. In addition to their role in cell adhesion, these junctions may be the sites of direct ionic and metabolic coupling between adjacent cells (Loewenstein, 1966[36]; Gilula *et al.*, 1972[37]) which some investigators have found to be deficient in tumour cells (Loewenstein and Kanno, 1967[38]; Jamakosmanovic and Loewenstein, 1968[39]; Kanno and Matsui, 1968[40]; Furshpan and Potter, 1968[41]; Sheridan, 1970[42]). This deficiency in coupling may be intimately related to control of cell motility though evidence on this point is conflicting (Flaxman *et al.*, 1969[43]; Harris, 1970[44]; Trinkaus *et al.*, 1971[45]). Clearly, the chemical and physical basis of the decreased mutual adhesiveness of tumour cells is still obscure.

Alterations in surface properties of tumour cells are exceedingly complicated. For example, concanavalin A agglutinates cells transformed by a variety of carcinogenic agents at concentrations which will not agglutinate untransformed cells; the latter can, however, be rendered agglutinable by treatment with proteases (Inbar and Sachs, 1969)[46]. The complexity of the changes in surfaces structure that accompany malignant transformation is illustrated by the work of Ben-Bassat *et al.* (1971)[47], who have produced evidence indicating that the alterations in the binding sites of concanavalin A following transformation can involve any or all of the following events: uncovering of sites buried in normal cells, a concentration of exposed sites by a decrease in cell size, and a rearrangement of exposed sites without a decrease in cell size. All of these factors may be influenced by culture condition and the type of serum used for growing the cells. No definite information is available at present concerning the relationship between the lectin-binding surface groups and reduced cell adhesion and motility except for the interesting observation by Friberg *et al.* (1971)[48] who found that migration of tumour cells was inhibited by concanavalin A. But with one exception, all the tumour cells examined were agglutinated by concanavalin A, and it cannot be excluded that the inhibition of migration of the cells, which were initially very close to each other, is a consequence of cross-linking of their surfaces rather than actual inhibition of migration by binding of the lectin to surface components involved in cell migration.

RELEASE OF LYTIC ENZYMES: LYSOSOMAL HYDROLASES, HYALURONIDASE, COLLAGENASES

A different approach to the problem of cell separation and facilitation of tumour invasion has been developed by Sylvén and his colleagues. It has long been known that invading tumours are frequently associated with the destruction of local connective tissues. Sylvén and Bois (1960)[49] developed a simple technique for sampling the interstitial fluid of different regions of tumours through fine capillary tubes and estimating the levels of activity of various enzymes present in the cell-free fluid. Comparing the enzyme content of the interstitial fluids of certain tumours in mice with that of plasma and peritoneal fluid, they found that the catheptic activity of the tumour fluid was three to four times higher than that of the plasma; the glutathione reductase and arginase activities could be as much as twenty-five times higher. Sylvén and his colleagues suggested that these enzymes originated from the tumour cells as a consequence of their increased membrane permeability; they proposed that the proteolytic cathepsins facilitated tumour cell detachment by weakening the adhesions between normal tissue cells at the periphery of tumours and degrading connective tissue structures such as collagen, all of which would contribute to the ability of tumour cells to invade. Much of the earlier work (Glenner *et al.*, 1959[50]; Mottet, 1961[51]; Pearse *et al.*, 1962[52]) on the associations of aminopeptidases with tumours gave conflicting results and utilized histochemical techniques which yielded qualitative rather than quantitative information. Furthermore, this approach provided information on the occurrence of these enzymes within cells rather than in the interstitial fluid. For example, Pearse *et al.* (1962)[52] made a histochemical study of aminopeptidase activity in forty-five human neoplasms and concluded that the tumour cells possessed little or no activity, whereas the activity of fibroblasts and macrophages in the surrounding stroma was high. They found no correlation between the invasiveness of these tumours and their level of stromal aminopeptidase activity, but it is the levels of activity of enzymes *outside* the cells that may be more relevant to invasion. These observations of high levels of enzymes in normal stromal cells did, however, raise the question of the origin of the interstitial enzymes within tumours; the relatively high intercellular levels of cathepsin activity of certain tumours could be derived from infiltrating macrophages which had released enzymes during phagocytosis or following cell death. The studies of Niemi and Sylvén (1968)[53] of the enzyme activities of interstitial fluids from talc-induced granulomas in rats indicated that leakage of cathepsins and other enzymes occurred from both intact and Irreversibiy damaged macrophages and fibroblasts in sterile and infected granulomas. Comparison of the patterns of activity of different enzymes present in the interstitial fluid of these granulomas with the interstitial fluids of tumours did, however, reveal distinct differences; and it was suggested that very large numbers of macrophages would have to be present to account for the levels and patterns of enzyme activities observed in tumour fluid (Sylvén, 1968)[54]. Sylvén considers that a trypsin-like cathepsin B, which is found in the interstitial fluid of tumours and is active at neutral pH, may be chiefly responsible for reduced cell adhesiveness in tumours and the degradation of structural proteins of normal tissues surrounding the tumour. This enzyme is believed to be lysosomal in origin, but it should be emphasized that tumour invasion is not invariably associated with the release of lysosomal enzymes. Brandes *et al.* (1967)[55] studied the invasion by L1210 mouse leukaemic cells of skeletal and smooth muscle and were unable to detect significant quantities of lysosomal enzymes by light or electron microscopic histochemistry in the invasion zone. Leukaemic cells are, however, derived from normal cells which are themselves invasive; for this reason they may possess special mechanisms of infiltration not involving the bulk secretion of cathepsin and other lysosomal enzymes.

A more serious criticism of the role played by extracellular lysosomal enzymes in tumour invasion is contained in the work of Gullino and Lanzerotti (1972)[56]. Gullino has devised an elegant technique for the continuous sampling of tumour interstitial fluid through membrane filter chambers implanted inside growing tumours. The membrane filters exclude the entry of cell but permit the passage of molecules of high molecular weight, and sampling of the extracellular fluid can be carried out continuously through the use of attached catheters without disturbing the tumour which encloses the chamber. Gullino and Lanzerotti observed that the extracellular fluids of primary (spontaneous) and transplantable rat mammary tumours contained negligible quantities of six characteristic lysosomal enzymes though their intracellular concentrations were quite high. Sylvén's technique of sampling extracellular fluid with capillaries does not completely exclude the possibility of damage to viable cells. Any damage to cells could result in the release of enzymes thus producing an artificially high enzyme level in the extracellular fluid. It is essential to apply Gullino's filter membrane method to the study of the enzyme composition of extracellular fluids of tumours of varying invasiveness in order to resolve these contradictions.

Most of the hydrolases of tumour interstitial fluid have strongly acid pH optima and measurement of the pH of tumours has yielded conflicting results, probably depending on the region sampled. Sylvén (1967)[57] found the pH of tumours to be the same as that of normal tissues, while Gullino *et al.* (1964)[58] found a slight acid shift. From consideration of the overall negative surface charge density of cells, Weiss (1967)[59] has suggested that certain regions of the cell periphery may have a much lower pH than the bulk phase of the extracellular fluid, and that proteases with low pH optima may be more active in the region of the cell periphery. The sequential making and breaking of adhesions between the surface of a migrating cell and the substrate which is necessary for cell locomotion may be governed by local and rhythmic fluctuations of surface pH in the regions of cell-substrate adhesion. These local alterations of pH could control the activity of enzymes which may be involved in the breaking of cell-substrate adhesions.

Other enzymes in addition to proteases have been considered. Hyaluronidase, by virtue of its ability to degrade ground substance and reduce its viscosity, is one obvious candidate for enzymic facilitation of tumour spread. Measurement of the levels of hyaluronidase activity in tumours and its relation to invasion has yielded conflicting results and has frequently been complicated by the presence of contaminating micro-organisms, a potent source of hyaluronidase (Kiriluk *et al.*, 1950)[60]. Recent work by Fiszer–Szafarz and Gullino (1970a[61], b[62]), in which they eliminated the possibility of microbial contamination, has provided firm evidence of significant increases in the levels of hyaluronidase in the interstitial fluids of the Walker carcinosarcoma in rats. The role of hyaluronidase in tumour invasion has been extensively reviewed by Cameron (1966)[63], who made the interesting suggestion that hyaluronidase secretion by tumour cells could have two opposing effects. Hyaluronidase may facilitate invasion by degradation of ground substance, but also retard it by stimulating fibroblastic hyperplasia and consequent collagenization and fibrosis which, in certain circumstances, may present a mechanical barrier to tumour infiltration. This suggestion is reminiscent of that of Santesson (1935)[64] who studied the infiltrative capacities of explants of mouse mammary tumours in tissue culture and found that the most actively infiltrating had negligible proteolytic activity while the least infiltrative tumours had greater proteolytic activity. He suggested that greater proteolysis by the more benign tumours caused collapse of connective tissue structures, the fibrous elements of which formed a meshwork barrier to tumour infiltration. These observations raise basic questions concerning the role of degradative enzymes present in the interstitial fluid of tumours. Although the work of Sylvén and others provides evidence of the presence of these enzymes in the interstitial fluid there is still little direct evidence for a causal relationship between the presence of such enzymes and the invasive ability of the tumour.

Some of the most convincing work on the presence of degrading enzymes in tumours has come from the work of Strauch and his colleagues. The invasive growth of cancer is frequently associated with extensive destruction of normal connective tissues; although it has frequently been suggested that this may be due to the presence of collagenolytic enzymes in the invasion zone, until recently, there has been little success in detecting these enzymes. Eisen *et al.* (1971)[56] have, however, produced immunochemical evidence for the presence of collagenases in extracts of human skin. The activity of these enzymes was almost completely inhibited by the presence of protein inhibitors, such as α_1-antitrypsin and α_2-macroglobulin. Similarly, Vaes (1972)[66] demonstrated that collagen protease is released from bone explants into the medium in the form of an inactive proenzyme which could be activated by the proteolytic action of added trypsin. Strauch (1972)[67] considers that there are at least two classes of collagenases—one splitting collagen into several high molecular weight constituents, and the other degrading these fragments into quite low molecular weight components. Strauch (1972)[67] and his colleagues found that in contrast with benign breast tumours, invasive mammary carcinomas possessed considerably increased levels of both types of collagenolytic enzymes; the highest levels of activity were present in the outer invading region of the tumour. In a detailed study, Keiditsch and Strauch (1970)[68] demonstrated that this increased activity of collagenases was due to the increased collagenase content per tumour cell and was not merely related to a high concentration of viable tumour cells at the periphery of the lesion. The presence of collagenases in other types of human tumours has also been reported by Taylor *et al.* (1970)[69] and by Strauch (1972)[67]. This increased activity of peptidases and proteases present in various tumours may be associated with a decreased concentration of the inhibitors of these enzymes rather than with an increased synthesis and release of enzymes by tumour cells (Blackwood *et al.*, 1965[70]). It would seem at present that there is good evidence of increased protease, and particularly collagenase, activity associated with the tumours; but formal demonstration that neoplastic invasion is caused primarily by the release of these enzymes by the tumour cells is still lacking.

THE RELEASE OF TOXINS

The release of diffusible toxic substances from tumour cells which selectively killed or harmed normal cells at a distance from the tumour periphery would certainly facilitate local invasion. Unfortunately, the evidence available indicates that such materials may equally inhibit or stimulate the growth of normal cells depending on the types of tumour and normal cells which are used. For example, Smith and Cress (1961)[71] and Holmberg (1962)[72] prepared extracts from tumour cells and their extracellular fluids which were harmful to normal fibroblasts. In a series of studies, Holmberg (1968a[73], b[74], c[75]) extracted fluids from tumours in both experimental animals and human patients and isolated a low molecular weight polypeptide in crystalline form: this material caused detachment of L cells from glass and inhibited the growth of (and eventually killed) cells from a number of cell lines. Initially, it was considered that the polypeptide was more toxic to normal fibroblasts than to tumour cells, but later work (Holmberg, 1968b) demonstrated no significant differences in its toxicity for normal or malignant cells in culture. Using parabiotic cultures, Katsuta and his colleagues (Katsuta and Takaoka, 1961[76], 1964[77], Katsuta *et al.*, 1968)[78] found that media from cultures of rodent sarcoma and hepatoma slightly inhibited the maintenance and growth of normal fibroblasts and epithelial cells, but stimulated the growth of tumour cells. Ludford and Barlow (1944[79], 1945[80]) and Foley *et al.* (1963)[81] found that the growth of fibroblasts was stimulated by diffusable agents released by carcinoma cells, while Ranadive and Bhide (1962)[82] concluded from studies of conjoint cultures that the growth-stimulating activity of tumour cells was closely related to the phase of tumour progression and the grade of malignancy. These conflicting results may be partly resolved by the observations of Rounds (1970)[83] who isolated a growth modifying factor from the culture media of three established lines of human malignant cells; this factor stimulated the growth of normal fibroblasts at low concentrations but was growth-inhibitory and cytotoxic when added to the same fibroblast cultures at higher concentrations. The growth-stimulating or cytotoxic effect of the tumour-derived material depended on its concentration. By contrast, *in vivo* there is direct contact between tumour cells and the normal cells of the host in addition to effects mediated by diffusable substances; and conflicting results have been obtained in culture systems where normal and tumour cells have been maintained in direct contact (Bürk and Williams, 1971[84], Rubin, 1966[85], 1970[86]; Abercrombie *et al.*, 1957[87]; Weiss, 1970[88]). These interactions between normal and tumour cells in culture which result in the stimulation or inhibition of growth of either type of cell may be mediated by the release of chemical substances or subcellular components, or by direct contact interactions; but their precise nature and relevance to the *in vivo* situation remain obscure.

CONTACT INHIBITION OF MIGRATION

A more direct approach to the problem of tumour invasion has been attempted by Abercrombie and others, using tissue culture methods. It is evident from the work of Wood *et al.* (1967)[8] on the behaviour of normal fibroblasts and epithelial cells in rabbit ear chambers, that these cells do not usually migrate *in vivo*. Abercrombie and Heaysman (1953[89], 1954[90]) and Abercrombie *et al.* (1967)[87] suggested from their studies on normal fibroblasts in culture that the absence of movement of these cells *in vivo* may be determined by the contact of the cell surfaces with each other. In sparse monolayer cultures of normal fibroblasts, the contact between the leading ruffled membranes of a migrating cell with the surface of another cell usually results in a cessation of activity of the ruffled membrane and a contraction of the migrating cell, which is then arrested. Another factor which may be involved in cessation of movement of cells following contact with other cells is that the cell surfaces may not be sufficiently adhesive to permit migration of one cell over another. Thus, normal endothelial cells, which *in vivo* are relatively non-adhesive, inhibit the migration of tumour cells (Barski and Belehradeck, 1965)[91] and macrophages (Abercrombie, 1970[92]) which are not inhibited by normal fibroblasts. A similar observation has been made by Bell (1972a[93]) who found that polyoma virus-transformed 3T3 cells, KB cells, Sarcoma 180 cells, and embryonic chick heart fibroblasts failed to spread and migrate on the upper surfaces of a variety of sheets of confluent normal chick embryo cells.

A consequence of contact inhibition of movement is that when a complete confluent monolayer of normal fibroblasts is formed, movement of individual cells is markedly restricted in all directions. The migration of cells from various sarcomas, particularly some highly anaplastic mouse sarcomas (Abercrombie *et al.*, 1967[87]) is not inhibited by contact with the normal fibroblasts; it is probable that this absence of contact inhibition is implicated in the local invasion of these sarcomas *in vivo*. Other sarcomas show an incomplete loss of contact inhibition when confronted with normal fibroblasts (Abercrombie, 1961[94]). Some of the problems involved in demonstrating a loss of contact inhibition of movement are emphasized by the work of Bell (1972b[95]) who found that contact inhibition occurred not only in cultures of normal cells but also in polyoma virus-transformed T3T3 cells. The transformed cells criss-crossed each other while the normal cells did not; neither cells moved over the surfaces of other cells but both were able to move underneath them, remaining in contact with the substrate.

The nature of the interactions involved in contact inhibition of cell migration are unknown. Flaxman *et al.* (1969)[43] studied the ultrastructure of surface contacts formed between pairs of cultured cells which had been fixed at varying times after contacts had formed between them. Tight junctions, obliterating intercellular spaces, were formed within minutes of contact being established between cells exhibiting contact inhibition. Wolpert and Gingell (1969)[96] have suggested that the close approach of two cell surfaces leads to an increase in surface potential; this may induce conformational changes in the surfaces which in turn activate adenyl cyclase resulting in increased production of cyclic AMP (adenosine 3′5′ monophosphate). This could alter the local concentration of calcium leading to changes in the activity and structure of the microfilaments and microtubules which, situated beneath the cell surface, are believed to be responsible for cell motility. The observations of Johnson *et al.* (1971)[97] of the restoration of ‘normal’ morphological and growth characteristics to sarcoma cells following treatment with cyclic AMP, and the pronounced increase of cellular cyclic AMP in normal cells following the establishment of maximal contacts in confluent cultures described by Heidrick and Ryan (1971)[98], both suggest that reduction of contact inhibition of tumour cells may be associated with reduced levels of adenyl cyclase (Bürk, 1968)[99].

Confrontations between types of normal and tumour cells in culture other than fibroblasts and sarcoma cells have not been investigated in such detail. Santesson (1935)[64] observed that the cells of ‘highly differentiated mammary tumours’ did not infiltrate normal fibroblasts but pushed them back, while the more anaplastic carcinomas actively infiltrated the fibroblasts. Wilbanks and Richart (1966)[100] examined the interaction of normal squamous epithelium, normal connective tissue and intraepithelial (*in situ*) neoplasia from the human uterine cervix in monolayer culture. They observed that normal epithelium caused retraction and detachment of normal fibroblasts and of the intraepithelial neoplastic cells. Invasion of the normal epithelial sheets by neoplastic cells was never observed. In this system there seems to be competition between different cell types for the substrate, and the dominant cells appear to be those of the normal cervical epithelium.

The profound influence of the nature of the substrate on the interactions between normal and tumour cells in monolayer culture has led many investigators to use three-dimensional *in vitro* systems for the study of tumour invasion (Leighton and Kline, 1954[101]; Leighton *et al.*, 1959[102]; Wolff and Schneider, 1956[10]; Easty and Easty, 1963[9]). Leighton *et al.* (1959)[102] confronted three-dimensional cultures of fibroblasts growing in sponges with a variety of tumour cells, and observed that the degree of neoplastic infiltration was related to the orientation of the fibroblasts to the tumour. Where the fibroblasts were arranged tangentially i.e. parallel to the tumour, invasion was minimal; with radially orientated fibroblasts, tumour invasion was maximal. This effect may be related to the phenomenon of contact guidance. Weiss (1958)[103] demonstrated that both normal and tumour cells grown in plasma clots tend to orientate themselves along the lines of tension within the clot, and also on microgrooves etched in a glass surface—i.e. the orientation of the substrate can influence the orientation of the cells. The polarization of the direction of movement of tumour cells may be influenced by other factors such as gradients of population density, metabolites, oxygen tension. One such gradient has been demonstrated by Weiss and Scott (1963)[104] who found that a pH gradient polarizes cell locomotion by stimulating cells to move from a region of high or low pH towards a region of neutral pH. If, as has been reported, the pH of the interstitial fluid of tumours is often significantly lower than that of surrounding normal tissue, this could provide a mechanism directing the movements of tumour cells outwards from the central tumour mass.

PHAGOCYTOSIS AND CHEMOTAXIS

Several workers have examined the role of phagocytosis of normal cells by tumour cells or the insertion of cytoplasmic probes by tumour cells into normal cells. The phagocytosis of portions of normal cells and of erythrocytes by some lymphomes has been reported by Diamondopolous and Smith (1964)[105] and Bernard and Leplus (1964)[106], but this may merely reflect the retention of the phagocytic properties of the original normal cells. A study of the invasion of rat liver by Novikoff Hepatoma cells has, however, revealed similar evidence of phagocytosis of hepatic cell debris by the infiltrating tumour cells (Babai and Tremblay, 1972[107]); the insertion of tumour processes into normal liver cells, with resulting damage, was also found. These observations may not be universal, however, since Kendrey and Nemeth (1967)[108] reported that cells of a tumour described as an invasive Küpffer-cell sarcoma in a rat had apparently lost the phagocytic capacity characteristic of normal Küpffer cells. The possible role of phagocytosis of the fibrous components of normal connective tissue in invasion has been examined by Gilfillan (1968)[109] who found that carcinoma and sarcoma cells in monolayer culture ingested and degraded chopped elastin fibres more vigorously than their normal epithelial and mesenchymal counterparts. It is not known whether this property of the tumour cells in culture is expressed *in vivo* against intact fibres of connective tissue though it is interesting that fragmentation of elastic fibres is sometimes seen in the vicinity of locally invasive mammary carcinomas in man.

Chemotaxis of tumour cells is not generally considered to play a role in invasion though a Japanese group (Hayashi *et al.*, 1970[110]; Yoshida *et al.*, 1970[111]; Ozaki *et al.*, 1971[112]) has recently isolated a factor from tumours which attracts tumour cells but not polymorphonuclear leucocytes; if injected intradermally, it promotes the extravascular migration of tumour cells at the site of injection without increasing vascular permeability. The authors consider that this factor may play an important role in tumour invasion, but while these observations are interesting it is difficult to see how the factor will in fact promote either local invasion from the primary tumour or from blood vessels into adjacent tissues. It might, indeed, be expected to have the opposite effect since tumour cells should be attracted towards the highest concentration of the substance, which presumably is within the tumour itself. One possibility is that tumours *in vivo* may release this material in an inactive form which is subsequently activated at some distance from the tumour, thereby providing a stimulus for the migration of tumour cells away from the primary tumour.

INFLAMMATORY AND IMMUNE RESPONSES OF THE HOST

The role of inflammatory and immune responses of the host on the growth of tumours has been extensively investigated, but until recently little attention has been paid to their possible activities in relation to the spread of cancer. Investigations of the spread of cancer have mainly been confined to examining the relationships between the antigenicity of the tumour, the immunological status of the host and the development of metastases (Kim, 1970[113]; Deodhar and Crile, 1969[114]; Vaage and Weiss, 1969[115]; Vaage *et al.*, 1971[116]; see also Chapters 5 and 12). The role of host responses on the local invasion of tumour cells has only been examined indirectly. The observations of Wood *et al.* (1961)[117] show that when tumour cells become lodged within capillaries a thrombus is formed which is eventually associated with damage to the adjacent vascular endothelium. Leucocytes migrate to the damaged site and their movement through the vessel wall is thought to create defects through which the tumour cells subsequently migrate. A similar role for host leucocytes has been proposed by Wheatley and Easty (1964)[118] from observations of the effects of stimulation and suppression of the response of leucocytes to the growth of an ascitic tumour of the mouse. Infiltration of the parietal peritoneum by leucocytes preceded tumour invasion and stimulation of leucocyte infiltration accelerated tumour invasion; suppression of leucocytes retarded it. The mechanisms involved are not known but Weiss (1967)[59] has suggested that the leucocytes migrate through normal tissues by releasing lysosomal hydrolases which weaken the cohesion of adjacent normal cells. Currie and Sime (1973)[119] have demonstrated that substances present in syngeneic immune serum of mice may strongly inhibit the *in vitro* motility of the specific tumour cells but not of normal spleen cells nor cells from other tumours. The nature of the substance responsible for this effect is at present unknown, though Currie and Sime suspect that it is tumour-specific antibody. If it operates similarly *in vivo* it could play an important role in inhibiting the the local invasion of tumour cells.

The proliferation of connective tissue surrounding tumours is considered by Vasiliev (1958)[120] to play an essential role in neoplastic invasion by providing mechanical support, essential nutrients and possibly chemotactic substances, all of which may favour the outward migration of tumour cells. *In vitro* studies support the view that substances may be elaborated by various normal and neoplastic cells which facilitate the growth of other cells, but there is little evidence that this property is specific to fibroblasts.

Hartweit and Halleraker (1970)[122] and Hartweit and Cater (1971)[123] investigated the role of inflammatory reactions in potentiating invasion of subcutaneous implants of the Ehrlich carcinoma in mice. Hartveit (1969)[121] observed that tumour growth was inhibited by treating the mice with polyethylene glycol. The local inflammatory response surrounding the tumour was suppressed, and tumour growth in these treated animals was expansive rather than infiltrative. Hartveit and Halleraker (1970)[122] subsequently found that treatment with the anti-inflammatory agent butazolidine did not suppress tumour growth (judged by the weights of subcutaneous tumours produced) but altered the orientation of the connective tissue surrounding the tumour; it appeared to encapsulate the tumour, converting the newly formed peripheral blood capillaries from a radial to a tangential orientation, and replacing the usual granulocytic infiltrate with one of lymphocytes and macrophages. The net result of these changes appeared to be the abolition of tumour infiltration and its replacement by purely expansive growth. Anti-inflammatory drugs such as butazolidine are potent inhibitors of proteolytic enzymes (Cowey and Whitehouse, 1966)[124], and it is possible that this property is involved in its anti-invasive effects. The work of Hartveit and her colleagues provides suggestive evidence for the role of local inflammation in potentiating the infiltration of subcutaneously implanted Ehrlich carcinomas. The factors responsible for the tumour associated inflammation are not established, but complement-mediated lysis of the tumour cells may be involved (Hartveit and Cater, 1971)[123].

References

1. Young, J. S., *J. Path. Bact.*, **77**, 321 (1959).
2. Warren, B. A. and Shubik, P., *Lab. Invest.*, **15**, 464 (1966).
3. Wood, S. Jr., *Archs. Path.*, **66**, 550 (1958).
4. Folkman, J., *New Engl. J. Med.*, **18**, 1182 (1971).
5. Folkman, J., Merler, E. and Abernethy, C. J. *J. Exp. Med.*, **133**, 275 (1971).
6. Waldeyer, R., *Virchows Arch. Path. Anat. Physiol.*, **55**, 67 (1872).
7. Willis, R. A. *Pathology of Tumours*, *4th Edition*, Butterworth, London (1967).
8. Wood, S. Jr., Baker, R. R. and Marzocchi, B. In *Mechanisms of Invasion in Cancer*, Editor P. Denoix, pp. 26. Springer-Verlag, Berlin (1967).
9. Easty, G. C. and Easty, D. M. *Nature*, **199**, 1104 (1963).
10. Wolff, St., and Schneider, N., *C.R. Soc. Biol.* (Paris), **159**, 845 (1956).

11. Wolff, Et. and Weniger, J. P., *J. Embryol. exp. Morph.*, **2,** 161 (1954).
12. Coman, D. R., *Cancer Res.*, **4,** 625 (1944).
13. McCutcheon, M., Coman, D. R. and Fontaine, B. M., *Cancer*, **1,** 460 (1948).
14. Tjernberg, B. and Zajicek, J., *Acta Cytol.*, **9,** 197 (1965).
15. Carruthers, C. and Suntzeff, V., *Science*, **19,** 245 (1944).
16. Hickie, R. A. and Kalant, H., *Cancer Res.*, **27,** 1053 (1967).
17. Coman, D. R., *Cancer Res.*, **21,** 1436 (1961).
18. Bangham, A. D. and Pethica, B. A., *Proc. Roy. Phys. Soc. Edinburgh.*, **28,** 43 (1960).
19. Patinkin, D., Zanitsky, A. and Doljanski, F. *Cancer Res.*, **30,** 498 (1970a).
20. Weiss, L., Ziegel, R., Jung, O. S. and Bross, I. D. J. *Exp. Cell Res.*, **70,** 57 (1972).
21. Ambrose, E. J., James, A. M. and Lowick, H. J. B. *Nature*, **177,** 576 (1956).
22. Purdom, L., Ambrose, E. J. and Klein, G. *Nature*, **181,** 1586 (1958).
23. Sakai, I., *Nagoya Med. J.*, **13,** 51 (1967).
24. Ohta, N., Pardee, A. B., McAuslan, B. R. and Burger, M. M. *Biochim. Biophys. Acta*, **158,** 98 (1968).
25. Wu, H., Meezan, E., Black, P. G. and Robbins, P. W. *Biochemistry*, **8,** 2509 (1969).
26. Vassar, P. S., *Lab. Invest.*, **12,** 1072 (1963).
27. Weiss, L. and Sinks, L. F., *Cancer Res.*, **30,** 90 (1970).
28. Cook, G. M. W. and Jacobson, W. *Biochem. J.*, **107,** 549 (1968).
29. Patinkin, D., Schlesinger, M. and Doljanski, F. *Cancer Res.*, **30,** 489 (1970b).
30. Frye, L. D. and Edidin, M. *J. Cell Sci.*, **7,** 319 (1970).
31. Easty, G. C. and Mercer, E. H. *Cancer Res.*, **20,** 1608 (1960).
32. Martinez-Palomo, A., Braislovsky, C. and Bernhard, W. *Cancer Res.*, **29,** 929 (1969).
33. Martinez-Palomo, A. *Lab. Invest.*, **22,** 605 (1970).
34. McNutt, N. S. and Weinstein, R. S. *Science*, **165,** 597 (1969).
35. McNutt, N. S., Herschberg, R. A. and Weinstein, R. S. *J. Cell Biol.*, **51,** 805 (1971).
36. Loewenstein, W. R., *Ann. New York Acad. Sci.*, **137,** 441 (1966).
37. Gilula, N. B., Reeves, O. R. and Steinbauch, A., *Nature*, **236,** 262 (1972).
38. Loewenstein, W. R. and Kanno, Y., *J. Cell Biol.*, **33,** 225 (1967).
39. Jamakosmanovic, A. and Loewenstein, W. R., *J. Cell Biol.*, **38,** 556 (1968).
40. Kanno, Y. and Matsui, Y. *Nature*, **218,** 775 (1968).
41. Furshpan, E. J. and Potter, D. D. In *Current Topics in Developmental Biology*, Editors A. A. Moscona and A. Monroy, **3,** 95. Academic Press, New York.
42. Sheridan, J. D. *J. Cell Biol.*, **45,** 91 (1970).
43. Flaxman, B. A., Revel, J. P. and Hay, E. D. *Exp. cell Res.*, **58,** 438 (1969).
44. Harris, A. *Amer. Zoologist* 10/3 *abstr.*, 324 (1970).
45. Trinkaus, J. P., Betchaku, T. and Krulikowski, L. S. *Exp. cell Res.*, **64,** 291 (1971).
46. Inbar, M. and Sachs, L. *Proc. Natn. Acad. Sci.*, **63,** 1418 (1969).
47. Ben-Bassat, H., Inbar, M. and Sachs, L. *J. Membrane Biol.*, **6,** 183 (1971).
48. Friberg, S., Cochran, A. J. and Golub, S. H. *Nature New Biol.*, **232,** 121 (1971).
49. Sylvén, B. and Bois, I., *Cancer Res.*, **20,** 831 (1960).
50. Glenner, G. G., Burstone, M. S. and Meyer, D. B., *J. Nat. Cancer Inst.*, **23,** 857 (1959).
51. Mottet, N. K., *Am. J. Path.*, **39,** 17 (1961).
52. Pearse, A. G. E., Hess, R. and Snyder, R., *Henry Ford Hospital Symposium*

on Biological Interactions in Normal and Neoplastic Growth, p. 657, Churchill, London (1962).
53. Niemi, M., and Sylvén, B., *Actapath. microbiol.*, Scand., **72,** 205 (1968).
54. Sylvén, B., *Europ. J. Cancer.*, **4,** 463 (1968).
55. Brandes, D., Anton, E. and Schofield, B. *Cancer Res.*, **27,** 2159 (1967).
56. Gullino, P. M. and Lanzerotti, R. H., *J. Natl. Cancer Inst.*, **49,** 1349 (1972).
57. Sylvén, B. In *Endogenous Factors influencing Host-Tumour Balance.* Editors, R. W. Wissler, T. L. Dao and S. Wood, Jr., p. 267. University of Chicago Press (1967).
58. Gullino, P. M., Clark, S. H. and Grantham, F. H. *Cancer Res.*, **24,** 780 (1964).
59. Weiss, L. *The Cell Periphery.* North Holland Publishing Co., Amsterdam (1967).
60 Kiriluk, L. B., Kremen, A. and Glick, D. *J. Nat. Cancer Inst.*, **10,** 993 (1950).
61. Fiszer-Szafarz, B. and Gullino, P. M., *Proc. Soc. exp. Biol. Med.*, **133,** 597 (1970a).
62. Fiszer-Szafarz, B. and Gullino, P. M. *Proc. Soc. exp. Biol. Med.*, **133,** 805 (1970).
63. Cameron, E. *Hyaluronidase and Cancer.* Pergamon Press (1966).
64. Santesson, L. *Act path. microbiol.* Scand. Suppl., **24,** 1 (1935).
65. Eisen, A. Z., Bauer, E. A. and Jeffrey, J. J. *Proc. Nat. Acad. Sci.*, **68,** 248 (1971).
66. Vaes, G., *Biochem.*, **126,** 275 (1972).
67. Strauch, L. 'The Role of Collagenases in Tumour Invasion'. In *Tissue Interactions in Carcinogenesis.* Editor D. Tarin, p. 399. Academic Press, London (1972).
68. Keiditsch, E. and Strauch, L. *Verh. Deut. Ges. Path.*, **54,** 438 (1970).
69. Taylor, A. C., Levy, B. M. and Simpson, J. W., *Nature*, **228,** 366 (1970).
70. Blackwood, C. E., Mandl, I. and Long, M. *Am. J. Obstet. Gynaecol.*, **91,** 419 (1965).
71. Smith, A. G. and Cress, H. R. *Lab. Invest.*, **10,** 898 (1961).
72. Holmberg, B. *Nature*, **195,** 45 (1962).
73. Holmberg, B. *Europ. J. Cancer*, **4,** 263 (1968a).
74. ————, *Europ. J. Cancer*, **4,** 271 (1968b).
75. ————, *Europ. J. Cancer*, **4,** 475 (1968c).
76. Katsuta, H. and Takaoka, T. *Jap. J. exp. Med.*, **31,** 307 (1961).
77. Katsuta, H. and Takaoka, T. *J. Nat. Cancer Inst.*, **32,** 963 (1964).
78. Katsuta, H. Takaoka, T. and Nagai, T. In *Cancer Cells in Culture.* Editor H. Katsuta, p. 157, University of Tokyo Press (1968).
79. Ludford, R. J. and Barlow, H. *Cancer Res.*, **4,** 694 (1944).
80. Ludford, R. J. and Barlow, H. *Cancer Res.*, **5,** 257 (1945).
81. Foley, J. F., Kennedy, B. J. and Ross, J. D., *Cancer Res.*, **23,** 368 (1963).
82. Ranadive, K. J. and Bhide, S. V. In *Biological Interaction in Normal and Neoplastic Growth.* Editors M. J. Brennan and W. L. Simpson, p. 337, Little, Brown and Co., Boston (1962).
83. Rounds, D. E. *Cancer Res.*, **30,** 2847 (1970).
84. Bürk, R. R. and Williams, C. A. In *Growth Control and Cell Cultures.* Ciba Foundation Symposium. Editors G. E. W. Wolstenholme and J. Knight, p. 107. Churchill, London (1971).
85. Rubin, H. *Exp. cell Res.*, **41,** 149 (1966).
86. Rubin, H. *Science*, **167,** 1271 (1970).

87. Abercrombie, M., Heaysman, J. E. M. and Karthauser, H. M. *Exp. cell Res.*, **13,** 276 (1957).
88. Weiss, R. A. *Exp. cell Res.*, **63,** 1 (1970).
89. Abercrombie, M. and Heaysman, J. E. M. *Exp. cell Res.*, **5,** 111 (1953).
90. Abercrombie, M. and Heaysman, J. E. M. *Exp. cell Res.*, **6,** 293 (1954).
91. Barski, G. and Belehradek, J. *Exp. cell Res.*, **37,** 464 (1965).
92. Abercrombie, M. *Europe. J. Cancer*, **6,** 7 (1970).
93. Bell, P. B., *J. Cell Biol.*, **55,** No. 2., 60A (1972a).
94. Abercrombie, M. *Canadian Cancer Conference*, **4,** 101 (1961).
95. Bell, P. B., *J. Cell Biol.*, **55,** No. 2., 16A (1972b).
96. Wolpert, L. and Gingell, D. In *Homeostatic Regulators.* Ciba Foundation Symposium. Editors, G. E. W. Wolstenholme and J. Knight, p. 241. Churchhill, London (1969).
97. Johnson, G. S., Friedman, R. M. and Pastan, I., *Proc. Nat. Acad. Sci.*, **68,** 425 (1971).
98. Heidrick, M. L. and Ryan, W. L. *Cancer Res.*, **31,** 1313 (1971).
99. Bürk, R. R., *Nature*, **219,** 1271 (1968).
100. Willbanks, G. D. and Richart, R. M. *Cancer Res.*, **26,** 1641 (1966).
101. Leighton, J. and Kline, I. *Texas Repts. Biol. Med.*, **12,** 868 (1954).
102. Leighton, J., Kalla, R. L., Kline, I. and Belkin, M. *Cancer Res.*, **19,** 23 (1959).
103. Weiss, P. *Int. Rev. Cytol.*, **7,** 391 (1958).
104. Weiss, P. and Scott, B. I. H. *Proc. Nat. Acad. Sci.*, **50,** 330 (1963).
105. Diamondopolous, G. T. and Smith, E. B. *Cancer*, **27,** 329 (1964).
106. Bernard, W. and Leplus, R. *Fine Structure of the Normal and Malignant Lymph Nodes*, p. 59, Pergamon Press, Oxford (1964).
107. Babai, F. and Tremblay, G. *Cancer Res.*, **32,** 2765 (1972).
108. Kendrey, G. and Németh, K. *Neoplasma*, **14,** 273 (1967).
109. Gilfillan, R. F. *Cancer Res.*, **28,** 137 (1968).
110. Hayashi, H., Yoshida, K., Azaki, T. and Ushijima, K. *Nature*, **227,** 174 (1970).
111. Yoshida, K., Ozaki, T., Ushijima, K. and Hayashi, H. *Int. J. Cancer*, **6,** 123 (1970).
112. Ozaki, T., Yoshida, K., Ushijima, K. and Hayashi, H., *Int. J. Cancer*, **7,** 93 (1971).
113. Kim, V. *Science*, **167,** 72 (1970).
114. Deodhar, S. D. and Crile, G., Jr., *Cancer Res.*, **29,** 776 (1969).
115. Vaage, J. and Weiss, D. W. *Cancer Res.*, **29,** 1920 (1969).
116. Vaage, J., Chen, K. and Merrick, S. *Cancer Res.*, **31,** 496 (1971).
117. Wood, S., Holyoake, E. D. and Yardley, J. H. *Canadian Cancer Conference*, **4,** 167 (1961).
118. Wheatley, D. N. and Easty, G. C. *Br. J. Cancer*, **18,** 743 (1964).
119. Currie, G. A. and Sime, G. C. *Nature, New Biol.*, **241,** 284 (1973).
120. Vasiliev, J. M. *Br. J. Cancer*, **12,** 524 (1958).
121. Hartveit, F. *Acta path. microbiol.*, Scand., **77,** 623 (1969).
122. Hartveit, F. and Halleraker, B. *Acta path. microbiol.* Scand., **78,** 516 (1970).
123. Hartveit, F. and Cater, D. B. *Acta path. microbiol.*, Scand., **79,** 423 (1971).
124. Cowey, F. K. and Whitehouse, M. W. *Biochem. Pharmacol.*, **15,** 1071 (1966).

Chapter 5

METASTASIS

R. L. CARTER, D.M., M.R.C.Path.
Member of the Institute of Cancer Research, London

Most malignant tumours grow, invade locally and disseminate, giving rise to separate tumours at distant sites. This process is known as metastasis and the new tumours formed are described as metastatic or secondary tumours. The capacity to metastasize is not unique to cancer but it is clinically the most significant characteristic of the neoplastic process. Patients who die of cancer generally do so as a consequence of disseminated disease. Metastatic spread is usually a late clinical feature but it may occur early, providing the first clue to the presence of cancer—an obscure anaemia, a pathological fracture, jaundice or an unexplained lymphadenopathy. The primary tumour is sometimes small and difficult to locate during life. Conversely, metastatic deposits may declare themselves many years after seemingly effective treatment of the primary tumour. Once they are clinically apparent, metastatic tumours usually grow progressively but exceptions are occasionally encountered: secondary deposits may stop growing, temporarily or permanently, and may even regress. Though rare, such occurrences illustrate the important point that metastatic growth is sometimes susceptible to control.

General pathology of metastasis*

The primary tumour itself provides a few clues to its metastatic potential. Poorly differentiated tumours are more likely to metastasize than well differentiated neoplasms but in several circumstances, notably with some tumours of the adrenal, ovary and thyroid, differentiation is an unreliable guide to metastatic behaviour. Primary tumours invade by infiltrating the surrounding tissues, extending preferentially along fascial planes. Certain structures are characteristically resistant to invasion, e.g. cartilage, compact bone and periosteum, and large arteries. One unusual form of local spread is seen in some cancers of the breast which extend into the epithelium of the nipple to produce a condition known as Paget's disease. Local invasion is commonly but not invariably the prelude to distant metastasis: basal cell tumours of the skin, thymomas and most astrocytomas are invasive tumours which almost never metastasize.

When tumours metastasize they disseminate from the primary focus via pre-existing channels, spaces and cavities of the body.

*For more detailed accounts see Willis, 1967[1], 1973[2]; and Boyd, 1970[3].

Lymphatic spread, initially to regional lymph nodes, is particularly characteristic of carcinomas. Tumour cells enter lymphatic vessels and grow either in solid cords (permeation) or as discrete cell clumps (embolization). The relative importance of spread by these two processes has been disputed unnecessarily since both occur. Permeation is uncommon but is sometimes strikingly seen in subpleural and subperitoneal lymphatics, and also in the thoracic duct. Embolic spread is the main mode of lymphatic dissemination, from the primary tumour to proximal lymph nodes and also from one group of nodes to another. The 'perineural lymphatics' described particularly in the vicinity of the prostate, bladder, breast and pancreas are now thought to be perineural spaces and not true lymphatic channels (Rodin *et al.*, 1967[4]).

Haematogenous spread is a feature of many sarcomas and some carcinomas (e.g. of kidney, prostate, thyroid, and liver); also choriocarcinoma. Tumour cells enter the blood stream either directly by penetrating small vessels near the primary tumour, or indirectly from the thoracic duct and possibly from other lymphatico-venous connections (p.77). They circulate as single cells or small clumps and are initially trapped in the pulmonary or hepatic capillaries, depending on their point of entry. The lungs and liver are the two commonest sites for blood-borne metastases but other organs are also involved—parts of the axial skeleton, brain, kidneys, adrenals and skin. Systemic metastases are not, however, distributed in an indiscriminate fashion. Some sites are commonly involved by metastatic tumour, others almost never; and metastases from certain primary tumours show consistent predilections for specific sites.

Spread in body cavities is not uncommon. Carcinomas of the stomach, colon and ovary may form secondary deposits in the peritoneal cavity. Carcinomas of the breast, lung and oesophagus sometimes spread similarly in the pleural and pericardial cavities. Choroid plexus tumours, ependymomas, pinealomas and medulloblastomas may seed along the cerebrospinal cavity though spread to sites outside the central nervous system is exceptional. Multiple tumours are sometimes encountered in the urinary and bronchial passages but it is rarely possible to distinguish between multiple primary neoplasms and true metastases.

Appearance of metastases

Metastatic tumours vary greatly in number and size. Usually multiple, they may be present in enormous numbers. Most of them reproduce fairly closely the histological structure of the primary tumour but their degree of differentiation is sometimes greater and occasionally less.

It will be apparent from this brief introduction that the metastatic process poses many problems including the mode of local invasion; the detailed mechanisms of metastatic spread; the distribution, establishment and development of metastases; and the vagaries of metastatic growth including dormancy and spontaneous arrest and regression. These topics are considered in the rest of this chapter.

Analysis of the metastatic process

One feature of the metastatic process must be stressed from the outset. Metastasis involves an orderly and cumulative sequence of events; each event has to be analysed separately and each involves a measure of interaction between tumour and host (Willis, 1967[1], 1973[2]; Leighton, 1967[5]; Foulds, 1969[6]).

Certain aspects of human metastatic tumours are amenable to study. Examples include their biosynthetic activities, particularly of hormone or hormone-like polypeptides (Bagshawe, 1969[7]; Croughs *et al.*, 1972[8]) and carcinoembryonic antigens (see Laurence and Neville, 1972[9]), changes in distribution of tissue isoantigens (Davidsohn *et al.*, 1973[10]), ploidy and karyotype analyses (Koller, 1956[11]; Rabotti, 1959[12]) growth rate and cell kinetics (Young and De Vita, 1970[13]; Charbit *et al.*, 1971[14]; Terz *et al.*, 1971[15]; Lee and Spratt, 1972[16]) and responses to hormones (Franks, 1958[17], 1960[18]; Mellette, 1970[19]). Studies in human patients have also provided much of the information available on tumour cells circulating in the blood (see Griffiths and Salsbury, 1965[20]).

But detailed analysis of the metastatic process is not feasible in man and recourse has to be made to experimental animals. Although human tumours have been transplanted successfully as xenografts, some of them metastasizing in their new hosts (Giovanella *et al.*, 1973[21]), most experimental work has involved animal tumours. The majority of autochthonous tumours in animals do not metastasize consistently and transplantable tumours are usually used. Some transplanted tumours which metastasize regularly are listed below:

Mice	Cloudman melanoma (DBA); Ehrlich carcinoma (BALB/c); sarcoma T 241 Lewis (C57BL); sarcoma S37 (BALB/c and DBA2).
Rats	Walker carcinosarcoma; Flexner–Jobling carcinoma; Jensen sarcoma; Yoshida sarcoma.
Rabbits	Brown–Pearce and V2 carcinomas.
Hamsters	Amelanotic melanomas (Fortner); metastasizing and non-metastasizing lymphomas (ML and NML).

The general objections to the use of transplanted tumours are familiar: their principal disadvantages as models for metastasis are their rapid growth rate and their failure to spread to certain locations, e.g. axial skeleton and brain which are commonly involved by metastases in man. As an alternative, tumour cells are frequently injected intravascularly, usually into peripheral veins or the hepatic portal system. This is a manifestly artificial procedure, which involves the sudden introduction of large numbers of tumour cells at one site, by-passing critical early stages of the metastatic process. It is, however, useful for studying some aspects of the metastatic process particularly as the dose of tumour cells can be measured. It is worth noting here that the difficulties of quantifying experimental metastasis are still considerable (see Wexler, 1966[22]; Boeryd *et al.*, 1966[23]).

Certain aspects of the metastatic process have been studied by injecting tumour cells into the chorioallantoic veins of chick embryos (Leighton, 1967[5]; Easty *et al.*, 1969[24]; Vlaeminck *et al.*, 1972[25]) but the present account will deal solely with metastasis in intact animals.

THE PRIMARY TUMOUR AND ITS LOCAL MILIEU: THE INITIAL STAGES OF INVASION AND METASTASIS

The mechanisms of detachment of tumour cells from the primary tumour and their local spread in the adjacent tissues have been discussed in Chapter 4. This section is confined to a brief comment on certain aspects of the tumour and its fibrovascular stroma on which growth and development of the primary tumour are directly dependent (Tannock, 1970[26]). The interaction between infiltrating tumour and local connective tissues is complex, involving tissue destruction (implicit in invasion) and also proliferation: scirrhous carcinomas (e.g. of breast, stomach and prostate) evoke an intense fibroblastic reaction, a feature which is usually retained by their metastatic tumours growing in lymph nodes or liver.

Blood vessels within tumours are sometimes strikingly abnormal and, in highly anaplastic neoplasms, consist of little more than irregular channels lined directly by tumour cells (Willis, 1967[1], 1973[2]). Many tumours have necrotic centres and the vessels are best preserved at the edges of the lesions. Vessels in the surrounding stroma are prominent and there is evidence that tumours may induce local vasoproliferation by releasing 'angiogenesis factors' (Folkman, 1971[27]). The endothelial cells lining blood vessels in experimental tumours proliferate rapidly (Tannock, 1970[26]) and it may be significant that vessels near tumours respond abnormally to vasomotor and inflammatory agents (Cater *et al.*, 1966[28]; Cater and Taylor, 1966[29]; Underwood and Carr, 1972[30]); they could well represent a weak and potentially exploitable link in tumour organization. This is illustrated by recent work with the dioxopiperazin compound ICRF 159 (see Le Serve and Hellmann, 1972[31]); the substance appears to prevent metastases by stopping haematogenous dissemination of cells from grafted tumours and it is thought to act directly on the tumour vasculature. It is doubtful whether tumours have lymphatics (Zeidman, 1957[32]) though dilated lymphatic vessels are commonly seen in the surrounding tissues.

DISSEMINATION IN LYMPHATICS; NON-IMMUNOLOGICAL (BARRIER) FUNCTION OF LYMPH NODES

The mechanisms by which tumour cells penetrate lymphatic endothelium are unknown but their subsequent mode of gross spread to regional lymph nodes is well documented. A number of connections between lymph nodes and veins have been described other than the thoracic duct (Pressman *et al.*, 1962[33], 1966[34]), and studies with Walker tumour cells, tagged with ^{51}Cr and injected intravascularly, show that cells can move between the vascular and lymphatic circuits across the extravascular space and emerge in the thoracic duct lymph (Fisher and Fisher, 1966[35]; Hilgard *et al.*, 1972[36]). Too rigid a distinction between lymphatic and blood vascular systems is thus misleading.

The time of lymph node involvement is impossible to determine accurately in human patients though theoretical considerations, based on tumour kinetics, suggest that it is likely to be early, i.e. before a primary has reached a size of 1 mm^3. (Igot and Le Gal, 1968[37]). Experimental studies (Plenk *et al.*, 1954[38]) have shown that cells from a transplanted neuroblastoma in ABC mice reach the regional lymph nodes 4 to 6 days after grafting. Incoming tumour cells in the afferent lymphatics localize first in the marginal sinuses; they then drift to the medullary sinuses and small organized clumps appear in the superficial parts of the pulp (Zeidman and Buss, 1954[39]; Ludwig and Titus, 1967[40]; see also Willis, 1973[2]).

It is disputed whether regional lymph nodes form an effective barrier to incoming tumour cells, a barrier consisting of the reticulin framework and the sinus macrophages. First proposed by Virchow in 1860, the filtering action of lymph nodes was accepted for many years. The experiments of Zeidman and Buss (1954[39]) indicated that popliteal nodes in the rabbit trapped V2 tumour cells, injected into the afferent lymphatics, for up to three weeks; but more recent work by Fisher and Fisher (1966[41], 1967[42]) has demonstrated that many tumour cells injected into afferent lymphatics or adjacent soft tissues traverse the popliteal nodes and emerge in the efferent lymph. Barrier function appears to be compromised by local irradiation (Fisher and Fisher, 1967[42]), prior lymphangiography (Engzell *et al.*, 1968[43]), passive exercise and treatment with cortisone (Stoker, 1969[44]); some of these observations are difficult to appraise as both irradiation and cortisone may suppress the local immune response (v.i.). Intrinsic properties of the tumour cells themselves are also likely to contribute to the efficacy (or otherwise) of trapping. Differences in membrane properties, for instance, could be responsible for the different proclivities of carcinomas and sarcomas to metastasize to regional nodes.

Once tumour cells are retained in lymph nodes, a number of consequences can be envisaged.

1. the cells may proliferate and replace the node. The flow of incoming lymph will be deflected and perhaps reversed, diverting new lymph-borne tumour cells to fresh nodes. The cancerous node will itself act as a focus for further ('tertiary') deposits (Crile *et al.*, 1971[45]), with malignant cells spreading along uninvolved lymphatics, adjacent veins, and lymphaticovenous communications.
2. the cells may die (cf. Ludwig and Titus, 1967[40]) either from metabolic causes or through the activities of local defences. Destruction of free tumour cells in regional lymph nodes by macrophages and lymphocytes has been observed experimentally (e.g. Carter and Gershon, 1966[46], 1967[48]) but it is doubtful whether anything comparable occurs in human nodes (Willis, 1973[2]).
3. the cells may persist, alive but dormant, *without* forming metastatic deposits. Such cells may give rise to palpable tumours if the nodes are transferred to syngeneic recipients (Gershon *et al.*, 1967[48]; Feldman and Nachtigal, 1967[45]), illustrating the point that demonstration of tumour cells in a node by bioassay is not synonymous with metastasis.

The immune reactions of lymph nodes to metastatic tumour are discussed on p. 86.

DISSEMINATION VIA THE BLOOD STREAM

The host vasculature into and through which tumour cells disseminate is unexpectedly varied. Such variation is expressed structurally by the presence of arteriovenous anastomoses and by intervenous communications such as those linking the hepatic portal and systemic circuits, and the paravertebral venous complexes which extend from the pelvis to the skull, communicating segmentally with the caval system (Batson, 1942[50]). There are also variations in haemodynamics: these may be generalized, such as the momentary alterations in venous blood flow following the Valsalva manoeuvre, or regional – for instance the low-pressure paravertebral veins, a system that 'is more of a lagoon with occasional ebb and flow than a channel of streaming blood' (Boyd, 1970[3]).

The mode of penetration of tumour cells into the blood is obscure. In anaplastic tumours, cells may enter directly from the disorganized vasculature of the tumour itself. Blood flow through many vessels within tumours is, however, precarious (Tannock and Steel, 1969[51]) and better preserved vessels at the edge of the tumour or in the surrounding stroma are more likely portals of invasion. In experimental systems, tumour cells have been shown to enter the blood stream early after inoculation of tumour. Romsdahl *et al.* (1961[52]) demonstrated viable tumour cells in blood only twenty-four hours after implanting the T241 sarcoma intramuscularly into C57BL mice; lung metastases were observed after seven days.

Freely circulating tumour cells

Many aspects of the presence of tumour cells in circulating blood have been described in human patients (Griffiths and Salsbury, 1965[20]; Malmgren, 1968[53]). They are most readily demonstrated in patients with sarcomas, fairly readily in patients with adenocarcinomas and least frequently in patients with epidermoid carcinomas; they are found singly or in small clumps and appear to be more numerous during the later stages of the disease. Features of the primary tumour that seem to favour the release of cells into the blood are a poor degree of cellular differentiation and the presence of necrosis. An interesting correlation between growth of the primary tumour and release of tumour cells in the blood was reported in patients with malignant melanoma by Romsdahl *et al.* (1960[54]).

There are several practical problems associated with the studies of circulating tumour cells in man. These include the site of sampling (venous effluent from the tumour or systemic venous blood), methods of concentration, and identification. And once identified, the significance of such cells is usually obscure. Most circulating tumour cells found in patients are probably post-mitotic and attempts to cultivate them *in vitro* have been largely unsuccessful (Malmgren, 1968[57]). Experimental studies indicate that few circulating tumour cells survive. A high death rate among intravenously injected tumour cells (admittedly a contrived situation) was described at a morphological level by Takahashi (1915[55]) and the process has subsequently been studied in detail in experiments with tumour cells labelled with radioisotopes: ^{3}H, (Baserga *et al.*, 1960[56]), ^{51}Cr (Fisher and Fisher, 1967[57]) and ^{125}I-IUDR (Hofer *et al.*, 1969[58]; Fidler, 1970[59]). The elegant investigations of Baserga and his colleagues indicate that as few as $\frac{8}{1,000}$ labelled Ehrlich tumour cells survive in the mouse after intravenous injection. Experiments involving labelled tumour cells sometimes pose problems of technique and interpretation; for a critical account of these, see Fidler (1970[59]).

The disappointing conclusion that emerges from clinical studies is that the demonstration of circulating tumour cells carries few practical implications: most workers agree that they have no prognostic significance. In experimental systems, it is possible to inject different numbers of tumour cells and obtain a rough dose-response relationship between number of cells injected and number of tumour deposits that eventually form (Zeidman *et al.*, 1950[60]; Romsdahl *et al.*, 1961[52]) but it is not uncommon to find animals with progressively growing primary tumours (transplanted or autochthonous), no visceral metastases, but many circulating tumour cells (Kim, 1966[61]; Gershon *et al.*, 1967[48]; Wexler *et al.*, 1969[62], 1971[63]; Crile *et al.*, 1971[64]). Such cells may, however, grow when transferred to syngeneic recipients and it is possible that their failure to form metastases may be due to immune and other host responses—see later.

Circulating tumour cells in experimental animals have been studied *in vivo* by cinemicrographic techniques, particularly in the ear chamber and in the mesentery; the investigations of Zeidman (1961[65]) and of Wood (1958[66] 1964[67], 1971[68]) are particularly valuable. Zeidman showed that V2 and Brown–Pearce carcinoma cells are strikingly deformable and squeeze readily through small capillaries. But eventually, tumour cells impact in small vessels—the first stage in their escape from the vascular system.

Arrested tumour cells

Tumour cell emboli arrested in capillaries have long been familiar to morphologists (Takahashi, 1915[55]; see also Willis, 1967[1], 1973[2]) but more detailed studies of their formation have come from the cinemicrographic work of Wood (q.v.): the following sequence of events is commonly accepted.

Small clumps of tumour cells, generally six to ten, stick to vascular endothelium. They are then enclosed in a clot of fibrin and platelets, entangled with polymorphs. Local endothelial defects develop through which, after about three to six hours, tumour cells escape. The initial site of adherence is not determined by capillary diameter, rate of blood flow, or vasomotor activity but the process is favoured by the natural stickiness of tumour cells and their capacity, in some instances, to release thromboplastin-like substances. The importance of local intravascular coagulation is suggested by several experimental studies indicating that the incidence of metastases is generally decreased by treatment with heparin, thrombocytopenic or fibrinolytic agents (see Rudenstam, 1968[69]; also Gasic *et al.*, 1968[70]; Pick and Cater, 1971[71]; Wood, 1971[68]).

The results of recent work have raised some objections to this scheme. Fisher and Fisher (1967[72]) observed no alteration in the retention or lodgement of tumour cells in the livers of rats treated with heparin, warfarin, fibrinolysins and ϵ-aminocaproic acid (EACA); they used ^{51}Cr-labelled Walker cells, injected intraportally. Tumour cell aggregates without fibrin clots are sometimes encountered (Jones *et al.*, 1971[73]; Vlaeminck *et al.*, 1972[25]) and a recent study by Weiss and his colleagues (Holyoke *et al.*, 1972[74]) failed to demonstrate thromboplastic activity in the vicinity of tumour cells. Hagmar (1970[75], 1972[76]) has found that metastases from a syngeneic sarcoma and melanoma were increased in mice treated with heparin and with the defibrinating agent Arvin. Many experiments with anticoagulants have involved large doses, sometimes given over a prolonged period, and the main effects have been seen when treatment has preceded the inoculation of tumour. The possibility of dual effects, on the tumour as well as on the host, has been proposed (Boeryd and Hagmar, 1972[77]; Hagmar 1972[78]; see also Gasic and Gasic, 1962[79]; Gasic *et al.*, 1968[70]) and it is now recognized that a highly charged polyanion like heparin may change cell volumes and cell membranes and alter cell adhesiveness and migratory patterns. Recent work by Hilgard *et al.* (1972[36]) is relevant here, in which ^{51}Cr-labelled Walker cells were injected into the aorta of rats with thoracic duct fistulae. Clearance of tumour cells from the blood of heparinized animals was unchanged but the usual effluent of tumour cells in thoracic duct lymph ceased; heparin appeared to block specifically the migration of Walker cells across the interstitial space. Again, changes in the surface charge (the ψ potential) may drastically alter a tumour cell's initial phase of contact with vascular endothelium (Weiss, 1967[80]) though such changes are easier to postulate than prove.

Clearly trapping of tumour cells in the circulation is a complex process to which several elements from both tumour and host—mechanical, thrombotic and electrostatic—contribute.

Circulatory factors and the distribution of metastases

The problem of the localization of metastatic tumour has already been noted; the difficulties are most obvious in relation to tumour disseminating in the blood stream. The relation between initial intravascular trapping of tumour cell emboli and subsequent metastatic growth is reasonably straightforward in two locations—the liver and lungs. Metastases in a third site, the axial skeleton, can also be explained to some extent as a consequence of trapping of tumour cells which have entered the paravertebral venous plexuses (v.s.). Some skeletal metastases, particularly from the prostate (Franks, 1956[81]) and breast, are thought to localize by this route, a mode of spread that has been reproduced experimentally (Coman and De Long, 1951[82]). But it is improbable that the axial skeleton is involved solely through the paravertebral venous plexuses (Willis, 1967[1], 1973[2]), and other mechanisms for such systemic spread, not only to the skeleton but also to other sites, have to be postulated. There are various possibilities to consider.

1. Cardiac anomalies such as a patent foramen ovále can be implicated in very rare instances.
2. Tumour cells may bypass some parts of the capillary bed by traversing arteriovenous shunts. They may also reach seemingly 'ectopic' sites by means of the structural and haemodynamic variants already described.
3. Tumour cells, despite their large size, are readily deformed and thus able to squeeze through capillary beds. Transpulmonary migration was implied by Takahashi in 1915 and was demonstrated experimentally by Zeidman and Buss (1952[83]) and, by means of ^{51}Cr-labelled cells, by Fisher and Fisher (1967[57]).
4. Pulmonary deposits may themselves act as foci for further dissemination of tumor cells (Wexler *et al.*, 1969[62]; Crile *et al.*, 1971[64]). Although this is usually regarded as a late effect associated with large pulmonary tumours, Willis (1952[1]) emphasizes that the pulmonary metastases may be minute, adequately accounting for the alleged paradox of no detectable lung metastases despite widespread systemic deposits.

Once viable tumour cells reach the arterial circulation, further difficulties arise. In particular, there is the question of the seemingly selective involvement of organs by metastatic growth; some organs (brain or adrenal) are frequently involved by metastatic deposits while others (skeletal muscle or spleen) are not. The problem is well illustrated in experiments where tumour cells have been injected directly into the left heart (Sugarbaker, 1952[84]; Coman, 1953[85]). Tumour deposits do not develop in all organs; different tumours give different and distinctive patterns of organ involvement; and some tissues apparently escape. 'Resistant' organs such as muscle do, however, readily support the growth of tumour fragments directly implanted into them (De Long and Coman, 1960[86]). It is difficult to imagine that 'resistant' organs are not exposed to circulating tumour cells and one possible explanation is that the tumour cells may be unable to penetrate blood vessels in certain locations. Special features of the vasculature are certainly known to occur in skeletal muscle and spleen, two tissues that are very rarely the site of secondary tumours. The alternative possibility, that some vessels may be particularly vulnerable to penetration by circulating tumour cells, has received little attention; some recent experimental work which favours this view is discussed in the next section.

It is clear that mechanical and circulatory factors help to determine the distribution of intravascular tumour cell emboli and, in some situations, the subsequent development of metastatic deposits. But they do not provide a complete explanation of the distribution of secondary tumours and other extravascular factors also appear to be involved.

EXTRAVASCULAR TUMOUR CELLS: THE ESTABLISHMENT OF METASTATIC DEPOSITS

The dangers posed by circulating tumour cells are potential rather than actual. But once such cells penetrate into the extravascular spaces a critical phase in the metastatic process has been reached.

The escape of tumour cells from blood vessels has been recorded in the cinemicrographic studies of Wood (v.s.); events at the ultrastructural level have been investigated by Ludatscher *et al.* (1967[87]), Jones *et al.* (1971[73]), and Vlaeminck *et al.* (1962[25]). Tumour cells appear to traverse vascular endothelium in a similar fashion to leucocytes migrating into a zone of inflammation; the endothelial defects observed in cinemicrographic studies do not appear to have been seen in the electron microscope. The unresolved controversy of the need for a co-existing clot of fibrin and platelets has already been mentioned. Ludatscher *et al.*[87] described healthy-looking tumour cells covered by endothelium, suggesting that penetration may sometimes be delayed. Jones *et al.*[73] found that Walker cells took twenty-four to forty-eight hours to penetrate the pulmonary vessels, a considerably longer time than that reported by Wood for V2 cells in vessels in rabbit ear chambers. Many arrested tumour cells fail to escape through the vessel wall. The aggregate of cells is fragile and easily broken and the wall itself may be impenetrable (cf. Coman, 1953[85]). On the other hand, some blood vessels seem to be infiltrated by tumour cells with particular ease: the liver sinusoids, for example, have a characteristic fenestrated arrangement and there is experimental evidence that this may favour the formation of intrahepatic metastases (Cotmore and Carter, 1973[88]).

The interaction between tumour cells and host in the extravascular compartment is ill-understood, but various elements can be pieced together. Free tumour cells, initially unorganized and lacking a stroma, must be extremely vulnerable. Many cells will die—mostly for metabolic reasons but some may be destroyed by local inflammatory and/or immune responses. The little evidence available (Brennan, 1968[89]) suggests that tumour cells persist and thrive in skin windows despite a brisk acute inflammatory reaction; but there could be regional variations in the inflammatory response and it may be impaired as a result of immune deficiencies in the host (v.i.). Thirdly, free tumour cells may traverse tissues spaces and enter lymphatics (Fisher and Fisher, 1966[35]; Wood, 1971[68]; Hilgard *et al.*, 1972[36]) a possibility discussed earlier. The process whereby extravascular tumour cells acquire their stroma must be different from that associated with the primary tumour in at least one respect. Primary tumours arise at a site of progressive and presumably long-standing disorganization; secondary tumours are derived from cells which are essentially implanted into hitherto normal tissues in which development of a fibrovascular stroma is less readily initiated. Special considerations operate in sites such as bone where stromal reactions may be osteolytic or osteoblastic varying, to some extent, with the type of tumour. Osteoblastic lesions are usually associated with metastases from carcinoma of the prostate; the more common osteolytic changes occur with several forms of metastatic tumour (breast, kidney, thyroid) but both osteolytic and osteoblastic changes may co-exist in the same patient, even in the same bone (Willis, 1967[1], 1973[2])—an interesting demonstration of the functional diversity of tumour cells (see also Franks, 1958[17], 1960[18]).

Once a focus of tumour cells acquires an adequate stroma, it is likely to grow progressively though it should be emphasised that little is known about the cell kinetics of early metastases (Lamerton, 1972[90]). There are, however several examples of anomalous growth in clinically apparent metastases. Metastatic tumours may stop growing, temporarily, or permanently; they may regress 'spontaneously' (the best documented examples are renal carcinoma, malignant melanoma, neuroblastoma and choriocarcinoma); and they may undergo a process of maturation, seen in neuroblastoma and also in teratomas and some embryonal sarcomas (Willis, 1967[1], 1973[2]; Everson and Cole, 1966[91]; Smithers, 1964[92], 1969[93]). A different variant of growth is exemplified by the phenomenon of *dormancy* where metastases from certain tumours—notably breast, kidney and uveal tract—manifest themselves twenty years or more after apparently successful treatment of the primary lesion (Gordon-Taylor, 1954[94]). Dormancy has been reproduced with some success in the experiments of Fisher and Fisher (1959[95], 1965[96]). Small numbers of Walker tumour cells (50–250) injected intraportally gave rise to few or no deposits for periods of up to twenty weeks, but numerous intrahepatic tumours developed after laparotomy and handling of the liver (sham hepatectomy), and also after treatment with a hepatotoxic agent such as chloroform. These results have been confirmed by Sugarbaker *et al.* (1971[97]), using larger doses of intraportal tumour cells in the same outbred system; but their attempts to repeat the observations in a syngeneic tumour-host model were unsuccessful. It is obvious that the basis of dormancy is still obscure. We do not know the proliferative or immunogenic capacity of dormant tumour cells, the nature of the host response to them, or the reason why dormant tumour cells can be activated by trauma.

EXTRAVASCULAR FACTORS AND THE DISTRIBUTION OF METASTASES

It was noted earlier that the localization of metastatic tumour cannot be explained solely on the basis of mechanical and circulatory factors. The local tissue environment—the 'soil' (Paget, 1889[98]; Willis, 1967[1], 1973[2])—also appears to be involved though the actual mechanisms are obscure and the evidence is often circumstantial. A few illustrative examples of 'soil' factors follow:

Lucké *et al.* (1952[99]) injected equal numbers of V2 tumour cells into systemic veins and the portal vein of rabbits; consistently more deposits developed in the liver than in the lungs. Kinsey (1961[100]) found that subcutaneous grafts of the S91 melanoma metastasized exclusively to the lungs. The selectivity persisted even when lung tissue was transplanted into the muscles of the thigh; grafts of several other tissues were not involved by metastatic tumour. Studies on the growth of Walker cells injected intraportally in rats (Fisher and Fisher, 1965[96], 1967[101]) indicate that procedures as diverse as trauma, reticuloendothelial blockade, administration of dextran and high fat diets all enhance the growth of tumour deposits *without* any increased trapping of ^{51}Cr-labelled cells. The hepatic changes brought about by these various manoeuvres are unclear but transaminase levels were often increased. Carter *et al.* (1971[102]) showed that lysosomal abnormalities in the liver and other host tissues were associated with enhanced metastatic growth of a transplanted lymphoma (ML) in hamsters. The lysosomal changes, which were induced with the non-ionic detergent Triton WR 1339, did not occur in the tumour but Triton may affect tumour cells in other ways, e.g. by altering membrane properties (Franchi *et al.*, 1971[103]). Finally, Pilgrim (1969[104]) has offered an ingenious interpretation of 'soil' function using a transplated lymphoma in C3H mice that metastasized exclusively to the spleen. A comparison of growth of tumour injected directly into a preferred site (spleen) and a non-preferred site (kidney) suggests a differential rate of cell loss with greater migration from the non-preferred site.

Regional variations in the inflammatory and immune responses may also impinge on the initial location and development of metastases. Thus, the metastatic process is sometimes altered in situations of sustained immunosuppression: not only is there more metastatic tumour but its *distribution* is also changed (see next section).

The contribution made by the tumour cells themselves ('the seeds') has to be considered. The putative role of the tumour cell membrane was stressed earlier and it is possible that membrane properties may be involved in extravascular localization. Surface charge, for instance, may contribute to the migratory properties of tumour cells in the extravascular spaces and possibly to the formation of cell-cell contacts, either with other tumour cells or with the inflammatory and immune cells of the host. Convincing experimental evidence is, however, difficult to obtain (see Weiss and Cudney, 1971[105]).

The localization of metastatic tumour is now seen to be the consequence of many interacting factors involving both tumour and host. Mechanical, circulatory and local tissue factors are all implicated and a fourth element—the immune response—has also to be considered.

IMMUNOLOGICAL FACTORS AND THE METASTATIC PROCESS

There is increasing evidence that some aspects of the metastatic process may be affected by the immune reactivity of the host. Complete analysis would require a knowledge of the immunogenicity (cf. Kim, 1971[106])—or tolerogenicity—of the tumour, together with full characterization of the host's cellular and humoral immune responses. This is impossible at present and the evidence available comes from a variety of sources.

It was noted some years ago that patients with carcinoma of the breast treated with cortisone were prone to develop metastases at unusual sites—the spleen and also heart, duodenum, pancreas, gall bladder and thyroid (Iversen and Hjort, 1958[107]; Sherlock and Hartmann, 1962[108]). More recently, enhanced metastasis has been observed in patients with Ewing's sarcoma, treated by combined radiation and cytostatic drugs (Marsa and Johnson, 1971[109]). Two remarkable cases have been reported where metastases developed from tumour cells inadvertently transplanted in homografts of kidney and liver; they resolved after withdrawal of immunosuppressive treatment[110]. In experimental animals, cortisone (and also cytostatic drugs and irradiation) has long been known to increase the incidence of metastases (Agosin *et al.*, 1952[111]; Kondo and Tsukui, 1959[112]) but the changes produced by such treatment are complex and difficult to interpret. Somewhat easier to appraise are the reports that treatment with anti-thymocyte or anti-lymphocyte sera (ATS, ALS) enhances metastasis from autochthonous and transplanted tumours (Fisher *et al.*, 1969[117]; Deodhar and Crile, 1969[114]; Gershon and Carter, 1970[115]): ATS is believed to act principally on thymus-processed lymphocytes (T cells) and it is logical to suggest that these cells are implicated in some way in the control of metastasizing tumour. T cells may act directly as cytotoxic lymphocytes; they may co-operate with bone-marrow-derived (B) lymphocytes in the synthesis of antibody; and they may function indirectly, stimulating macrophages and other inflammatory cells by releasing soluble materials such as lymphokines (cf. Mackler, 1971[116]). Weston *et al.* (1972)[117] have shown that subcutaneous grafts of the EL4 lymphoma, normally a non-metastasizing tumour, evoked proliferation of T cells in the regional lymph nodes; the full implications of such proliferation are not entirely clear but it is striking that the EL4 lymphoma, grafted into T-cell *deficient* mice, metastasized in about half the animals. Methods for distinguishing T and B cells in man are now available and Stjernswärd *et al.* (1972)[118] have reported that the lymphopenia following irradiation for mammary carcinoma mainly involves T cells. Follow-up of these patients should establish whether a deficiency of T cells can indeed be linked with the development of metastases (cf. Hagen *et al.*, 1972[119]).

The role of antibody in the host response to metastasizing tumour is difficult to assess. It is clear that humoral immune responses to tumours are complex and involve specific antitumour antibodies, blocking antibodies that enhance tumour growth, and antiblocking antibodies that counteract blocking antibodies (Hellström and Hellström, 1971[120]). These antibodies are discussed fully in Chapter 12, but their probable relevance to metastasis may be illustrated with the following examples. Patients with early or localized malignant melanoma develop specific antitumour antibodies: when the disease disseminates the antibodies disappear and a blocking antibody has been implicated which is believed to act against the original antitumour antibody as an anti-antibody (Lewis *et al.*, 1969[121], 1971[122]). More commonly, blocking antibodies act directly against tumour cells from which they can sometimes be eluted. Blocking antibodies have been demonstrated in sera from patients with many different malignant tumours and their correlation with progressively disseminating disease is close (Hellström *et al.*, 1971[123]). Conversely, patients whose malignant disease remits may develop unblocking antibodies; these have been found in sera from some cases of neuroblastoma and malignant melanoma. The full implications of blocking and unblocking antibodies in disseminating malignant disease have, however, still to be clarified and it should be noted that some of the Hellströms' findings have been challenged (Currie *et al.*, 1971[125]); in particular there is controversy as to whether the blocking activity of sera is indeed due to antibodies. The problem is discussed in detail in Chapter 12.

There is a little experimental support for the view that the immune reactions evoked by disseminating tumour, cellular or humoral, are expressed with varying effectiveness at different anatomical locations—immunological factors may thus contribute to the eventual localization of metastatic tumour. Mice immunized intramuscularly with methylcholanthrene-induced sarcomas show different degrees of resistance when challenged at different sites (Vaage *et al.*, 1971[125]; Wexler *et al.*, 1971[126]; see also Chapter 12). EL4 cells injected intravenously into normal mice and into specifically T-cell deficient mice (cf. Weston *et al.*, 1972[117]) give rise to different patterns of tumour deposits in the two sorts of recipients (Weston, 1974[127]). Mice deficient in T cells die early with massive visceral involvement; normal mice die later with few deposits (sometimes none), occurring almost exclusively in soft tissues rather than parenchymatous organs.

One anatomical site that merits particular attention is the group of lymph nodes draining a malignant tumour.

Immunological events in regional lymph nodes

Nodes near malignant tumours undergo various reactive changes before they are replaced by metastatic growth. The functional significance of such changes is uncertain and it is difficult to link them with any one property of the tumour such as its metastasizing potential. This has, however, been feasible with two lymphomas in hamsters, one of which metastasizes while the other does not. The metastasizing lymphoma (ML) evokes a medullary plasmacytosis in the regional lymph nodes with immunoglobulin production before they are replaced by secondary tumour. The non-metastasizing lymphoma (NML) stimulates a homograft-like response with proliferation of paracortical blast cells; there is also follicular enlargement and activation of sinus macrophages (Carter and Gershon, 1966[46]; 1967[47]; Gershon and Carter, 1967[128]; Carter *et al.*, 1968[129]). It is important to note that viable NML cells *are* present in these reactive regional lymph nodes but they do not form discrete deposits. With both tumours, morphological changes also occur in more distant nodes and in the spleen—i.e. the reactive changes are concentrated in the regional nodes but are not confined there. If the regional nodes are excised before grafting, ML and NML evoke the same changes in the new 'proximal' nodes and their metastatic potential is unaltered. On the other hand, NML will metastasize in animals with a systemic immune paresis brought about by treatment with ATS or whole-body irradiation (Gershon and Carter, 1970[115]). Other features of NML emphasize the close relationship between the immune response and suppression of metastasis. NML evokes a specific cell-mediated immune response but, despite the strength of this reaction, the immunizing tumour graft continues to grow—a paradoxical situation known as concomitant immunity (Gershon *et al.*, 1967[48]; 1968[130]; Gershon and Kondo, 1969[131], 1971[132]; Nomoto *et al.*, 1970[133]). Procedures that induce NML to metastasize do so by breaking concomitant immunity so that hitherto immune animals now accept challenging grafts of NML. This effect is seen in irradiated or ATS-treated hamsters and it also occurs, within certain limits of time, after the primary tumour graft has been excised—see p. 18.

The morphological and immunological changes associated with ML and NML suggest that the response associated with ML mainly involves B cells and that NML stimulates a mixed reaction in which T cells predominate. Unfortunately, it is difficult to apply these conclusions to the lymph node response observed in man. Reactive changes in uninvolved lymph nodes draining human tumours have long been familiar and the prognostic significance of features such as sinus histiocytosis or follicular and paracortical hyperplasia continue to be disputed; but the functional significance of such changes has received little attention and morphological findings need to be supplemented by additional investigations such as immunofluorescence Burtin *et al.*, 1969[134]) and *in vitro* investigations of cultured lymphocytes (Vánky *et al.*, 1973[135]). This information is urgently needed to settle the question of the role of uninvolved regional lymph nodes in cancer. If intact and reacting nodes impede the growth and/or metastasis of a local tumour, such nodes should presumably be retained. But if the regional nodes have no protective value—and indeed may represent favoured locations for metastatic growth—they should be removed. Do the regional nodes represent barriers (in a general sense) to tumour cells, or oases?

The problem is compounded by the fact that excision of the primary tumour alone may affect the development of metastases. In most experimental situations, ablation of a primary tumour or tumour graft is followed by a reduced incidence of metastasis—the source of metastatic tumour has been removed (Ketcham *et al.*, 1961[136]; 1966[137]). But there are also well-documented reports where excision of the tumour has been followed by *increased* metastasis (Lewis and Cole, 1958[138]; Schatten, 1958[139]; Greene and Harvey, 1960[140]; Gershon *et al.*, 1968[130]); a similar sequence may occur in clinical practice, notably with osteosarcomas. Non-specific factors such as trauma and shock can be excluded and the operation of immune factors is likely, particularly in view of the findings of Gershon *et al.* (1968[130]) with NML. These workers showed that removal of the normally non-metastasizing lymphoma (NML) between seven and nineteen days after grafting resulted in a loss of concomitant immunity and a swing in the immune response away from a predominantly cell-mediated process to one involving enhancing antibody. This observation illustrates the importance of maintaining a given balance between humoral and cellular components of the immune response, a balance that in turn seems to be related to the intensity of antigenic stimulation—there is perhaps an analogy here with the alterations in the immune response following rejection of a skin allograft. Equally interesting was the demonstration of metastatic deposits from NML only twelve days after removal of the primary tumour graft, too soon for such tumours to have developed from cells liberated at the time of surgery. It thus appears that immunological factors may also contribute to the activation of dormant tumour cells (see p. 83).

The findings in experiments where regional nodes were included or excluded in excisions of primary tumours are predictably confusing. Crile, in particular, has investigated the problem in both allogeneic and syngeneic systems in mice (Crile, 1965[141], 1968[142], 1969[143]; Crile and Deodhar, 1971[144]). He has found that, within certain time limits after implantation of tumour, ablation of the tumours and contiguous lymph nodes leads to an increased incidence of metastasis and increased susceptibility to rechallenge with the same tumour—i.e. there is an impairment of concomitant immunity. Removal of the regional lymph node alone also enhanced metastatic growth. Some of these findings have been challenged, e.g. by Hammond and Rolley (1970)[145], who could not confirm that excision of a tumour and the regional nodes increased metastatic growth. Controversy also surrounds the observation that if, instead of excising the primary tumour, the graft is lethally irradiated and left *in situ*, concomitant immunity is temporarily maintained and the incidence of metastasis is accordingly not increased (Crile and Deodhar, 1971[144]). Vaage *et al.* (1971)[125] were unable to demonstrate prolongation of the immune response while a lethally irradiated tumour remained in place.

It is not possible to resolve these difficulties until more information is available, but a few general comments may be made. There is sufficient evidence to propose that the growth and distribution of metastatic tumour is, in some systems, at least partly determined by the host's immune response. T cells are probably involved. The host response may for a time be concentrated in the regional nodes but it is eventually systematized. Immunological factors are likely to be most effective in preventing metastatic growth; once metastases are established the immune reactivity of the host will be increasingly irrelevant. While the general immunological aspects of the metastatic process need to be explored in more detail, it may also be prudent to examine tumour-lymph node interactions in more specific instances. The morphological and functional responses in axillary lymph nodes draining a carcinoma of the breast are not necessarily the same as those mounted by mesenteric nodes draining a colonic carcinoma. The point is strengthened by therapeutic esperience: while the value of removing uninvolved axillary lymph nodes in mammary carcinoma is still disputed, the case for irradiating pelvic and abdominal nodes draining a testicular seminoma is now widely accepted.

Addenda

ANTICOAGULANTS AND ENHANCED METASTASIS

Discussion continues over the mode of action of anticoagulants in the metastatic process. In a detailed study with[125] I-labelled KHT sarcoma cells in syngeneic C3H mice, Brown (1973)[146] was unable to demonstrate that Warfarin produced any cytotoxic or cytostatic effects on the tumour cells. The lowered incidence of metastases was shown to be due to increased clearance of tumour cells from the lungs of anticoagulated mice between 6 and 24 hours after injection, and Brown concluded that the effect was the consequence of interference with thrombus formation. The use of ^{51}Cr as an isotopic label is criticised (cf. Fisher and Fisher 1967).[57]

OSTEOLYTIC METASTASES

Some light on the mode of development of osteolytic metastases stems from the experiments of Powles *et al.* (1973).[147] These workers have shown that certain human breast cancers (and also the Walker carcinosarcoma tumour in rats) release an osteolytic agent, the effects of which can be demonstrated in mouse calvarial bones maintained *in vitro*. This activity is inhibited by aspirin and it is thought that the osteolytic agent may be a prostaglandin. It will be important to examine other human tumours which are associated with osteolytic secondary deposits in this system.

HOST IMMUNITY AND THE LOCALIZATION OF INTRAVASCULAR TUMOUR CELLS

Evidence that immune factors may influence the eventual localization of circulating tumour cells is provided in a paper by Weiss *et al.* (1974).[148] Using ^{125}IUDR-labelled cells from a fibrosarcoma and a lymphosarcoma, these workers compared their distribution in three groups of syngeneic mice: normal animals, tumour-bearing animals and animals immunized with the appropriate X-irradiated cells. They found that cells from the two tumours, though initially given by the same route, had a different anatomical location in normal animals one hour later, and that the pattern of distribution of each tumour was changed in sensitized and tumour-bearing mice. These observations provide complementary information to that obtained from the study by Weston *et al.* (1972),[11] though the mechanisms involved remain wide open for investigation.

GENERAL IMMUNOLOGICAL COMPETENCE AND THE INCIDENCE OF METASTASES

Carnaud *et al.* (1974)[149] examined the incidence of pulmonary metastases from the Lewis carcinoma in C57BL and C3H mice rendered immunoparetic by sublethal irradiation, or adult thymectomy plus irradiation, or neonatal thymectomy. Treated animals showed a greater incidence of lung deposits. These experiments are notable for two reasons: the 'primary' Lewis tumour was established in the subcutaneous tissues as a solid implant and not injected intravenously; secondly, the effects of immunological restitution (with injections of spleen cells or with thymic implants) were studied and shown to reduce the number of metastases.

LOCAL IRRADIATION AND METASTASES

In some experimental systems, irradiation of a transplanted tumour has enhanced its metastatic spread (van den Brenk and Sharpington, 1971;[150] Sheldon and Fowler, 1973)[151] and there is evidence that *prior* irradiation of sites such as the lungs, liver and kidneys (van den Brenk *et al.* 1973;[152] van den Brenk and Kelly, 1973;[153] Withers and Milas, 1973)[154] may render these tissues more susceptible to metastatic involvement when tumour cells are subsequently injected. The situation is, however, complex—growth of tumours in other sites such as the subcutaneous tissues is *impaired* by prior irradiation (Hewitt and Blake, 1968)[155]—and the underlying mechanisms are ill-understood. The enhanced growth of tumour cells in irradiated lungs is inhibited by treatment with anti-inflammatory corticosteroids and it has been suggested that inflammatory and granulation tissue reactions may be growth-promoting (van den Brenk *et al.*, 1974);[156] but other factors are almost certainly involved. The clinical implications of these various experiments are uncertain.

T LYMPHOCYTES AND METASTASIS

Although several lines of evidence continue to indicate that T cells are sometimes implicated in the host response to metastasising tumour, it is important to note that this effect is generally most marked in relation to allografted neoplasms (e.g. Weston *et al.* 1974).[127] One can anticipate a good deal of variation between tumour systems but Woodruff *et al.* (1973),[157] using three murine syngeneic tumours, found that severe depletion of thymus-derived lymphocytes did not undermine resistance; indeed, in some instances T cell depletion led to a significant increase in resistance.

'BLOCKING ANTIBODIES'

The notion of 'blocking antibodies' has changed radically. The subject is complex but, in brief, most investigators now regard blocking antibodies as antigen-antibody complexes (Sjögren *et al.* 1971;[158] Hellström and Hellström, 1972;[159] Baldwin *et al.* 1972).[160] There is growing evidence that tumours shed tumour-specific antigen into the circulation and it is probable that antigen and antigen-antibody complexes interfere with host defences such as cytotoxic lymphocytes, thus facilitating metastatic growth (Currie and Basham, 1972,[161] Currie 1973).[162] A recent account of the role of circulating antibodies in malignant melanoma is given by Lewis (1974).[163]

THE REGIONAL LYMPH NODE

Fisher *et al.* (1973)[164] have compared the *in vitro* responses of blood lymphocytes and regional lymph node cells to PHA in patients with cancers of the breast and colon. Broadly similar results were obtained in both groups. Responsiveness to PHA was demonstrable in cells from uninvolved nodes and was also present, albeit at reduced levels, in cells from local nodes partially replaced by metastatic tumour. A greater response was usually evoked in blood lymphocytes than in lymph node cells from the same patient. Comparisons between blood lymphocytes and regional lymph node cells in their *specific* reactivity against autochthonous tumours have been studied in modified mixed lymphocyte tests (Vánky *et al.* 1974).[135] Cells from nodes draining large long-standing sarcomas were found to be non-reactive against autochthonous tumour cells though they could still be stimulated with PHA; blood lymphocytes obtained from these same patients responded to the autochthonous tumour in most instances. Animal experiments are giving diverse results. The studies of Fisher *et al.* (1974)[165] in mice indicated that cells from regional nodes draining a syngeneic transplanted mammary tumour were active against the tumour in both *in vivo* and *in vitro* test systems until the animals were moribund. No comparable activity was demonstrated at any stage in cells from more distant lymphoid tissues. On the other hand, work with a syngeneic squamous carcinoma in rats (Flannery *et al.*; 1973)[166] showed that antitumour activity, measured by *in vitro* microcytotoxity, reached a peak in the draining nodes 2 weeks after the tumour was transplanted; activity then declined in the local node but cytotoxic cells were subsequently demonstrable in more distal lymphoid structures. The anergic phase in the regional node coincided with the appearance of overt metastases.

The effects of excision of the regional lymph nodes on experimental metastasis are no clearer, and studies both supporting and contesting Crile's original observations continue to appear. Practical details such as the size of the tumour and, above all, the time of its excision are critical. It is well established that in the initial phase following tumour transplantation, immune reactivity remains localized to the regional nodes as shown by successful adoptive transfer experiments with immune lymph node cells; later, adoptive transfer of immunity from the local node is increasingly ineffective (Mitchison, 1954).[167] Do Crile's 'early cases' have any clinical counterparts? Given the slow cell kinetics of most human tumours, it is difficult to imagine that any immune response, even though initiated in the regional nodes, has not systematized throughout the immune system by the time that a patient presents clinically.

References

1. Willis, R. A. *Pathology of Tumours*, *4th Edn.*, Butterworth, London (1967).
2. Willis, R. A. *The spread of Tumours in the Human Body*. Second Edition, Butterworths, London, 1973.
3. Boyd, W. *A Textbook of Pathology*, *8th Edn.*, Kimpton, London (1970).
4. Rodin, A. E., Larson, D. L. and Roberts, D. K. *Cancer*, **20,** 1772 (1967).
5. Leighton, J. *The Spread of Cancer*, Academic Press, New York and London, (1967).
6. Foulds, L. *Neoplastic Development*, Vol. I. Academic Press, London and New York (1969).
7. Bagshawe, K. *Choriocarcinoma*, E. Arnold, London (1969).
8. Croughs, R. J. M., Eastham, W. N., Hackeng, W. H. L., Schopman, W., Feltkamp-Vroom, T. M., Dolman, A. and Hennemann, G. *Clin. endocrinol.*, **1,** 157 (1972).
9. Laurence, D. J. R. and Neville, A. M. *Br. J. Cancer*, **26,** 335 (1972).
10. Davidsohn, I., Norris, H. J., Stejkal, R. and Lill, P. *Arch. Path.*, **95,** 132 (1973).
11. Koller, P. C. *Ann. N.Y. Acad. Sci.*, **63,** 793 (1956).
12. Rabotti, G. *Nature*, **183,** 1276 (1959).

13. Young, R. C. and DeVita, V. T. *Cell Tissue Kinet.*, **3,** 285 (1970).
14. Charbit, A., Malaise, E. P. and Tubiana, M. *Europ. J. Cancer*, **7,** 307 (1971).
15. Terz, J. J., Curutchet, H. R. and Lawrence, W. *Cancer*, **28,** 1100 (1971).
16. Lee, Y-T. N. and Spratt, J. S., Jr. *Cancer*, **29,** 344 (1972).
17. Franks, L. M. *Br. J. Urol.*, **30,** 383 (1958).
18. Franks, L. M. *Cancer*, **13,** 490 (1960).
19. Mellette, S. J. *Clin. Orthopaed.*, **73,** 73 (1970).
20. Griffiths, J. D. and Salsbury, A. J. Circulating Cancer Cells. Thomas, Springfield, Illinois (1965).
21. Giovanella, B. C., Yim, S. O., Morgan, A. L., Stenlin, J. S., and Williams, L. J. *J. nat. Cancer Inst.*, **50,** 1051 (1973).
22. Wexler, H. *J. nat. Cancer Inst.*, **36,** 641 (1966).
23. Boeryd, B., Ganelius, T., Lundin, P. and Mellgren, J. *Int. J. Cancer*, **1,** 497 (1966).
24. Easty, G. C., Easty, D. M. and Tchao, R. *Europ. J. Cancer*, **5,** 287 and 295 (1969).
25. Vlaeminck, M. N., Adenis, L., Mouton, Y. and Demaille, A. *Int. J. Cancer*, **10,** 619 (1972).
26. Tannock, I. F. *Cancer Res.*, **30,** 2470 (1970).
27. Folkman, J. New England J. Med., **285,** 1182 (1971).
28. Cater, D. B., Adair, H. M. and Grove, C. A. *Br. J. Cancer*, **20,** 504 (1966).
29. Cater, D. B. and Taylor, C. R. *Br. J. Cancer*, **20,** 517 (1966).
30. Underwood, J. C. E. and Carr, I. *J. Path.*, **108,** 157 (1972).
31. Le Serve, A. W. and Hellmann, K. *Br. med. J.*, **1,** 597 (1972).
32. Zeidman, I. *Cancer Res.*, **17,** 157 (1957).
33. Pressman, J. J., Simon, M. B., Hand, K. and Miller, J. *Surg. Gynec. Obstet.*, **115,** 207 (1962).
34. Pressman, J. J., Burtz, M. B. and Shafer. L. *Surg. Gynec. Obstet.*, **119,** 984 (1964).
35. Fisher, B. and Fisher, E. R. *Surg. Gynec. Obstet.*, **122,** 791 (1966).
36. Hilgard, P., Beyerle, L., Hohage, R. and Hiemeyer, V. and Kübler, M. *Europ. J. Cancer*, **8,** 347 (1972).
37. Igot, J. P. and le Gal, Y. *Ann. Anat. path.* (*Paris*), **13,** 449 (1968).
38. Plenk, H. P., Sorenson, F. M. and Eichwald, E. J. *Cancer Res.*, **14,** 580 (1954).
39. Zeidman, I. and Buss, J. M. *Cancer Res.*, **14,** 403 (1954).
40. Ludwig, J. and Titus, J. L. *Archs. Path.*, **84,** 304 (1967).
41. Fisher, B. and Fisher, E. R. *Science*, **152,** 1397 (1966).
42. Fisher, B. and Fisher, E. R. *Cancer*, **20,** 1907 and 1914 (1967).
43. Engzell, U., Rubio, C., Tjernberg, B. and Zajicek, J. *Europ. J. Cancer*, **4,** 305 (1968).
44. Stoker, T. A. M. *Br. J. Cancer*, **23,** 132 and 136 (1969).
45. Crile, G., Isbister, W. and Deodhar, H. *Cancer*, **28,** 657 (1971).
46. Carter, R. L. and Gershon, R. K. *Amer. J. Path.*, **49,** 637 (1966).
47. Carter, R. L. and Gershon, R. K. *Amer. J. Path.*, **50,** 203 (1967).
48. Gershon, R. K., Carter, R. L. and Kondo, K. *Nature*, Lond., **213,** 674 (1967).
49. Feldman, M. and Nachtigal, D. *U.I.C.C. Monograph*, **6,** 118 (1967).
50. Batson, O. *Ann. Int. Med.*, **16,** 38 (1942).
51. Tannock, I. F. and Steel, G. G. *J. nat. Cancer Inst.*, **42,** 771 (1969).
52. Romsdahl, M. D., Chu, E. W., Hume, R. and Smith, R. R. *Cancer*, **14,** 883 (1961).
53. Malmgren, R. A. Circulating Cancer Cells and their Significance—a

Reappraisal. In *The Proliferation and Spread of Neoplastic Cells.* Williams and Williams, Baltimore (1968).
54. Romsdahl, M. M., Potter, J. F., Malmgren, R. A., Chu, E. W., Brindley, C. O. and Smith, R. R. *Surg. Gynec. Obstet.*, **111**, 675 (1960).
55. Takahashi, M. *J. Path. Bact.*, **20,** 1 (1915).
56. Baserga, R., Kisieleski, W. E. and Halvorsen, K. *Cancer Res.*, **20,** 910 (1960).
57. Fisher, B. and Fisher, E. R. *Cancer Res.*, **27,** 412 (1967).
58. Hofer, K. G., Prensky, W. and Hughes, W. L. *J. nat. Cancer Inst.*, **43.** 763 (1969).
59. Fidler, I. J. *J. nat. Cancer Inst.*, **45,** 773 (1970).
60. Zeidman, I., McCutcheon, M. and Coman, D. R. *Cancer Res.*, **10,** 351 (1950).
61. Kim, U. *Cancer Res.*, **26,** 461 (1966).
62. Wexler, H., Ryan, J. J. and Ketcham, A. S. *Cancer*, **23,** 946 (1969).
63. Wexler, H., Kenady, D. E. and Ketcham, A. S. *Cancer*, **27,** 56 (1971).
64. Crile, G., Isbister, W. and Deodhar, S. V. *Cancer*, **28,** 655 (1971).
65. Zeidman, I. *Cancer Res.*, **21,** 38 (1961).
66. Wood, S. *Archs. Path.,* **66,** 550 (1958).
67. Wood, S. *Bull. Schweiz. Acad. med. Wiss.*, **20,** 92 (1964).
68. Wood, S. Mechanisms of Establishment of Tumour Metastases. In *Pathobiology Annual Vol.* 1. Ed. H. L. Joachim. Butterworth, London (1971).
69. Rudenstam, C-M. *Acta chir. scand.* Suppl., 391 (1968).
70. Gasic, G. J., Gasic, T. B. and Stewart, C. S. *Proc. Nat. Acad. Sci.*, **61,** 46 (1968).
71. Pick, C. R. and Cater, D. B. *Br. J. exp. Path.,* **52,** 14 (1971).
72. Fisher, B. and Fisher, E. R. *Cancer Res.*, **27,** 421 (1967).
73. Jones, D. S., Wallace, A. C. and Fraser, E. E. *J. nat. Cancer Inst.*, **46,** 493 (1971).
74. Holyoke, E. D., Frank, A. L. and Weiss, L. *Int. J. Cancer*, **9,** 258 (1972).
75. Hagmar, B. *Acta path. microbiol. scand.* (*A*), **78,** 131 (1970).
76. Hagmar, B. *Europ. J. Cancer,* **8,** 17 (1972).
77. Boeryd, B. and Hagmar, B. *Acta path. microbiol. scand.* (*A*), **80,** 303 (1972).
78. Hagmar, B. *Acta path. microbiol. scand.* (*A*), **80,** 357 (1972).
79. Gasic, G. and Gasic, T. *Proc. Nat. Acad. Sci.*, **48,** 1172 (1962).
80. Weiss, L. *The Cell Periphery, Metastasis and other Contact Phenomena.* Amsterdam, North Holland, 1967.
81. Franks, L. M. *J. Path. Bact.*, **72,** 603 (1956).
82. Coman, D. R. and deLong, R. P. *Cancer Res.*, **14,** 610 (1951).
83. Zeidman, I. and Buss, J. M. *Cancer Res.*, **12,** 731 (1952).
84. Sugarbaker, E. D. *Cancer*, **5,** 606 (1952).
85. Coman, D. R. *Cancer Res.*, **13,** 397 (1953).
86. deLong, R. P. and Coman, D. R. *Cancer Res.*, **10,** 513 (1950).
87. Ludatscher, R. M., Luse, S. A. and Suntzeff, V. *Cancer Res.,* **27,** 1939 (1967).
88. Cotmore, S. F. and Carter, R. L. *Int. J. Cancer*, **11,** 725 (1973).
89. Brennan, M. J. Host/cell tumour Cell Interactions Influencing establishment of Metastases: Clinical and Experimental Observations. In *The Proliferation and Spread of Neoplastic Cells.* Williams and Wilkins, Baltimore, 1968.
90. Lamerton, L. F. *Br. J. Radiol.* **45,** 161 (1972).
91. Everson, T. C. and Cole, W. H. *Spontaneous Regression of Cancer.* Saunders Philadelphia and London, 1966.
92. Smithers, D. W. *On the Nature of Neoplasia in Man.* E. & S. Livingstone, Edinburgh and London, 1964.
93. Smithers, D. W. *Lancet*, **ii,** 949 (1969).

94. Gordon-Taylor, G. *Br. Med. J.,* **1,** 455 (1959).
95. Fisher, B. and Fisher, E. R. *Ann. Surg.,* **150,** 731 (1959).
96. Fisher, E. R. and Fisher, B. *Acta cytol.*, **9,** 146 (1965).
97. Sugarbaker, E. D., Ketcham, A. S. and Cohen, A. M. *Cancer*, **28,** 545 (1971).
98. Paget, S. *Lancet*, **i,** 571 (1889).
99. Lucké, B., Breedis, C., Woo, Z. P., Berwick, L. and Nowell, P. *Cancer Res.*, **12,** 734 (1952).
100. Kinsey, D. L. *Cancer*, **13,** 674 (1960).
101. Fisher, B. and Fisher, E. R. *Proc. soc. exp. Biol. Med.*, **124,** 881 (1967).
102. Carter, R. L., Birbeck, M. S. C. and Stock, J. A. *Int. J. Cancer*, **7,** 34 (1971).
103. Franchi, G., Morasca, L., Reyers-Degli-Innocenti, I. and Garattini, S. *Europ. J. Cancer*, **7,** 523 (1971).
104. Pilgrim, H. I. *Cancer Res.*, **29,** 1200 (1969).
105. Weiss, L. and Cudney, T. L. *Int. J. Cancer*, **7,** 187 (1971).
106. Kim, U. *Science*, **157,** 72 (1970).
107. Iversen, H-G. and Hjort, G. H. *Acta path. microbiol., scand.*, **44,** 205 212 (1958).
108. Sherlock, P. and Hartmann, W. H. *J. Am. med. Assn.*, **181,** 103 (1962).
109. Marsa, G. W. and Johnson, R. E. *Cancer*, **27,** 1051 (1971).
110. *Editorial. Br. med. J.*, **3,** 713 (1972).
111. Agosin, M., Christen, R., Badinez, O., Gasic, G., Neghome, A., Pizarro, O. and Jarpar, A. *Proc. Soc. exp. Biol. Med.*, **80,** 128 (1952).
112. Kondo, T. and Tsukui, K. *Proc. Soc. exp. Biol. Med.*, **112,** 384 (1959).
113. Fisher, B., Soliman, O. and Fisher, E. R. *Proc. Soc. exp. Biol. Med.*, **131,** 16 (1969).
114. Deodhar, S. D. and Crile, G., Jr. *Cancer Res.*, **29,** 776 (1969).
115. Gershon, R. K. and Carter, R. L. *Nature*, **226,** 368 (1970).
116. Mackler, B. F. *Lancet*, **ii,** 297 (1971).
117. Weston, B. J., Cheers, C., Carter, R. L., Leuchars, E., Wallis, V. J. and Davies, A. J. S. *Int. J. Cancer*, **9,** 66 (1972).
118. Stjernswärd, J., Jondal, M., Vánky, F., Wigzell, H. and Sealy, R. *Lancet*, **i,** 1352 (1972).
119. Hagen, C., Frøland, A. and Weberg, E. *Lancet*, **i,** 1340 (1972).
120. Hellström, I. and Hellström, E. *Cancer*, **28,** 1269 (1971).
121. Lewis, M. G., Ikonopisov, R. L., Nairn, R. C., Phillips, T. N., Fairley, H. G., Bodenham, D. C. and Alexander, P. *Br. med. J.*, **3,** 547 (1969).
122. Lewis, M. G., Phillips, T. N., Cook, K. B. and Blake, J. *Nature*, **232,** 52 (1971).
123. Hellström, I., Sjögren, H. O., Warner, G. and Hellström, K. E. *Int. J. Cancer*, **7,** 226 (1971).
124. Currie, G. A., Lejeune, F. and Fairley, G. H. *Br. med. J.*, **2,** 305 (1971).
125. Vaage, J., Chen, K. and Merrick, S. *Cancer Res.*, **31,** 496 (1971) and *Cancer Res.,* **33,** 1957 (1973).
126. Wexler, H., Chretien, P. B. and Ketcham, A. S. *Cancer, Res.* **28,** 641 (1971).
127. Weston, B. J., Carter, R. L., Easty, G. C., Connell, D. I., and Davies, A. J. S. *Int. J. Cancer*, **14,** 176 (1974).
128. Gershon, R. K. and Carter, R. L. *Amer. J. Path.*, **50,** 137 (1967).
129. Carter, R. L., Gershon, R. K. and Kondo, K. *Transplantation*, **6,** 313 (1968).
130. Gershon, R. K., Carter, R. L. and Kondo, K. *Science*, **159,** 646 (1968).
131. Gershon, R. K. and Kondo, K. *J. nat. Cancer Inst.*, **43,** 545 (1969).
132. Gershon, R. K. and Kondo, K. *J. nat. Cancer Inst.*, **46,** 1169 (1971).

133. Nomoto, K., Gershon, R. K. and Waksman, B. *J. nat. Cancer Inst.*, **44,** 739 (1970).
134. Burtin, P., Loisillier, F., Buffe, D., Guillerm, M. and Gluckman, E. *Cancer*, **23,** 80 (1969).
135. Vánky, F., Stjernsward J., Nilsonne, U. and Sundblad, R. *J. nat Cancer Inst.*, **51,** 17 (1973).
136. Ketcham, A. S. Kinsey, D. L., Wexler, H. and Mantel, N. *Cancer*, **14,** 875 (1961).
137. Ketcham, A. S., Wexler, H. and Minton, J. P *J. Am. Med. Assn.*, **198,** 157 (1966).
138. Lewis, M. R. and Cole, W. H. *Archs. Surg.*, **77,** 621 (1958).
139. Schatten, W. E. *Cancer*, **11,** 455 (1958).
140. Greene, H. S. N. and Harvey, E. K. *Cancer Res.*, **20,** 1094 (1960).
141. Crile, G. Jr., *Surg. Gynec. Obstet.*, **120,** 975 (1965).
142. Crile, G. Jr. *Surg. Gynec. Obstet*, **126,** 1270 (1968).
143. Crile, G. Jr. *Cancer*, **24,** 1283 (1969).
144. Crile, G. Jr. and Deodhar, S. D. *Cancer*, **27,** 629 (1971).
145. Hammond, W. G. and Rolley, R. T. *Cancer*, **25,** 368 (1970).
146. Brown, J. M. *Cancer Res.*, **33,** 1217 (1973).
147. Powles, T. J., Clark, S. A., Easty, D. M., Easty, G. C. and Neville, A. M. *Br. J. Cancer*, **28,** 316 (1973).
148. Weiss, J., Glaves, D. and Waite, D. A. *Int. J. Cancer*, **13,** 850 (1974).
149. Carnaud, C., Hoch, B., and Trainin, N. *J. Nat. Cancer Inst.*, **52,** 395 (1974).
150. van den Brenk, H. A. S. and Sharpington, C. *Br. J. Cancer*, **25,** 812 (1971).
151. Sheldon, P. W. and Fowler, J. F. *Br. J. Cancer*, **28,** 508 (1973).
152. van den Brenk, H. A. S., Burch, W. M., Orton, C. and Sharpington, C. *Br. J. Cancer*, **27,** 291 (1973).
153. van den Brenk, H. A. S. and Kelly, H. *Br. J. Cancer*, **28,** 349 (1973).
154. Withers, H. R. and Milas, L. *Cancer Res.*, **33,** 1931 (1973).
155. Hewitt, H. B. and Blake, E. R. *Br. J. Cancer*, **22,** 808 (1968).
156. van den Brenk, H. A. S., Kelly, H. and Orton, C. *Br. J. Cancer*, **29,** 365 (1974).
158. Sjögren, H. O., Hellström, I., Bansal, S. C. and Hellström, K. E. *Proc. Nat. Acad. Sci.*, **68,** 1372 (1971).
159. Hellstrŏm, K. E. and Hellstrŏm, I. *Ann. Rev. Med.*, **23,** 19 (1972).
160. Baldwin, R. W., Price, M. R. and Robins, R. A. *Nature New Biol.*, 238, 185 (1972).
161. Currie, G. A. and Basham, C. *Br. J. Cancer*, **26,** 467 (1972).
162. Currie, G. A. *Br. J. Cancer*, **28,** 25 (1973).
163. Lewis, M. G. *J. Clin. Path.*, **27,** *Suppl.* (*Roy. Coll. Path.*), **7,** 83, (1974).
164. Fisher, B., Saffer, E. A. and Fisher, E. R. *Cancer*, **30,** 1202 (1972).
165. Fisher, B., Saffer, E. A. and Fisher, E. R. *Cancer*, **33,** 631 (1974).
166. Flannery, G. R., Chalmers, P. J., Rolland, J. M. and Nairn, R. C. *Br. J. Cancer*, **28,** 118 (1973).
167. Mitchison, N. A. *Proc. R. Soc. Lond. D.*, **142,** 72 (1954).

Chapter **6**

DEVIANT METABOLIC PATTERNS IN MALIGNANT DISEASE

K. R. HARRAP, Ph.D. F.R.I.C.

Senior Lecturer, Department of Applied Biochemistry, Institute of Cancer Research, London

---

The failure of malignant cells to respond to the homeostatic controls of the host, their ability to invade surrounding tissues, and their frequent propensity for metastasis has persuaded many observers that unique molecular explanations must underlie such abberrant biological behaviour. This belief has inspired many of the biochemical investigations in chemotherapy and carcinogenesis. Selective cancer chemotherapy depends, of course, on the existence of a unique metabolic lesion in the tumour cells, against which a chemical attack could be mounted. However, extensive biochemical studies have failed to reveal the existence of such qualitative metabolic defects and the agents in current use remain crude 'chemical sledgehammers', exerting their cytotoxic effects primarily on dividing cells, and deriving a marginal selectivity from kinetic differences in cell cycle time between tumour and normal cell populations.

The outcome of biochemical studies in experimental carcinogenesis has been more rewarding. A major stumbling block hitherto has been the need to discriminate between those metabolic events which are associated with tumour initiation, and those which accompany tumour progression and tissue de-differentiation. With the advent of a spectrum of experimental hepatomas it has been possible to discriminate between these effects and to lay down biochemical guidelines which assist in defining how the malignant phenotype differs from the normal and to suggest why this confers upon the malignant cell its ability to grow, apparently without restraint.

It is now understood that the requirements for meaningful interpretation of biochemical differences between tumour cells and 'normal' cells are most stringent. It is critical that tumour metabolism be related to that of its tissue of origin: much of the earlier work was concerned with comparisons between tissues possessing totally disparate functional activity, and it is difficult to correlate such observations. There are, however, further requirements: where alterations in genetic function are implicated it becomes necessary to relate

---

Footnote: The following abbreviations are used in this chapter. [See p. 38].

ADP, Adenosine diphosphate; ATP, Adenosine triphosphate; G6P, glucose-6-phosphate; F1P, fructose-1-phosphate; F16P, fructose 1, 6-diphosphate; nRNA, nuclear RNA; rRNA, ribosomal RNA; tRNA, transfer RNA; mRNA, messenger RNA.

enzyme changes recorded in neoplasia to those occurring when a normal tissue adapts to stress conditions (such as starvation, hormonal imbalance, regeneration). Moreover, enzymatic changes occurring during neoplasia must also be related to those occurring during development for a full definition of those alterations which may be related selectively to the neoplastic state.

It is impossible, within the space available, to record faithfully all the biochemical deviations which have been reported in tumour cells. A more profitable exercise might be to examine how the intensive study of one area of metabolism, in one well characterized tumour system, has gradually led to a molecular definition of the malignant phenotype which may now be used as a biochemical yardstick of comparison for further enquiries in other systems. Accordingly, the first part of this chapter will discuss the molecular basis for the deviant carbohydrate metabolism in experimentally induced hepatomas. The conclusions emerging from such studies, which are corroborated by work in other areas of metabolism, indicate that gene expression is modified during the development of malignant disease. The last part of the presentation will summarize the information, obtained from a wide range of cell types, which indicates that abnormal gene expression may involve changes in both the transcription and translation of genetic information.

Carbohydrate metabolism in tumour cells

The present era of tumour biochemistry may be considered to have evolved from the pioneering studies of Otto Warbug, who observed that many established transplantable tumours possess a highly elevated glycolysis in comparison with a range of normal tissues (Warburg[242]). Warburg's proposal that this elevated glycolysis represents the single unifying characteristic of tumour cells (Warburg[243]), required modification when other workers pointed out that many normal replicating tissues may also possess a high glycolytic activity. Moreover, Warburg's interpretation of his data, that elevated tumour glycolysis was attributable to an irreversible impairment of respiration, was subsequently disproved in a series of careful investigations (see Weinhouse[263] for review). But in spite of these reservations on Warburg's findings, the elevated glycolysis of tumour cells remains their most striking biochemical characteristic.

With the discovery of the 'minimum deviation hepatomas' by Harold Morris, an experimental model became available which permitted the *systematic* study of those factors which underlie elevated tumour cell glycolysis. These tumours were induced by controlling feeding of low doses of carcinogens to inbred rats (Morris *et al.*[126], Morris[126], Lea *et al.*[106], Lea *et al.*[107]). The slower growing hepatomas were well differentiated, with a morphology scarcely different from that of the tissue of origin; with increasing growth rate they became less well differentiated. The initial problem was to identify those metabolic changes which were essential to the carcinogenic process and those which were coincidental, (i.e. attributable to the extensive tissue dedifferentiation which occured in the time interval between tumour initiation and the ultimate appearance of a palpable tumour mass). For this purpose biochemical changes were related to growth rate as a parameter of malignancy, it being difficult technically to quantitate invasion and metastasis: it was assumed that the changes which were observed in the well differentiated slowly growing hepatomas, and persisted throughout the hepatoma spectrum, were associated with tumour initiation. By contrast, those changes which occurred only in the rapidly growing, extensively dedifferentiated tumours, and which were not detectable in the slow-growing tumours, were described as coincidental to tumourigenesis. The significance of elevated tumour glycolysis was an early question which could be investigated in this model system. It was soon apparent that slow growing, well-differentiated hepatomas, possessed a glycolytic capacity comparable to that of normal control liver; glycolysis was elevated only in the more rapidly growing members of the series. Hence while a high aerobic and anaerobic glycolysis was a dominant biochemical feature of the extensively dedifferentiated hepatomas, it seemed unlikely that it was associated with the initiating events in carcinogenesis, but that it developed in relation to tissue dedifferentiation. Subsequent studies have concentrated on attempting to define the molecular basis for the elevated glycolysis of hepatoma cells.

Regulation of carbohydrate metabolism in liver

The conversion of glucose into pyruvate (the glycolytic pathway) is opposed by the conversion of pyruvate into glucose (the gluconeogenic pathway) in normal liver tissues. The existence in the same cell of active catabolic and anabolic pathways responsible for glucose degradation and biosynthesis predicates the existence of control mechanisms which govern the relative balance between these opposing activities. The glycolytic and gluconeogenic pathways are shown in *Fig. 6.1.* Some enzymes, the so-called 'bifunctional enzymes', are common to both pathways. They include: phosphohexose isomerase (EC.5.3.1.9*), aldolase (EC.4.1.2.13), glyceraldehyde phosphate dehydrogenase (EC.1.2.1.13), phosphoglycerate kinase (EC.2.7.2.3), phosphoglyceromutase (EC.2.7.5.3), and phosphopyruvate hydratase (EC.4.2.1.11). These bifunctional enzymes have relatively high specific activities and an equilibrium point roughly mid-way in the reactions they catalyse.

The direction of glycolysis or gluconeogenesis is determined by enzymes which are essentially undirectional and are common only to the respective catabolic or anabolic pathway in which they operate. These so-called 'key enzymes' exert a pacemaker function by virtue of their low specific activities, and the fact that the equilibrium of the various reactions which they catalyse lies essentially in the direction of pyruvate (for the glycolytic pacemakers) or of glucose (for the gluconeogenic pacemakers). They include (for glycolysis) glucokinase (EC.2.7.1.2), phosphofructokinase (EC.2.7.1.11), pyruvate kinase (EC.2.7.1.40); (for gluconeogenesis) pyruvate carboxylase (EC.6.4.1.1), phosphoenolpyruvate carboxykinase (EC.4.1.1.32), fructose diphosphatase (EC.3.1.3.11), glucose-6-phosphatase (EC.3.1.3.9) (Krebs[97], Weber *et al.*[260],

*These and subsequent 'E.C. numbers' represent the terminology proposed by the International Commission on Enzyme Nomenclature. See Comprehensive Biochemistry Vol. 13. Enzyme nomenclature. eds. M. Florkin and E. H. Stotz. Second Edition. Elsevier, Amsterdam, 1965.

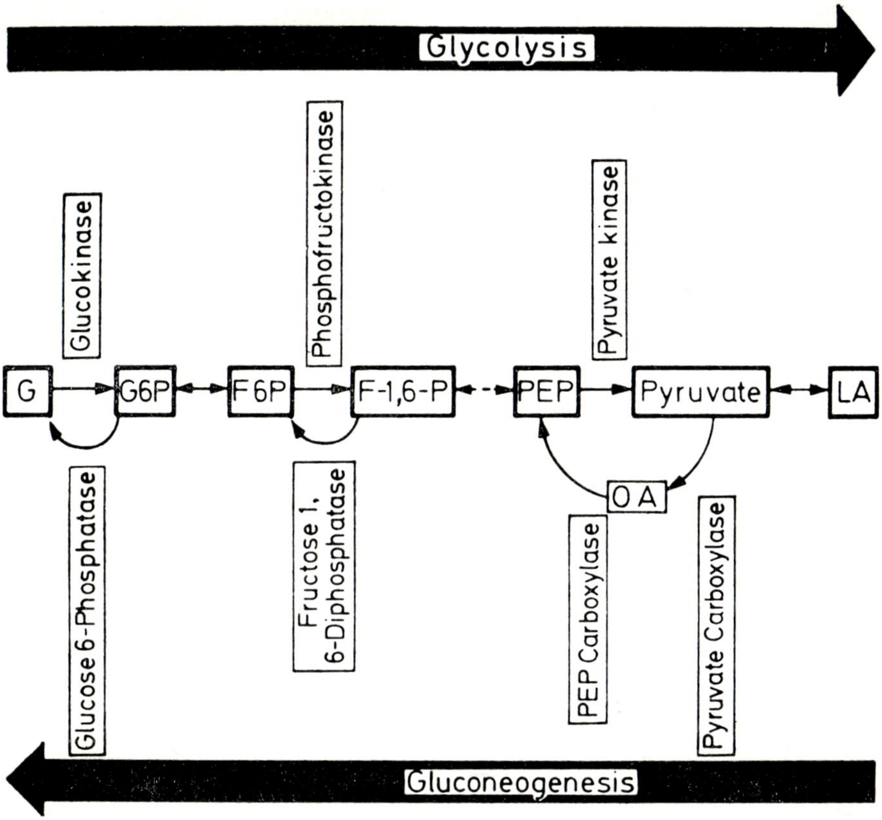

Fig. 6.1. The rate-controlling enzymes in the opposing pathways of glycolysis and gluconeogenesis (From Weber[247]).

Weber *et al.*[261], Weber [247]). These key pacemaker enzymes are the control points at which various rate controlling effectors operate.

The rate at which substrates are converted into products in an enzyme-catalysed reaction is determined by the concentration of enzyme present and its specific activity. The quantity of enzyme present in a tissue is determined by the relative rates of synthesis (which depends on the successful transcription and translation of genetic information) and degradation; its specific activity is determined by the relative concentrations of substrates, products, and rate controlling effectors. The rate of an intracellular enzyme-catalysed reaction is thus determined both by the genotype and by the intracellular molecular environment. The environmental controls which regulate the opposing pathways of glycolysis and gluconeogenesis are shown in *Fig. 6.2* (Weber[247]). In the glycolytic pathway, glucokinase and phosphofructokinase are activated by ATP, and the products of these reactions, G6P, G16P, ADP in turn activate pyruvate kinase. ADP is also inhibitory to fructose 6-phosphatase and fructose 1-6-diphosphatase, so that the gluconeogenic pathway is suppressed in presence of elevated levels of the nucleotide. ATP is an inhibitor of pyurvate

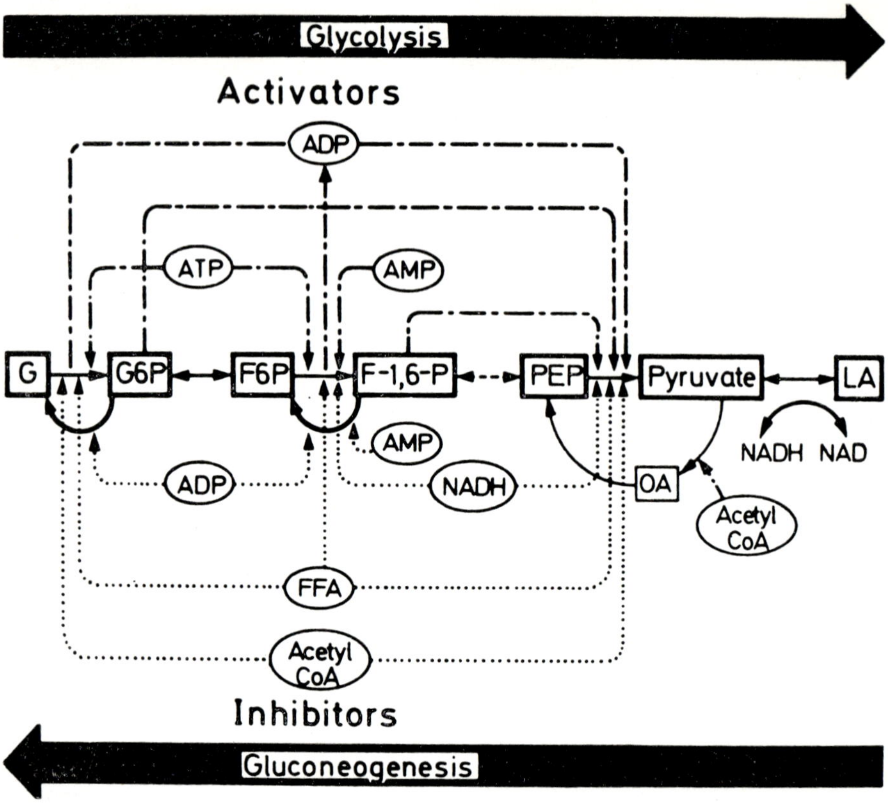

Fig. 6.2. Regulation of the opposing pathways of glycolysis and gluconeogenesis. ATP activates the phosphorylation of G and F6P, but inhibits pyruvate kinase. AMP activates phosphofructokinase but inhibits fructose 1, 6-diphosphatase. G6P and F16P activate pyruvate kinase. Hence glycolysis is 'triggered' by selective activation of the rate controlling enzymes of this pathway. Gluconeogenesis is favoured by selective inhibition of the glycolytic regulatory enzymes, all of which are inhibited by a rise in the free fatty acid level; acetyl CoA inhibits glucokinase and pyruvate kinase; NADH inhibits pyruvate kinase and phosphofructokinase. Acetyl CoA is also an activator of pyruvate carboxylase (From Weber[247]).

kinase, and hence this enzyme is suppressed in presence of elevated ATP levels, until triggered by rising G6P and F16P levels. The operation of the gluconeogenic pathway is achieved by selective inhibition of the glycolytic pathway by effectors associated with gluconeogenesis. Thus, free fatty acids inhibit all the key glycolytic enzymes, acetyl CoA inhibits glucokinase and pyruvate kinase, and selectively activates pyruvate carboxylase, while NADH inhibits pyruvate kinase and phosphofructokinase.

Glycolysis in the minimum deviation hepatomas

It is now possible to return to a more quantitative evaluation of the high glycolytic activity of tumour tissues referred to above, using as a test system the spectrum of minimum deviation hepatomas. It was shown unambiguously that elevated glycolysis was related directly to growth rate. In the slow-growing hepatomas, glycolysis was comparable to that of normal liver, becoming measurably increased only in the faster growing members of the series (Aisenberg and Morris[4], Burk *et al.*[31], Elwood *et al.*[53], Lin *et al.*[110], Sweeney *et al.*[200], Weber [246], Weber[247], Weber and Morris[255]). In attempting to establish the molecular basis for this behaviour, it became apparent that the activities of the key glycolytic enzymes, hexokinase, phosphofructokinase and pyruvate kinase *increased* in parallel with the heptoma growth rate

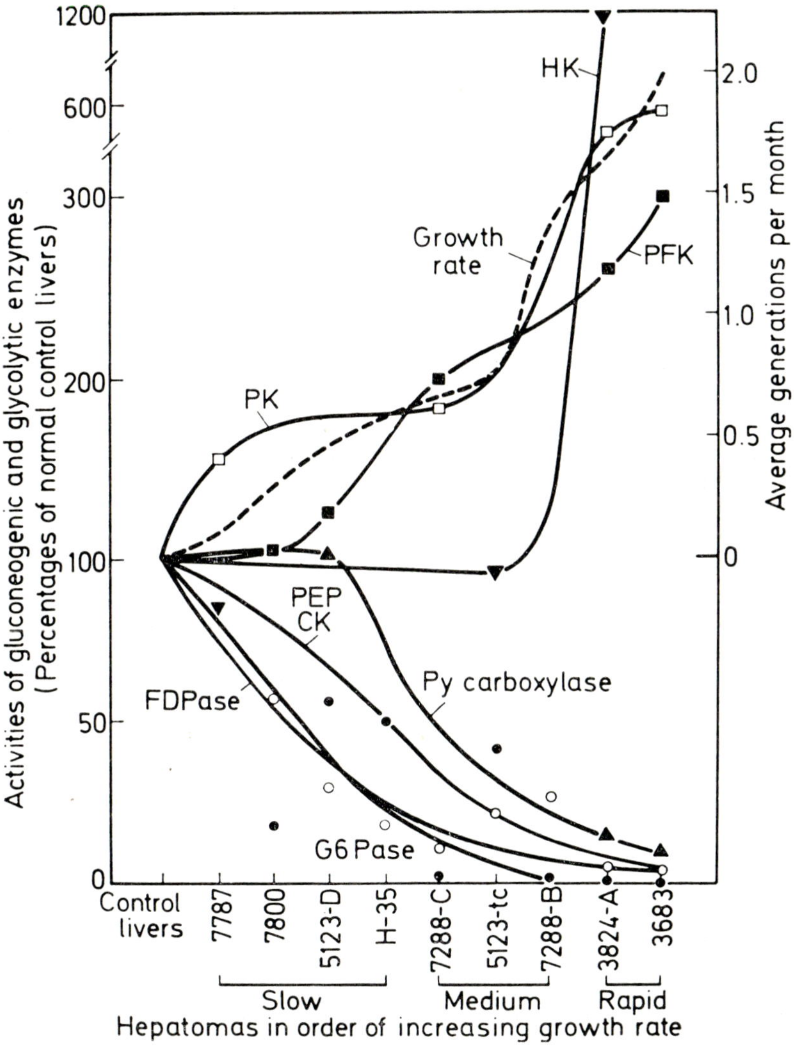

Fig. 6.3. Changes in the activities of the regulatory enzymes of glycolysis and gluconeogenesis in relation to hepatoma growth rate (From Weber[247]).

(Manjesh war *et al.*[115], Sharma *et al.*[187], Weber and Lea[254]). These changes were accompanied by *decreases* in the levels of the key gluconeogenic enzymes (Weber and Lea[254]), see *Fig. 6.3*. On the other hand, no correlation could be detected between the levels of the bifunctional enzymes and growth rate (Shonk *et al.*[187], Weber[244], Weber[245], Weber *et al.*[256], Weber and Cantero[251, 252], Weber and Lea[254], Weber and Morris[255]). Since the conditions adopted for assay of these separate enzymes were optimal, ensuring the absence of interference from extraneous intracellular effectors, these phenotypic changes are thought to reflect the altered functional activity of the genome in the tumours examined.

This pattern of coordinated changes in the levels of key glycolytic and gluconeogenic enzymes in the hepatoma spectrum has been contrasted by Weber with those changes which occur during normal hepatic differentiation: during the post-natal period the high levels of key gluconeogenic enzymes fall, accompanied by increases in the levels of key glycolytic enzymes until the adult steady-state balance is achieved (Weber *et al.*[258]).

Isoenzyme patterns in neoplasia

In addition to these alterations in the levels of rate controlling enzymes there also appears to be a changed isoenzymic distribution of carbohydrate metabolizing enzymes in hepatomas: isozymes in the adult liver which respond to nutritional or hormonal regulation are replaced by other modifications which are not subject to such controls and the overall effect is to shift the balance between glycolysis and gluconeogenesis markedly in favour of the former. This is no place for an exhaustive consideration of deviant isozyme patterns in tumours. The present discussion will be restricted to those changes which are relevant to abnormal glycolysis, gluconeogenesis and glycogen synthesis in a range of tumour types. For a more extensive account the reader is referred to several excellent reviews (Criss[44], Knox[95], Weinhouse[266], Weinhouse and Ono[267]).

Hexokinase isozymes

Four isozymes with hexokinase activity have been characterized in mammalian tissues (Grossbard and Schimke[73], Katzen and Schimke[86], Sharma *et al.*[180, 181]; Viñuela *et al.*[234]). These forms have been designated I, II, III, IV in order of increasing electrophoretic mobility. The first three forms occur predominantly in extrahepatic tissues: they have a relatively low Km for glucose (in the range 10^{-4} to 10^{-6}M) and are inhibited equally by G6P and ADP (Grossbard and Schimke[73]). The type IV enzyme has been classed as a glucokinase (Vinuela[234]). It is the predominant form in mammalian liver, has a high Km for glucose (10^{-2}M) and is inhibited by ADP but not by G6P. Further, this enzyme is closely controlled by the hormonal environment and by the dietary status of the animal: activity is low in the livers of fasted rats but increases five-fold on carbohydrate feeding. Glucokinase activity is also extremely low in the diabetic rat, being increased greatly after insulin treatment (Salas *et al.*[160, 161]). The hexokinases do not respond similarly to dietary or hormonal manipulation, though during liver regeneration the hexokinase levels rise markedly without any corresponding increase in glucokinase (Sharma *et al.*[181], Sillero *et al.*[189]). Hexokinase/glucokinase isozyme patterns have been measured in several malignant and premalignant tissues. During azo-dye induced hepatocarcinogenesis the glucokinase levels showed a tendancy to decrease while the hexokinases increased (Shatton *et al.*[184, 185]). On the other hand, in a number of human primary malignant hepatomas, hexokinase III was replaced by hexokinase II, without any apparent change in glucokinase level (Balinsky *et al.*[15]). In the minimum deviation hepatomas, glucokinase activity fell accompanied by elevation in hexokinase: the extent of these associated changes appeared to be related to the degree of de-differentiation of the neoplasm and to its growth rate: furthermore, it was impossible to restore to normal the low glucokinase levels by the administration of insulin or by the feeding of carbohydrate (Sato *et al.*[163], Shatton *et al.*[185]). Weinhouse has drawn attention to the similarities between this situation and that of foetal tissues where hexokinase activity is high and glucokinase absent (Ballard and Oliver[16], Walker[138], Weinhouse[266]). It is apparent that the glucokinase of the adult liver (which has a low affinity and high specificity for glucose, which is not inhibited by G6P, and whose level is strictly regulated by diet and hormones) is replaced in hepatomas by a hexokinase isozyme having a high affinity and low specificity for glucose. This modification is inhibited by G6P, and its level cannot be altered by changes in diet or hormonal status.

Phosphofructokinase

Four multimolecular forms of this enzyme have been separated by DEAE-cellulose chromatography (Tanaka *et al.*[208]). Type I predominates in muscle, heart and brain, and type IV in liver and kidney; other tissues contain mixtures of types II and III. No systematic studies of the distribution patterns of these isozymes have yet been carried out in hepatomas. For most other tumours tested, types II, III and IV are present, the latter predominating. The isozymes differ in the extent to which they are inhibited by ATP, and the degree to which this inhibition is reversed by adenine mono- and di-nucleotides. They are also activated to varying degrees by 3′,5′–cyclic AMP. It seems reasonable therefore to suspect that an alteration in the phosphofructokinase isozyme patterns of a tissue would have extensive effects on its glycolytic activity (Tanaka *et al.*[209]).

Pyruvate kinase isozymes

The existence of multimolecular forms of pyruvate kinase has been reported by a number of authors (Bailey *et al.*[11, 12], Bailey and Walker[13], Cottam *et al.*[41], Koler *et al.*[96], Pogson[142], Tanaka *et al.*[206, 207]). The pyruvate kinases from rat liver and muscle have been purified and characterized: the L form, but not the M form, is activated by F16P, while both forms are inhibited by ATP (Bailey *et al.*[11], Wood[270]). The liver form, but not the muscle enzyme, is responsive to dietary and hormonal stimuli: enzyme activity is enhanced when animals are fed a high carbohydrate diet; the level is low in the liver of diabetic rats and increases following insulin treatment (Krebs and Eggleston[28], Weber *et al.*[260, 262]).

It should be noted that the pyruvate kinase isozyme pattern may be more complicated than indicated here: several authors have detected up to four modifications of this enzyme in liver (Criss *et al.*[45], Tanaka *et al.*[207]). In the minimum deviation hepatomas the liver type enzyme predominates in the slow growing well differentiated tumours, but is almost totally replaced by the muscle type enzyme in the rapidly growing, extensively dedifferentiated neoplasms (Bailey *et al.*[12] Farina *et al.*[52], Lo *et al.*[112]). However, Criss observed the presence of a fifth pyruvate kinase isozyme in extensively dedifferentiated hepatomas which was absent from normal liver, muscle, and the slow growing tumours (Criss[43]). This moiety is thought to be identical to the enzyme which was distinguishable in its properties from both the normal liver and muscle types and which was isolated from an extensively de-differentiated tumour (Taylor *et al.*[210], Weber[248]).

In summary, the evidence for changes in pyruvate kinase isozyme distribution in fast-growing hepatomas would indicate that there is an absolute increase in activity of the muscle type enzyme, but in addition a new enzyme species appears. There is much circumstantial evidence to suggest that this new enzyme species has characteristics in common with the predominant type in foetal liver (Weinhouse[266]). Again this would appear to be an example of the expression in poorly differentiated tumours of foetal genes which are normally repressed in adult liver.

Aldolase isozymes

Three isoenzymic modifications of aldolase occur in mammalian tissues, forms A, B, C. C has been isolated from brain (Penhoet *et al.*[139]); B predominates in liver; A in skeletal muscle, spleen, heart; other tissues contain a mixture of A and B forms. The A and B forms are most pertinent to the present discussion: both isozymes catalyse the cleavage of F16P and F1P to the corresponding triose phosphates. However, the two isoenzymic modifications differ both in their substrate specificity and catalytic efficiency. The ratio of F16P to F1P cleavage activity is fifty for muscle aldolase and one for liver aldolase; further, muscle aldolase cleaves F16P at about ten times the rate of the liver enzyme (which cleaves both substrates with comparable efficiency (Blostein and Rutter[24], Rutter[154], Shonk *et al.*[187]). Michaelis constants have been reported for the muscle enzyme: F16P, $6{\cdot}1 \times 10^{-5}$M; F1P, $1{\cdot}2 \times 10^{-2}$M; and for the liver enzyme: F16P, $1{\cdot}2 - 2{\cdot}3 \times 10^{-6}$M; F1P, $8{\cdot}3 - 8{\cdot}7 \times 10^{-4}$M (Rutter *et al.*[155]).

The presence of muscle aldolase has been reported in a wide range of human and animal hepatomas (Balinsky *et al.*[15], Nordman and Schapira[130], Schapira *et al.*[168], Schapira [169], Schapira *et al.*[170]). In the highly differentiated minimum deviation hepatomas, the liver B enzyme is the sole form present: as the growth rate increases and the degree of tissue differentiation decreases, the B form is gradually replaced by the muscle (A) enzyme (Adelman *et al.*[3]). Again, Weinhouse has noted that this is reminiscent of the distribution in foetal liver where the A form predominates (Rutter and Weber[156], Weinhouse[266]). The shift in the aldolase isozyme pattern in hepatomas leads to the more efficient scission of F16P which is advantageous to actively glycolysing cells.

Fructose 1–6 diphosphatase

One modified form of fructose 1-6 diphosphatase has been isolated from liver and kidney (Bonsignore *et al.*[26], Pontremoli[143], Mendicino and Vasarhely[119]), and a second from skeletal muscle (Krebs and Woodford[99], Opie and Newsholme[133, 134], Sato and Tsuiki[165]). The notable difference between these two forms is that the muscle enzyme is far more sensitive than the liver enzyme to inhibition by AMP. The Ki for this inhibition in the case of the muscle enzyme is in the range 0·1 to 2·0μM, while for the liver form the Ki varies between 130 to 200μM. It is interesting that this inhibition could be obviated in the case of the liver type enzyme by pyridoxal-5′ phosphate (Krulwich[100, 101], Marcus and Hubert[116], Sato and Tsuiki[165, 166] Taketa and Pogell[205]). Slow growing hepatomas retain the liver isozyme, but this is replaced in faster growing tumours by the AMP-sensitive muscle form (Sato and Tsuiki[166], Takeda *et al.*[203], Weber and Morris[255]). While the liver isozyme responds to cortisone (Weber *et al.*[260], Weber and Lea[253]) and is present in the slower growing Morris hepatomas, the increase in level following cortisone administration is considerably reduced compared with that achieved in normal liver (Weber and Lea[253]). Hence the high Ki (AMP) cortisone-inducible modification of fructose 1-6 diphosphatase which predominates in normal liver has been replaced in rapidly growing tumours by the AMP-sensitive muscle form of the enzyme. This results in an overall decrease of fructose 1-6 diphosphatase activity and an associated loss of gluconeogenic capacity.

Glycogen Synthetase

Uridine diphosphate glucose, α-1, 4-glucan α-4-glucosyl transferase (EC 2.4.1.11) catalyses the reaction: UDP-glucose + glucan (n)-glucose units $\rightarrow$ glucan (n + 1) glucose units + UDP. Glycogen levels are generally low in tumours, but in a number of hepatomas this could not be accounted for in terms of the gross levels of glycogen synthetase present in these tissues (Tsuiki and Saheki[225], Saheki *et al.*[158], Saheki and Tsuiki[159], Takeda *et al.*[203], Takeda and Tsuiki[204]).

Accordingly attention has been given to identifying the form of glycogen synthetase present in these tissues. The enzyme exists in multimolecular forms. Two are present in muscle: D, which is dependent on G6P for activity, and I which is G6P independent (Villar-Palasi[233]). These two forms are interconvertible according to the following scheme.

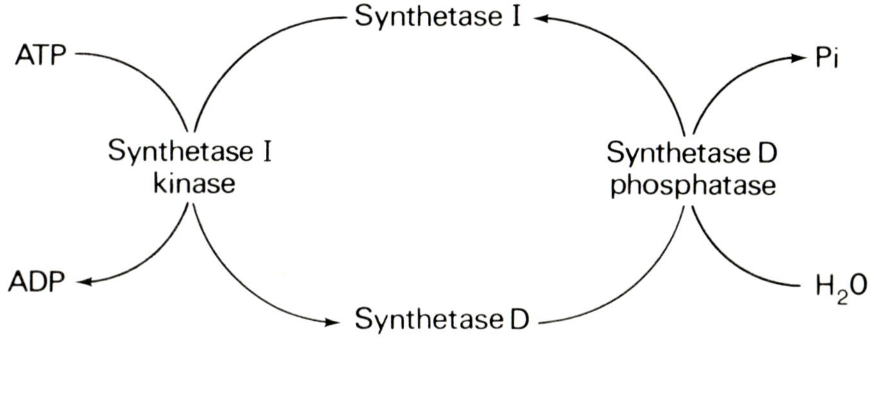

Only form I occurs in Liver. Perhaps the most striking difference between I and D forms of this enzyme is that in the presence of inorganic phosphate, sulphate, or maleate the activity of the D form is very low, even in presence of high levels of G6P, due to the high Km of the enzyme for UDP-glucose under these conditions (De Wulf and Hers[47], Tsuiki *et al.*[224], Gold and Segal[65]). The typical liver glycogen synthetase was replaced by the muscle type enzyme in two rapidly growing rat hepatomas (Tsuiki *et al.*[224]). In a study of glycogen synthetase isozymes in a range of Morris hepatomas, Sato *et al.* have shown that slow growing well differentiated tumours retained the liver type isozyme, while in the fast-growing extensively de-differentiated tumours this was replaced by the muscle isozyme (Sato *et al.*[164]). The latter authors have also shown that the liver form of glycogen phosphorylase [α-1, 4-glucan: ortho- phosphate glucosyl transferase (EC.2.4.1.1.)], an enzyme which is predominantly involved in glycogen degradation, is replaced by a foetal-type isozyme in rapidly growing tumours (Ryman and Whelan[157]).

It should be noted that the occurrence of multimolecular forms of enzymes is not restricted to those examples mentioned herein. For a more extensive summary of changes in isozyme patterns, in a range of neoplasias, the reader is referred to the recent review by Criss[44]. However, it is hoped that the present discussion has been sufficient to indicate that in the case of the Morris hepatomas, and in à number of other tumours, there is a general tendancy for enzymes which respond to homeostatic regulation to be deleted and to be replaced by modifications which are not influenced by dietary, hormonal or metabolite control. Many of these isozymes are found only in foetal tissues, for example hexokinase (Farina *et al.*[56], Knox *et al.*[94] Shatton *et al.*[185]), pyruvate kinase (Taylor *et al.*[210]), aldolase (Schapira *et al.*[170], Sugimura[198]), glutaminase (Linder-Horowitz *et al.*[111]), adenylate kinase (Criss *et al.*[45]), indicating the expression in the tumour of genetic information which is normally repressed in adult cells. The mechanism responsible for this misprogramming of genetic information has not been identified. Many authors have implied that this reversion to a foetal phenotype takes place by an ordered mechanism, and such terms as 'disdifferentiation' (Sugimura[199]) 'derepressive dedifferentiation' (Gold[66]) 'retrogenetic expression' (Gold[66], Gold and Friedman[67], Stonehill and Bendich[196]) 'retrodifferentiation' (Anderson and Coggin[6]) and 'blocked ontogeny' (Potter[146], Walker and Potter[240]) have been used in its description. However, Weinhouse concludes that, while there is circumstantial evidence in carcinogenesis that certain genes must be switched off before others are switched on, in general the alterations which occur are more suggestive of a disordered rather than an ordered mechanism of gene activation (Weinhouse[265, 266]). In the case of the Morris hepatomas, it seems unlikely that transcription of foetal genes is causal to the tumorigenic process, since foetal-type isozymes appear only in the faster-growing tumours, the adult isozyme pattern being retained in the slow-growing neoplasms. In this situation it would seem reasonable to ascribe the changes to the extensive tissue de-differentiation which has occurred (Weinhouse[266]). As evidence of the general degree of disagreement in this area, Weber contends that the metabolic situation of the hepatoma cell is distinguishable both from the normal adult hepatocyte and the foetal liver cell (Weber[250]).

There remains a cautionary note concerning the use of the Morris hepatomas in investigating the relevance of metabolic changes to the initiating events in carcinogenesis. This is implicit in the proposal that initiating events coincide with metabolic changes which are detectable in the morphologically well differentiated tumours and persist throughout the hepatoma spectrum, in parallel with increasing growth rate. It has already been pointed out above that an essential conclusion emerging from work with this model is that aberrant glycolysis in tumour cells is not determined by molecular events which are causal to the process of carcinogenesis. It could be claimed, therefore, that a great deal of information has been established concerning the molecular basis for a biochemical lesion (glycolysis) which is peripheral to oncogenesis. Nonetheless, the general pattern of changes in tumour glycolysis is reflected by changes in other metabolic pathways. The overall impression of a partial reversal to an embryonic phenotype is unavoidable and it remains to decide unambiguously whether these changes are causal to or peripheral to the carcinogenic process.

Alterations in isozyme distribution occur also in human tumour tissues and are not confined solely to experimental hepatomas (Balinsky *et al.*[15]). The identification of α-foetal protein (Abelev[2], Kahan and Levine[83], Stanislawski–Birenewajg *et al.*[195]) and of other foetal-type proteins in tumour tissues and secretions is occurring with increasing regularity and may provide an additional means of tumour diagnosis, or the possibility to monitor residual malignant disease following treatment (Laurence and Neville[105]). However, elucidation of the molecular mechanisms responsible for this reversion to foetal phenotype must await further study.

Enzyme changes in metabolic pathways other than glycolysis

Weber has proposed that the modification of key rate controlling enzymes is a general phenomenon in tumour cells and one might predict that changes such as those detected in the opposing pathways of glycolysis and gluconeogenesis would occur in other opposing metabolic pathways. As an example he has compared the balance between UMP synthesis and degradation in hepatomas and normal liver (Weber *et al.*[258]).

These pathways are illustrated below:

aspartate + carbamyl phosphate ⟶ ureido succinate ⟶ dihydro orotate ⟶ orotate ⟶ OMP ⟶ UMP

UMP ⟶ Uridine ⟶ Uracil ⟶ dihydro uracil ⟶ β-ureido propionate ⟶ β-Alanine + CO_2 + NH_3

The rate-limiting enzyme of the catabolic pathway is dihydrouracil dehydrogenase (4, 5 dihydrouracil: NADP oxidoreductase (EC.1.3.1.2) (Cannallekis[33]), the activity of which decreased progressively in parallel with increasing growth rate in a range of hepatomas: the activity in regenerating liver was comparable to that of normal adult liver (Queener *et al.*[148]). Thymidine is also a substrate for this enzyme, and is degraded by a range of hepatoma tissues at a rate which decreases in parallel with the growth rate of the tumour (Weber *et al.*[258]). On the other hand, the activities of the enzymes involved in the first two steps of *de novo* pyrimidine biosynthesis increased in parallel with the growth rate in a spectrum of hepatomas (Sweeney *et al.*[201, 202]). There would appear, therefore, to be a progressively enhanced activity of anabolic enzymes in association with a decreased activity of catabolic enzymes of pyrimidine metabolism, correlating with growth rate in a spectrum of experimental hepatomas. Other workers have shown that the activities of a number of enzymes essential for DNA biosynthesis increase in accordance with hepatoma growth rate, for example ribonucleotide reductase (EC 1.17.4.1) (Elford *et al.*[52]), DNA polymerase (EC.2.7.7.7.) (Ove *et al.*[136]),. thymidylate synthetase (EC.2.1.1.b) (Elford *et al.*[52], Ove *et al.*[135, 136]), thymidylate kinase (EC.2.7.4.9.) (Labow *et al.*[104], Sneider *et al.*[190]), thymidine kinase (EC.2.7.1.21) (Elford *et al.*[52]), deoxycytidylate deaminase (EC.3.5.4.12) (Sneider *et al.*[190]) aspartate transcarbamylase (EC.2.1.3.2.) (Bresnick[29], Sweeney *et al.*[202]), dihydroorotase (EC.3.5.2.3.) (Sweeney *et al.*[202]). Changes also occurred in the adenylate cyclase-(EC.4.6.1.1)-cyclic AMP phosphodiesterase (EC.3.1.4.17) enzyme system, in association with the development of malignancy. The response of the former enzyme to glucagon stimulation decreased progressively in a range of hepatomas in relation to increased growth rate (Allen *et al.*[5]). Further the activity of the high Km AMP phosphodiesterase decreased in association with an increase in activity of the low Km enzyme in experimental hepatomas (Clark *et al.*[40]).

Weber has pointed out that many of these changes are the converse of those that occur during liver differentiation, thus distinguishing the hepatoma from both adult liver and foetal liver (Weber *et al.*[258]): during differentiation the activities of the anabolic enzymes associated with DNA metabolism progressively decrease, accompanied by increases in the activities of catabolic enzymes.

Although this discussion has concentrated on the Morris hepatomas there is evidence from other systems that tumour related enzyme aberrations occur in proportion to the growth rate of the neoplasm (Knox *et al.*[92, 93], Lea *et al.*[107]).

Theories of carcinogenesis

A number of hypotheses have emerged, and continue to emerge, from the ever expanding body of data on tumour cell metabolism. While most of these theories have subsequently proved to be inadequate, they have provided a stimulus to further thought and experimentation in search of acceptable theories of carcinogenesis. The earlier proposal of Warburg[242], that an irreversible respiratory impairment represented an all-embracing characteristic of tumour cell metabolism, while not being substantiated by subsequent investigation, nevertheless provided the stimulus for the systematic studies described above. In a later proposal, (Greenstein[72]) observed that there was a certain uniformity in the enzyme patterns of tumour cells compared with the variant patterns observed in differentiated tissues. Greenstein postulated that as a precancerous tissue de-differentiated morphologically, so it de-differentiated biochemically, approaching a median pattern for a range of tumours examined. This theory was purely descriptive and took no account of the important changes in the regulation of enzyme systems which accompany carcinogenesis. Further, it was incompatible with the aberrant biological properties of tumour cells. Regulatory aspects were embraced in the 'deletion hypothesis' of Potter[144], which suggested that exposure of cells to carcinogens produced a series of somatic mutations leading to loss of control of those enzyme systems required for cell division.

These and other older theories were discussed in the first edition of this book. They are mentioned again for completeness and in order that the theories which presently receive support from various authorities are seen in some perspective.

The molecular correlation concept of carcinogenesis

Weber has studied anabolic and catabolic pathways in carbohydrate and DNA metabolism in the Morris hepatomas and has concluded that changes in certain key enzymes (summarized above) correlate with the degree of malignancy of the neoplasm. Moreover he claims that the progressive imbalance in enzyme profiles in the hepatoma spectrum is distinguishable from the enzyme pattern in differentiating and adult liver and is specific to malignancy. When the analysis is restricted to 'key' rate-limiting enzymes in antagonistic pathways, then an orderliness is perceived in these changes, while conversely there appears to be no relationship between the levels of bifunctional enzymes and malignancy. An important outcome of this philosophy is that it should be possible to predict for enzyme changes associated with malignancy (Weber[249, 250]).

The 'blocked ontogeny' hypothesis

In this theory, Potter[145, 146, 147, 240], proposes that the process of liver carcinogenesis is associated with the expression of an embryonic genotype. Two principal mechanisms are envisaged to explain how this could occur: either there pre-exists in adult liver a population of foetal cells which are able to divide and replace cells killed by the carcinogen; or hepatocytes may have the capacity to revert to a foetal phenotype under the influence of the carcinogen.

There is clearly a deep element of controversy between these two hypotheses, which centres around Weber's contention that the Molecular Correlation Concept encompasses a description of tumour cell metabolism which is distinct from that of foetal or adult tissues. Whichever of these theories is correct, there is unequivocal evidence that neoplasia is associated with a reprogramming of genetic information: the elucidation of this relationship is clearly dependent on an improved understanding of the regulation of normal cell differentiation. It is thought that at each stage of differentiation one set of genes is being actively transcribed while the remainder are switched off. This view has evolved from the knowledge that all cells of an organism contain identical genomes, that much of the genome is inactive, and that different ribonucleic acids are synthesized in different cell types (Britten and

Davidson[30]). The maintenance of the cell phenotype is additionally dependent on the translational events in protein biosynthesis, where mRNA on emerging from the nucleus associates with cytoplasmic ribosomes and provides a unit for the assembly of protein chains from amino acids carried on specific transfer RNA's.

There are several steps in this chain of events where regulatory processes may become modified. Structural changes could occur in the DNA; the DNA available for transcription could be altered; could regulation of transcription become modified; the mRNA could be excessively degraded in the nucleus and fail to reach the cytoplasm; and there could be modified control of translation or aberrent synthesis of tRNA's.

Results of hybridization studies have led to the proposal that controls operate on gene expression at three discrete levels: at the level of genome transcription; at the transfer of nuclear RNA moieties to the cytoplasm; at the level of translation of mRNA sequences into protein (Harris[75], Penman[141], Shearer and McCarthy[186]). The remainder of this presentation will be devoted to a brief consideration of the evidence of modification of these events in tumour cells. Further details will be found in Chapter 10.

Changes in transcription

There is much evidence that changes in transcription occur during development: the regulation of this component of the protein biosynthetic process in eukaryotic cells has been thoroughly reviewed recently (MacGillivray *et al.*[114]). The present discussion will be confined to those reports of modified transcriptional activity in tumour cells based on studies of DNA/RNA hybridization. This technique relies on measurements of the association of radioisotopically-labelled RNA's with dissociated single-stranded DNA, the latter generally immobilized in cellulose, agar, or on nitrocellulose filters (Bautz and Hall[22], Bolton and McCarthy[25], Gillespie and Spiegelman[64] Nygaard and Hall[131]). By allowing other RNA species to compete with labelled RNA for hybridization it is possible to assess the relative concentration of repetitive DNA transcripts in the RNA population. When interpreting data from such studies it is important to bear in mind that changes are detected only in the transcription of repetitive DNA sequences; no information is provided concerning unique sequences. The specificity and details of the techniques have received extensive consideration in recent reviews (MacGillivray *et al.*[114], Walker[239], Winocour[269]).

While it is accepted that all cells of the same animal have an identical DNA content, there is evidence from hybridization studies that the pattern of transcription varies from tissue to tissue of the same species (McCarthy and Hoyer[113]). Further, transcriptional changes occur during tissue differentiation (Church and McCarthy[38, 39], Denis[46], Turkington[224]) and during liver regeneration (Church and McCarthy[38, 39]). Comparable studies have been carried out in tumour cells in a search for impaired regulation of transcription, as evidenced by the appearance of aberrant RNA species. Much attention has been devoted to the functional activity of the viral genome in virus transformed cells, and the presence of viral mRNA has been demonstrated in a number of hybridization studies (Winocour[269]). A number of authors have detected an altered transcription in tumour cells as compared with the tissues of origin, or with other normal cells: primarily, differences have been detected in the species of rapidly labelled nuclear RNA transcribed from the repetitive sequences of DNA.

The nRNA hybridization patterns in a spectrum of tumours exhibit broadly three types of behaviour:

1. Deletion of certain species of nRNA in the tumour in comparison with the reference tissues. Thus in a rat ascites hepatoma (Ono *et al.*[132]) and in several Morris hepatomas (Drews *et al.*[48], Mendecki *et al.*[118]) the hepatoma cell nuclei were found to lack RNA species present in normal liver cell nuclei, while the latter contained all the RNA modifications present in the tumour. Drews *et al.* also noted that cytoplasmic RNA competed ineffectively with nuclear RNA in hybridization studies, suggesting that only a small proportion of nuclear RNA's are transported to the cytoplasm. They proposed that the mechanism governing the transport of nuclear RNA species is deranged in hepatomas.
2. A deletion in the tumour of nRNA present in the reference tissue, accompanied by the appearance in the tumour of a nRNA species not usually found in normal cells. Chiarugi[36] found that a Yoshida hepatoma differed from normal liver both in the absence of certain hepatic RNA messengers, and also in the presence of certain species usually absent from normal liver. This is comparable to the earlier observations of Kidson and Kirby on cytoplasmic RNA's made with a counter current technique (Kidson and Kirby[91]).
3. The appearance of new hybridizable sequences in the tumour cells. Church *et al.*[37] working with the transplantable Taper hepatoma, Turkington and Self[228] with transplantable mammary carcinomata, Neiman and Henry[129] with lymphocytes from patients with chronic lymphocytic leukaemia, all showed that species of nRNA were present in the tumour cells which were absent from the reference tissues. Further, Turkington and Self have shown that the overall progression of neoplastic disease from normal mammary gland cells to the development of spontaneous carcinomata is associated with discrete increments in the nRNA species present. Sawada *et al.*[167] have shown that RNA products synthesized from human acute lymphoblastic leukaemia chromatin contained additional RNA species which were not present in the transcripts from chronic lymphocytic leukaemia chromatin or from a line of cultured 'normal' lymphocytes. The question remains whether these altered transcriptional patterns were associated with the initiating events of carcinogenesis, or whether they emerged in relation to the extensive de-differentiation which occurs during tumour progression. In an attempt to answer this question Muramatsu and colleagues studied the transcriptional patterns in a line of hamster fibroblasts transformed in vitro with a chemical carcinogen (Muramatsu *et al.*[127]). They found that certain segments of repetitive DNA which had not been transcribed in the 'normal' cells were activated in the transformed cells. However, Levine *et al.*[109] had issued an earlier caution concerning the interpretation of such data from in vitro transformation studies. They used the hybridization-competition technique to compare transcription patterns

in primary hamster embyro cultures, in established hamster cell lines, and in SV 40 transformed hamster cell lines. They found that primary hamster embryo cells lack rapidly hybridizing RNA sequences that are transcribed in *both* transformed and untransformed established cell lines: it would appear that transcriptional changes occur during the process of obtaining an established cell line in vitro. Levine *et al.* therefore suggest that oncogenesis is not necessarily associated with the transcription of additional rapidly hybridizing RNA sequences.

This brief survey indicates that changes in transcriptional patterns are a characteristic feature of normal differentiating cells and of preneoplastic tissues. However, the exact relationship of these changes in neoplasia to the initiating events in carcinogenesis remains to be defined. The problem is complicated by the necessary technologies involved, where only RNA hybridizing rapidly to reiterated DNA sequences is measured. It is possible that the adoption of methods which are reported to discriminate between unique and reiterated DNA sequences (Gelderman *et al.*[63], Hahn and Laird[74]) and the separation of rapidly hybridizing RNA from the slowly hybridizing fraction (Pagoulatos and Darnell[137]) may assist in clarifying the picture. But there remains an unequivocal case for pursuing further studies devoted to elucidating the controls operating on genome transcription in order to interpret the relevance of the changes reported above to the development of neoplastic disease.

DNA-DEPENDENT RNA POLYMERASES AS DETERMINANTS OF GENE FUNCTION

The mammalian RNA polymerases form tight complexes with their chromatin templates, and definitive studies on the possible regulatory role of these enzymes in transcription have only become possible relatively recently with the availability of solubilization procedures which yield polymerases free of contaminating DNA (Jacob *et al.*[81]). Five forms, AI, AII, AIII, BI, BII have been described (Kedinger *et al.*[87]). Forms AI and AII are located in rat liver nucleoli and are insensitive to α-amanitin. The B forms are inhibited by this drug (Jacob *et al.*[81]) and with form AIII occur in the nucleoplasm. Only the B forms are able to transcribe rat liver chromatin, while form AI is probably involved in rRNA synthesis. (Butterworth *et al.*[32], Tocchini-Valentini and Crippa[220]). In one recent study the DNA-dependant RNA polymerases of regenerating rat liver have been compared with those extracted from a line of the Reuber H-35 hepatoma (Chesterton *et al.*[35]). Forms AI, AII, BI and BII were isolated from both sources: no new modification of the enzymes was found in the hepatoma. The relative activities of the AII, BI and BII enzymes in the hepatoma were approximately twice that of liver, while form AI was eightfold higher in the hepatoma. Only the latter observation was held to be of significance by the authors, by virtue of the errors inherent in the analytical method. It seems likely that the AI enzyme binds specifically to nucleolar ribosomal DNA (Tocchini-Valentini and Crippa[220]) and the elevated level in the hepatoma may therefore reflect an enhanced capacity for rRNA synthesis. The significance of these observations awaits further enquiry.

RNA-DIRECTED DNA POLYMERASE

The involvement of RNA-directed DNA polymerase in the modulation of transcriptional activity has been the focal point of studies related to the mode of action of the oncogenic RNA viruses in recent years. The essence of the problem has been to determine how the viral genetic information was incorporated into the host genome. The subject has been reviewed by several authors recently (Gallo[59], Green[71], Scolnik[178], Temin and Baltimore[218]). The initial guidelines were established by Temin[212] in 1963 when he proposed that viral RNA was used as a template for the synthesis of DNA, which could then be integrated into the host genome. This concept derived initially from experiments in which Actinomycin D (which specifically inhibits DNA-templated RNA synthesis) stopped the production of *all* RNA in cells infected with Rous sarcoma virus (Bader[10], Baluda and Nayak[20], Temin[213]). This was an unexpected result, since other RNA viruses can synthesize new RNA using as template the viral RNA genome: if the same mechanism persisted in the Rous sarcoma virus, it should not have been affected by Actinomycin D. The inference was that RNA synthesis in the Rous sarcoma virus was dependent on the prior assembly of a DNA template [called the provirus by Temin[215]]. Further evidence in support of this proposal was provided by the ability of antimetabolites to prevent the synthesis of provirus in stationary populations of chick embryo fibroblasts inoculated with Rous Sarcoma virus: infection was dependant on the synthesis of viral DNA directed by the viral RNA genome at a time when the fibroblasts were not affected by the antimetabolite, since they were not synthesizing DNA (Bader[10], Temin[217, 215, 217], Vigier and Golde[232]). The validity of the provirus hypothesis was enhanced by the demonstration that new DNA synthesized in cells transformed by Rous Sarcoma virus hybridized with 70S viral RNA (Baluda and Nayak[21], Temin[214]).

Although RNA polymerases had been reported in the virions of animal viruses—for example in vaccinia (Kates and McAuslan[85]) in reovirus (Shatkin and Sipe[183]) and in vesicular stomatitis virus (Baltimore *et al.*[19]), until 1970 no enzyme which synthesized DNA from an RNA template had been found in any type of cell. In 1970, two groups working independently reported the presence of an RNA dependent DNA polymerase in RNA tumour viruses: Baltimore[17] in Rous sarcoma virus and in Rauscher mouse leukaemia virus, and Temin and Mizutani[219] in Rouse sarcoma virus. The presence of a 'reverse transcriptase' as this enzyme was dubbed, in RNA tumour viruses was quickly confirmed, notably by Spiegelman *et al.*[193, 197] and by Green *et al.*[70].

While this enzyme will catalyse the synthesis of DNA from endogenous viral RNA (Temin *et al.*[219], Baltimore[17], Duesberg and Canaani[51]), it will also accept exogenous natural DNA (Mizutani *et al.*[122], Riman and Beaudreau[151], Spiegelman *et al.*[193]), synthetic DNA, DNA-RNA hybrids, or double stranded RNA (Mizutani *et al.*[122], Spiegelman *et al.*[193]) as template. Synthetic homopolymer RNAs were found to be poor templates for the enzyme (Mizutani *et al.*[122], Spiegelman *et al.*[193]) unless present with a complementary oligodeoxynucleotide primer (Baltimore and Sinoler[18]). Oligo (dT) or oligo (dC) enhanced the template activity of natural RNA's and it would appear that RNA-dependent and DNA-dependent synthesis occurs at the same site of the enzyme, since Poly (dAT) competed with viral RNA for purified DNA polymerase during DNA synthesis (Duesberg *et al.*[50]). When endogenous viral 70S RNA was used as template all the RNA was transcribed (Duesberg[49]).

The initial product of the polymerase reaction in presence of endogenous 70S viral RNA was a covalently bonded DNA-RNA molecule: the DNA was joined to the 70S RNA through the 3'-OH group of primer RNA (Verina *et al.*[231]). Before viral DNA could be incorporated into the host genome, the RNA-DNA complex had to be converted to double stranded DNA; the overall reaction sequence appears to be as follows:

$$\text{70S RNA} \longrightarrow \text{DNA-RNA} \longrightarrow \text{DNA-DNA}$$

While the exact details of this process remain unclear, it seems that Rous sarcoma virus contains a DNA'ase (endonuclease), an exonuclease, and a DNA ligase (Mizutani *et al.*[122, 123]), so that in theory, all the machinery is available for replication of the viral genome and its integration with that of the host. With the single exception of the Foamy virus, RNA-directed DNA polymerase activity is ubiquitously distributed in all known RNA tumour viruses (Baltimore[17], Gallo[59], Schlom *et al.*[171], Temin and Mizutani[219]).

RNA viruses related to those causing tumours in chickens and mice have been found in many other species; in the cat, for example, there is evidence that such particles may be oncogenic (Heubner and Todaro[80], Jarrett *et al.*[82], Richard *et al.*[149], Sneider and Theilen[191]). These observations have raised the possibility that viruses of a comparable nature may prove to be associated with neoplasias in man. So far, virus-type particle have been detected in association with acute leukaemia (Todaro *et al.*[221]), Burkitt lymphoma (Epstein *et al.*[54, 55]), breast carcinoma (Feller and Chopra[57], Moore *et al.*[124], Seaman *et al.*[179]) and in human milk (Moore *et al.*[124]). The detection of reverse transcriptase activity in some of these particles and in tumour cells suggested that the particles might be of a type similar to the oncogenic RNA sarcoma viruses, and reinforced speculation for a possible viral aetiology of some human neoplastic diseases (Schlom *et al.*[172, 173], Moore *et al.*[124], Gallo *et al.*[60, 61], Kufe *et al.*[103], Viola[235]). The causative effect of a virus in inducing cancers in animals is demonstrated by innoculating the virus into healthy recipients and monitoring the appearance of tumours. Clearly this approach is not permissable in cases of human disease and less direct methods have been adopted to investigate the possible aetiologic relationship between the human particles and the tumours with which they were found to be associated. Hybridization techniques were used to determine whether human tumours contained RNA molecules homologous to the supposedly human viral particles or to analogous animal viruses. Radioisotopically labelled DNA was prepared from mouse mammary tumour virus and used in hybridization experiments against a range of RNA species isolated from normal and neoplastic tissues. By such means it was possible to show that human leukaemias, sarcomas, and lymphomas contained RNA homologous to that of the mouse leukaemia virus (Hehlman[77, 78], Kufe *et al.*[102]). However it became apparent that the presence of reverse transcriptase activity in tumour cells could not be taken as a reliable indicator of oncogenic RNA-virus intrusion: activity was found in non-oncogenic animal RNA viruses (Scolnik *et al.*[174]) and in normal uninfected cells (Kang and Temin[84], Penner *et al.*[140], Scolnik *et al.*[176]). Subsequently, it proved possible to differentiate between viral and cellular RNA-dependent DNA polymerases isolated from virus infected cells by chromatographic and immunological techniques (Goodman and Spiegelman[69], Robert *et al.*[152], Ross *et al.*[153], Scolnik *et al.*[175]): two cellular DNA polymerases could be separated and distinguished from the viral reverse transcriptase. Antibody to purified viral enzymes was prepared and was found to inhibit selectively the activity of viral reverse transcriptase without affecting either of the two cellular polymerases. Further, viral 70S RNA was found to be an effective template only for the viral transcriptases, and did not interact with the cellular polymerases (Aaronson *et al.*[1], Parks *et al.*[138], Ross *et al.*[153]).

Leucocytes from patients with acute leukaemia contained reverse transcriptase associated with 70S RNA which was homologous with viral RNA (Baxt *et al.*[23], Sarngadharan *et al.*[162]). Further, Todaro and Gallo[222] have shown that a reverse transcriptase isolated from human acute myeloid leukaemia cells is closely related both biochemically and immunologically to a primate type C virus reverse transcriptase. In this work it was not possible to determine whether the leukaemic reverse transcriptase was coded for by viral genes, or whether the presence of enzyme was attributable to endogenous information, or whether it arose from exogenous infection by an external virus. In relation to tumour aetiology it becomes important, now that cellular and viral reverse transcriptase are distinguishable, to determine to what extent type C virus specific marker information occurs in human cells, whether this occurs specifically in tumour cells, and whether this information is expressed in differentiating or regenerating tissues.

Translational control of gene expression

There is mounting evidence that post-transcriptional controls are important in the regulation of protein biosynthesis in higher organisms, particularly in relation to the involvement of tRNA's. Wainwright and Wainwright[237] found that haemoglobin biosynthesis could be initiated in excised chick blastodiscs by providing a mixture of tRNA's extracted from the organism at a stage when haemoglobin was being actively synthesized. Anderson and Gilbert[8], working with a cell free rabbit reticulocyte system in *vitro*, showed that the relative proportions of α- and β-chain haemoglobins synthesized were related to the tRNA species present. Other workers have shown that structural modifications in tRNA molecules can affect their role in translation (Capra and Peterkofsky[34], Fitter and Hall[58], Gefter and Russell[62]). The most common structural modification found in the base components of tRNA's is the presence of a methyl group, which is inserted into the preformed macomolecule in a reaction catalysed by a range of tRNA-specific methylases. Up to ten methyl groups have been detected in mammalian tRNA's. Methylated t-RNA's have been shown to play a role in recognition by the amino acid transferring enzymes, in codon recognition, and in transfer of the carried amino acid to the ribosome (Capra and Peterkofsky[34], Gefter and Russell[62],

Shugart *et al.*[188]). It is recognized, however, that these remain incomplete descriptions of the functions of tRNA's. tRNA's and tRNA methylases have been the subject of several recent reviews, and the reader is referred to these for a more comprehensive account (Borek and Kerr[27, 28], Kerr and Borek[90], Sueoka and Kano-Sueoka[197]).

Chromatography elution profiles of tRNA's from tumour cells and normal cells have been reported by a number of workers. It would appear that the phenylalanyl-tRNA, tyrosyl-tRNA and aspartyl-tRNA are the most frequently altered moities in tumour cells. Baliga *et al.*[14] compared the elution profiles of eighteen aminoacyl-tRNA's from the Novikoff hepatoma with those of normal liver. The results indicated the emergence of new species of tRNA's specific for tyrosine, histidine and asparagine in the hepatoma and a shift in the elution profiles of six other amino-acid-specific tRNA's. Volkers and Taylor[236] detected the presence of new species of phenylalanyl tRNA and seryl tRNA in a Morris hepatoma, while the same tumour contained only one of the three modifications of histidyl-tRNA present in normal liver. Holland *et al.*[79] and Taylor *et al.*[211] demonstrated the presence of a new modification of tyrosyl tRNA in several cultured tumour cell lines. Aberrant tyr-tRNA elution patterns were also obtained by Hayashi *et al.*[76] for the Novikoff hepatoma and for three SV-40 induced hamster tumours.

The present restricted knowledge of the control mechanisms operating on translation makes it impossible to assess the relevance of these changes in tRNA patterns to the initiating events or to the progress of carcinogenesis. They imply however that translational controls may well be modified in tumour cells and indicate the urgency of continued studies designed to elucidate the significance of changes in tRNA profiles.

THE tRNA METHYLASES

The importance of tRNA methylation to translation has been indicated above. There is good evidence that the tRNA methylases are subject to regulatory control: the activity of these enzymes is modified in fully differentiated tissues by a naturally occurring protein inhibitor which is absent from differentiating and neoplastic tissues (Kerr[88, 89]). On the other hand tRNA methylases are activated in vitro by polyamines (Leboy[108]) and the correlation between polyamine levels and enhanced cell division has led to the proposal that changes in polyamine levels may be important in regulating tRNA methylation in differentiation and in response to hormones (Mays and Borek[117], Munns and Katzman[128], Riddick and Gallo[150], Sharma *et al.*[182], Turkington[226]). Polyamines have also been implicated in the regulation of tRNA methylation in tumour cells (Leboy[108]).

tRNA methyltransferase activities have been shown to be elevated in a wide range of tumours of both human and animal origin (Borek and Kerr[27]): there is both an overall increase in tRNA methyltransferase activity and the appearance of enzymes with new or altered specificities (Mittelman *et al.*[121]). It is possible that the tRNA methyltransferase patterns found in tumour cells represent a partial expression of foetal genotype, since tRNA species, which occur normally only in embryonic tissues and are absent from adult tissues, have been detected in tumours (Holland *et al.*[79], Yang [271]).

rRNA METHYLASES

In contrast to the extensive studies on the tRNA methylases, much less attention has been devoted to the methylation of rRNA. It seems that methylation of precursor rRNA is essential for rRNA maturation (methylation of 45S rRNA precedes its cleavage to the 28S and 18S forms): failure to methylate 45S RNA results in an inhibition of ribosome synthesis (Ascione and van de Woude[9], van de Woude *et al.*[229], Vaughan *et al.*[230]).

rRNA methylases do not appear to be elevated during chemically-induced hepatocarcinogenesis (Craddock[42]): an increased methylation of rRNA was detected in this study, but this was attributed to a gross increase in RNA synthesis. Torelli *et al.*[223] have shown in blast cells from acute leukaemia patients that under-methylation of 45S and 32S RNA's occurs: a substantial proportion of the former fails to undergo cleavage at the normal rate and remains unprocessed.

Conclusions

The results of extensive biochemical studies in the minimum deviation hepatomas have provided a molecular rationale for the aberrant glycolysis of these tissues. A pattern emerges of the systematic deletion of key rate-limiting enzymes in the opposing pathways of glycolysis and gluconeogenesis and their replacement by modifications which are less subject to regulatory control. Notably there is an increased tendancy for the synthesis of foetal type proteins in the highly malignant tumours. Similar patterns are apparent in other metabolic pathways and in other systems. It seems that these changes may be attributable to a general reprogramming of genetic information in malignant and premalignant tissues, though the data are as yet insufficient to decide to what extent this represents an emergence of foetal phenotype.

There is now an urgent requirement to elucidate the mechanisms responsible for this altered programming of genetic information. Many investigations have revealed that transcriptional and translational events are modified in a wide range of animal and human neoplasms. However, progress in interpreting the relevance of these data to oncogenesis is impeded by the inadequacy of present knowledge concerning the regulation of gene expression in normal developing and adult tissues. In this situation it may prove a wise investment to concentrate on this aspect of the problem in the immediate future.

References

1. Aaronson, S. A., Parks, W. P., Scolnik, E. M. and Todaro, G. J. *Proc. Nat. Acad. sci.* (*U.S.*), **68**, 920 (1971).
2. Abelev, G. I. *Adv. Cancer Res.*, **14**, 295 (1971).

3. Adelman, R. C., Morris, H. P. and Weinhouse, S. *Cancer Res.*, **27**, 2408 (1967).
4. Aisenberg, A. C. and Morris, H. P. *Nature*, Lond., **191,** 1314 (1961).
5. Allen, D. O., Munshower, J., Morris, H. P. and Weber, G. *Cancer Res.*, **31,** 557 (1971).
6. Anderson, N. G. and Coggin, J. H. *Proc. of 1st Conf. and Workshop on Embryonic and Fetal Antigens in Cancer*, Oak Ridge Nat. Lab., p. 7 (1971).
7. Anderson, N. G. and Coggin, J. H. Eds. *Proc. of 1st Conf. and Workshop on Embryonic and Fetal antigens in Cancer*, Oak Ridge Nat. Lab. (1971).
8. Anderson, W. F. and Gilbert, J. M. *Biochem. Biophys.*, Res. Comm. **36,** 456 (1969).
9. Ascione, R. and van de Woude, G. F. *J. Virol.*, **4,** 727 (1969).
10. Bader, J. P. *Virology*, **22,** 462 (1964).
11. Bailey, E. Stripe, F. and Taylor, C. B. *Biochem. J.*, **108,** 427 (1968).
12. Bailey, E., Taylor, C. B., and Bartley, W. *Nature*, Lond., **217,** 471 (1968).
13. Bailey, E. and Walker, P. R. *Biochem. J.*, **111,** 359 (1969).
14. Baliga, B. S. Borek, E., Weinstein, I. B. and Srinivasen, P. R. *Proc. Nat. Acad. Sci.*, U.S., **62,** 899 (1969).
15. Balinsky, D., Cayanis, E., Geddes, E. W. and Bersohn, I. *Cancer Res.*, **33,** 249 (1973).
16. Ballard, F. J. and Oliver, I. T. *Biochem J.*, **90,** 261 (1964).
17. Baltimore, D. *Nature*, Lond., **226,** 1209 (1970).
18. Baltimore, D. and Smoler, D. F. *Nucleic Acid-Protein Interactions. Nucleic Acid Synthesis in Viral Infection. Proc. Miami Winter Symposia*, Ed. Ribbons, D. W., Woessner, J. F. and Schultz, J. January 1971. North Holland.
19. Baltimore, D., Huang, A. S. and Stampfer, M. *Proc. Nat. Acad. Sci.*, U.S., **66,** 572 (1970).
20. Baluda, M. A. and Nayak, D. P. *J. Virol*, **4,** 554 (1969).
21. Baluda, M. A. and Nayak, D. P. in: *Biology of Large RNA Viruses*, Ed. Barry R. D. and Mahy, W. J. Acad. Press London (1970).
22. Bautz, E. K. F. and Hall, B. D. *Proc. Nat. Acad. Sci.*, U.S., **48,** 400 (1962).
23. Baxt, W., Hehlmann, R. and Spiegelman, S. *Nature New Biol.*, **240,** 72 (1972).
24. Blostein, R. and Rutter, W. J. *J. Biol. Chem.*, **238,** 3280 (1963).
25. Bolton, E. T. and McCarthy, B. J. *Proc. Nat. Acad. Sci*, U.S., **48,** 1390 (1962).
26. Bonsignore, A., Mangiarotti, M. A., Mangiarotti, A. De F. and Pontremoli, S. *J. Biol. Chem.*, **238,** 3151 (1963).
27. Borek, E. and Kerr, S. J. *Adv. Cancer Res.*, **15,** 163 (1972).
28. Borek, E. and Kerr, S. J. *Adv. Enz. Regln.*, **11,** 63 (1973).
29. Bresnick, E. *Cancer Res.*, **22,** 1246 (1962).
30. Britten, R. J. and Davidson, E. H. *Science*, **165,** 349 (1969).
31. Burk, D. Woods, M. and Hunter, J. *J. Nat. Cancer Inst.,* **38,** 839 (1967).
32. Butterworth, P. H. W , Cox, R. F. and Chesterton, C. J. *Eur. J. Biochem.*, **23,** 229, (1971).
33. Canellakis, E. S., *J. Biol. Chem.*, **221,** 315 (1956).
34. Capra, J. D. and Peterkofsky, A. *J. Mol. Biol.*, **33,** 591 (1968).
35. Chesterton, C. J., Humphrey, S. M. and Butterworth, P. H. W. *Biochem. J.*, **126,** 675 (1972).
36. Chiarugi, V. P. *Biochim. Biophys. Acta*, **179,** 129 (1969).
37. Church, R. B., Luther S. W. and McCarthy, B. J. *Biochim. Biophys. Acta*, **190,** 30 (1969).
38. Church, R. B. and McCarthy, B. J. *J. Mol. Biol.,* **23,** 477 (1967).
39. Church, R. B. and McCarthy, B. J. *Proc. Nat. Acad. Sci.*, **58,** 1548 (1967)

40. Clark, J. F., Morris, H. P. and Weber, G. *Cancer Res.,* **33,** 356 (1973).
41. Cottam, G. L. Hollenberg, P. F. and Coon, M. J. *J. Biol. Chem.*, **244,** 1481 (1969).
42. Craddock, V. M. *Biochim. Biophys Acta*, **195,** 351 (1969).
43. Criss, W. E. *Biochem. Biophys. Res. Comm.*, **35,** 901 (1969).
44. Criss, W. E. *Cancer Res.*, **31,** 1523 (1971).
45. Criss, W. E. Litwack, G. Morris, H. P. and Weinhouse, S. *Cancer Res.*, **30,** 370 (1970).
46. Denis, H. *J. Mol. Biol.*, **22,** 285 (1966)
47. De Wulf, H. and Hers, H. G. *Eur. J. Biochem*, **6,** 552 (1968).
48. Drews, J., Brawerman, G. and Morris, H. P. *Eur. J. Biochem.*, **3,** 284 (1968).
49. Duesberg, P. H. in: *The Biology of Oncogenic Viruses*, Amsterdam North Holland p. 154. Lepetit Colloquium on biology and medicine. Ed. Silvestri, L. G. (1971).
50. Duesberg, P., Helm, K. V. and Canaani, E. *Proc. Nat. Acad. Sci.*, **68,** 2505 (1971).
51. Duesberg, P. H. and Canaani, E. *Virology*, **42,** 789 (1970).
52. Elford, H. L., Freese, M. Passamani, E. and Morris, H. P. *J. Biol. Chem.*, **245,** 5228 (1970).
53. Elwood, J. C., Lin, Y. Cristofalo, V. J., Weinhouse, S. and Morris, H. P. *Cancer Res.*, **23,** 906 (1963).
54. Epstein, M. A., Achong, B. G. and Barr, Y. M. *Lancet*, **1,** 702 (1964).
55. Epstein, M. A. Henle, G., Achong, B. G. and Barr, Y. M. *J. Exp. Med.*, **121,** 761 (1965).
56. Farina, F. A., Adelman, R. C., Lo, C. H. Morris, H. P. and Weinhouse, S. *Cancer Res.*, **28,** 1897 (1968).
57. Feller, W. F. and Chopra, H. C. *Cancer*, **28,** 1425 (1971).
58. Fittler, F. and Hall, R. H. *Biochem. Biophys. Res. Comm.*, **25,** 441 (1966).
59. Gallo, R. *Blood*, **39,** 117 (1972).
60. Gallo, R., Sarin, P. S., Allen, P. T., Newton, W. A., Priori, E. S., Bowen, J. M. and Dmochowski, L. *Nature New Biol.*, **232,** 140 (1971).
61. Gallo, R. Yang, S. S. and Ting, R. C. *Nature*, **228,** 927 (1970).
62. Gefter, M. L., and Russell, R. *J. Mol. Biol.*, **39,** 145 (1969).
63. Gelderman, A. H., Rake, A. V. and Britten, R. J. *Proc. Nat. Acad. Sci.*, **68,** 172 (1972).
64. Gillespie, D. and Spiegelman, S. *J. Mol. Biol.*, **12,** 829 (1965).
65. Gold, A. H. and Segal, H. *Arch. Biochem. Biophys.*, **120,** 359 (1967).
66. Gold, P. *Prog. Exp. Tumour Res.*, **14,** 43 (1971).
67. Gold, P. and Freedman, S. *J. Exp. Med.,* **122,** 467 (1965).
68. Gonzalez, C., Babul, J., Rabajille, E. and Niemeyer, H. *Biochemistry*, **6,** 460 (1967).
69. Goodman, N. C., and Spiegelman, S. *Proc. Nat. Acad. Sci.*, **68,** 2203 (1971).
70. Green, M., Rokutanda, M., Fujinaga, K., Ray, R. K., Rokutanda, H. and Gurgo, C. *Proc. Nat. Acad. Sci.*, **67,** 385 (1970).
71. Green, M. *Ann. Rev. Biochem.*, **39,** 701 (1970).
72. Greenstein, J. P. *Cancer Res.*, **16,** 641 (1956).
73. Grossbard, L. and Schimke, R. J. *J. Biol. Chem.*, **241,** 3546 (1966).
74. Hahn, W. E. and Laird, C. D. *Science*, **173,** 158 (1971).
75. Harris, H. in *Progress in Nucleic Acid Res.*, **2,** 20, Ed. Davidson, J. N. and Cohn, W. E. Academic Press London and New York (1963).
76. Hayashi, M., Griffin, A. C., Duff, R. and Rapp, F. *Cancer Res.*, **33,** 902 (1973).

77. Hehlman, R., Kufe, D. and Spiegelman, S. *Proc. Nat. Acad. Sci*, U.S., **69,** 435 (1972).
78. Hehlman, R., Kufe, D. and Spiegelman, S. *Proc. Nat. Acad. Sci.*, U.S., **69,** 1727 (1972).
79. Holland, J. J., Taylor, M. W. and Buck, C. A. *Proc. Nat. Acad. Sci.*, U.S., **58,** 2437 (1967).
80. Huebner, R. J. and Todaro, G. *Proc. Nat. Acad. Sci.*, U.S., **64,** 1087 (1969).
81. Jacob, S. T., Sajdel, E. M. and Munro, H. N. *Adv. Enz., Regln.*, **9,** 169 (1971).
82. Jarrett, O., Laird, H. M., Hay, D. and Crighton, G. W. *Nature*, London, **219,** 521 (1968).
83. Kaham, B. and Levine, L. *Cancer Res.*, **31,** 930 (1971).
84. Kang, C. Y. and Temin, H. M. *Proc. Nat. Acad. Sci.*, **69,** 1550 (1972).
85. Kates, J. R. and McAuslan, B. R. *Proc. Nat. Acad. Sci.*, U.S., **58,** 134 (1967).
86. Katzen, H. M. and Schimke, R. T. *Proc. Nat. Acad. Sci.*, U.S., **54,** 1218 (1965).
87. Kedinger, C., Nuret, P. and Chambon, P. *FEBS Letter*, **15,** 169 (1971).
88. Kerr, S. J. *Biochemistry*, **9,** 690 (1970).
89. Kerr, S. J. *Proc. Nat. Acad. Sci.*, U.S., **68,** 406 (1971).
90. Kerr, S. J. and Borek, E. *Adv. in Enzymol.*, **36,** 1 (1972).
91. Kidson, C. and Kirby, K. S. *Cancer Res.*, **24,** 1604 (1964).
92. Knox, W. E., Horowitz, M. L. and Friedell, G. H. *Cancer Res.*, **29,** 669 (1969).
93. Knox, W. E., Linder, M. and Friedell, G. H. *Cancer Res.*, **30,** 283 (1970).
94. Knox, W. E., Jamdar, S. C. and Davis, P. A. *Cancer Res.*, **30,** 2240 (1970).
95. Knox, W. E. *Enzyme Patterns in Fetal, Adult and Neoplastic Rat Tissues*, S. Karger, Basel, München, Paris, London, New York, Sydney (1972).
96. Koler, R. D., Bigley, R. H., Jones, R. T., Rigas, D. A., Vanbellinghen, P. and Thompson, P. *Cold Spring Harbor Symp. Quant. Biol.*, **29,** 213 (1964).
97. Krebs, H. A. *Bull. Johns Hopkins Hospital*, **95,** 19 (1954).
98. Krebs, H. A. and Eggleston, L. V. *Biochem. J.*, **94,** 3c (1965).
99. Krebs, H. A. and Woodford, M. *Biochem J.*, **94,** 436 (1965).
100. Krulwich, T. A., Enser, M. B., Traniello, S. and Horecker, B. L. *Fed. Proc.*, **28,** 412 (1969).
101. Krulwich, T. A., Enser, M. and Horecker, B. L. *Arch. Biochem, Biophys.*, **132,** 331 (1969).
102. Kufe, D., Hehlman, R. and Spiegelman, S., *Science*, **175,** 182 (1972).
103. Kufe, D., Magrath, I. T., Zeigler, J. L. and Spiegelman, S. *Proc. Nat. Acad. Sci.* U.S., **70,** 737 (1973).
104. Labow, R., Maley, G. F. and Maley, F. *Cancer Res.*, **29,** 366 (1969).
105. Laurence, D. J. R. and Neville, A. M. *Br. Jnl. Cancer*, **26,** 335 (1972).
106. Lea M. A., Morris, H. P. and Weber, G. *Cancer Res.*, **26,** 465 (1966).
107. Lea, M. A., Morris, H. P. and Weber, *G. Cancer Res.*, **28,** 71 (1968).
108. Leboy, P. S. *Biochemistry*, **9,** 1577 (1970).
109. Levine, A. S., Oxman, M. N., Eliot, H. M. and Henry, P. H. *Cancer Res.*, **32,** 506 (1972).
110. Lin, Y. C., Elwood, J. C., Rosado, A. Morris, H. P. and Weinhouse, S. *Nature* (Lond), **195,** 193 (1962).
111. Linder-Horowitz, M., Knox, W. E. and Morris, H. P. *Cancer Res.*, **29,** 1195 (1969).
112. Lo, C., Cristofalo, V. J., Morris, H. P. and Weinhouse, S. *Cancer Res.*, **28,** 1 (1968).
113. McCarthy B. J. and Hoyer, B. H. *Proc. Nat. Acad. Sci.*, **52,** 915 (1964).

114. MacGillivray, A. J., Paul, J. and Threlfall, G. *Adv. Cancer Res.*, **15,** 93 (1972).
115. Mankeshwar, R., Sharma, C., Morris, H. P., Donnelly, A. J. and Weinhouse, S. *Adv. Enz. Regln.*, **3,** 317 (1965).
116. Marcus, F. and Hubert, E. *J. Biol. Chem.,* **243,** 4923 (1968).
117. Mays, L. L. and Borek, E. *Biochem.*, **10,** 4612 (1971).
118. Mendecki, J. Minc, B. and Chorazy, M. *Biochim. Biophys. Res. Comm.*, **36,** 494 (1969).
119. Mendicino, J. and Vasarhely, F. *J. Biol. Chem.*, **238,** 3528 (1963).
120. Milman, L. S. and Yurowitski, Yu G. *Biochim. Biphys. Acta.*, **146,** 301 (1967).
121. Mittelman, A., Hall, R. H., Yohn, D. S. and Grace, J. J. *Cancer. Res.*, **27,** 1409 (1967).
122. Mizutani, S., Boettiger, D. and Temin, H. M. *Nature*, Lond., **228,** 424 (1970).
123. Mizutani, S., Temin, H. M., Kodama, M. and Wells, R. T. *Nature, New Biol.*, **230,** 232 (1971).
124. Moore, D. H., Charney, J., Kramarsky, B., Las Fargues, E. Y., Sarkar, N. H., Brennan, M. J. Burrows, J., Sirsat, S. M. Paymaster, J. C. and Vaidya, A. B. *Nature*, Lond., **229,** 611 (1971).
125. Morris, H. P., Dyer, H. M., Wagner, B. P., Miyaji, H. S. and Rechcigl, M. *Adv. Enz. Regn.*, **2,** 321 (1964).
126. Morris, H. P. *Adv. Cancer Res.*, **9,** 227 (1965).
127. Muramatsu, M., Nemoto, N., Inui, N. and Takayama, S. *Cancer Res.*, **33,** 739 (1973).
128. Munns, T. W. and Katzman, P. *Biochemistry*, **10,** 4949 (1971).
129. Neiman, P. E. and Henry, P. H. *Biochemistry*, **8,** 275 (1969).
130. Nordmann, Y. and Schapira, F. *Europ J. Cancer*, **3,** 247 (1967).
131. Nygaard, A. P. and Hall, B. D. *J. Mol. Biol.*, **9,** 125 (1964).
132. Ono, T. Kawamura, M. and Wakabayashi, K. *Gann*, **62,** 31 (1971).
133. Opie, L. H. and Newsholme, E. A. *Biochem. J.,* **103,** 391 (1967).
134. Opie, L. H. and Newsholme, E. A. *Biochem. J.*, **104,** 353 (1967).
135. Ove, P., Jenkins, M. D., Laszlo, J. *Biochem. Biophys. Acta*, **174,** 629 (1969),
136. Ove, P., Laszlo, J., Jenkins, M. D. and Morris, H. P. *Cancer Res.*, **29,** 1557. (1969).
137. Pagoulatos, G. N. and Darnell, J. E. *J. Mol. Biol.*, **54,** 517 (1970).
138. Parks, W. P., Scolnik, E. M. and Ross, J. J. *Virol.*, **9,** 110 (1972).
139. Penhoet, E., Rajkumar, T. and Rutter, W. J. *Proc. Nat. Acad. Sci.*, **56,** 1275 (1966).
140. Penner, P. E., Cohen, L. H. and Loeb, L. A. *Nature New Biol.*, **232,** 58, (1971).
141. Penman, S. *J. Mol. Biol.*, **17,** 117 (1966).
142. Pogson, C. I. *Biochem. Biophys. Res. Comm.*, **30,** 297 (1968).
143. Pontremoli, S., Traniello, S. Luppis, B. and Wood, W. A. *J. Biol. Chem.*, **240,** 3459 (1965).
144. Potter, V. R. *15th Ann. Symp. Fund., Cancer Res.*, pp. 219–268. Ed: T. C. Hsu, Texas Univ. Press Austria (1962).
145. Potter, V. R. *Canadian Cancer Conf.*, **8,** 9 (1969).
146. Potter, V. R. *Miami Winter Symp.*, **2.** 291. Amsterdam North Holland Pub. Co. (1970).
147. Potter, V. R., Walker, P. R. and Goodman, J. I. *Gann Monograph*, No. 13, 121 (1972).
148. Queener, S. F., Morris, H. P. and Weber, G. *Cancer Res.*, **31,** 1004 (1971).

149. Rickard, C. G., Post, J. E., Noronha, F. and Barr, L. M. *J. Nat. Cancer Inst.*, **42,** 987 (1969).
150. Riddick, D. H. and Gallo, R. C., *Cancer Res.*, **30,** 2484 (1970).
151. Ríman, J. and Beaudreau, G. S. *Nature*, Lond., **228,** 427 (1970).
152. Robert, M. S., Smith, R. G., Gallo, R. C., Sarin, P. S. and Abrell, J. W. *Science*, **176,** 798 (1972).
153. Ross, J., Scolink, E. M., Todaro, G. J. and Aaronson, S. A. *Nature New Biol.*, **231,** 163 (1971).
154. Rutter, W. J. in 'The Enzymes' Ed. Boyer, P. D., Lardy, H. and Myrbäck, K. Acad. Press (1961). p. 341
155. Rutter, W. J., Woodfin, B. M. and Blostein, R. E. *Acta Chem.* Scand., **17,** S226 (1963).
156. Rutter, W. J. and Weber, G. *Developmental and Metabolic Control Mechanisms and Neoplasia*, Univ. of Texas M. D. Anderson Hospital and Tumour Institute at Houston Baltimore. The Williams and Wilkins Co. (1965), p. 195.
157. Ryman, B. E. and Whelan, W. J. *Adv. Enzymol.*, **34,** 285 (1971).
158. Saheki, R., Sato, K., and Tsuiki, S. *Biochim. Biophys., Acta* 230, 571 (1971).
159. Saheki, R. and Tsuiki, S. *Biochem. Biophys. Res. Comm.*, **31,** 32 (1968).
160. Salas, M., Viñuela, E. and Sols, A. *J. Biol. Chem.*, **238,** 3535 (1963).
161. Salas, J. Salas, M., Viñuela, E. and Sols, A. *J. Biol. Chem.*, **240,** 1014 (1965).
162. Sarngadharan, M. G., Sarin, P. S. and Gallo, R. C. *Nature New Biol.*, **240,** 67 (1972).
163. Sato, S., Matsushima, T. and Sugimura, T. *Cancer Res.*, **29,** 1437 (1969).
164. Sato, S., Morris, H. P. and Weinhouse, S. *Cancer Res.*, **33,** 724 (1973).
165. Sato, K. and Tsuiki, S. *Biochim. Biophys. Acta*, **159,** 130 (1968).
166. Sato, K. and Tsuiki, S. *Arch. Biochem. Biophys.*, **129,** 173 (1969).
167. Sawada, H., Gilmore, V. H., and Saunders, G. F. *Cancer Res.*, **33,** 428 (1973).
168. Schapira, F., Dreyfus, J. and Schapira, G. *Nature*, Lond., **200,** 995 (1963).
169. Schapira, F. *Pathol. Biol.*, **18,** 309 (1970).
170. Schapira, F., Reuber, M. D. and Hatzfeld, A. *Biochem. Biophys. Res. Comm.*, **40,** 321 (1970).
171. Schlom, J., Harter, D. H., Burny, A. and Spiegelman, S. *Proc. Nat. Acad. Sci*, U.S., **68,** 182 (1971).
172. Schlom, J. Spiegelman, S. and Moore, D. H. *J. Nat. Cancer Inst.*, **48,** 1197 (1972).
173. Schlom, J., Spiegelman, S. and Moore, D. *Nature*, Lond., **231,** 97 (1971).
174. Scolnik, E., Rands, E., Aaronson, S. A. and Todaro, G. J. *Proc. Nat. Acad. Sci.*, **67,** 1789 (1970).
175. Scolnik, E. M., Parks, W. P., Todaro, G. J. and Aaronson, S. A. *Nature New Biol.*, **235,** 35 (1972).
176. Scolnik, E. M., Aaronson, S. A., Todaro, G. J. and Parks, W. P. *Nature* Lond., **229,** 318 (1971).
177. Scolnik, E. M., Parks, W. P., Todaro, G. J. and Aaronson, S. A. *Nature New Biol.*, **235,** 35 (1972).
178. Scolnik, E. M. In: *Current Topics in Biochemistry*, p. 47. Ed. Anfinson, C. B. Goldberger, R. F. and Scechter, A. N. Academic Press, New York (1972).
179. Seaman, G., Gallagher, H. S., Lukeman, J. M. and Dmochowski, L. *Cancer*, **28,** 1431 (1971).
180. Sharma, C., Manjeshwar, R., and Weinhouse, S. *J. Biol. Chem.*, **238,** 3840 (1963).

181. Sharma, R. M., Sharma, C., Donnelly, A. J., Morris, H. P. and Weinhouse, S. *Cancer Res.*, **25,** 193 (1965).
182. Sharma, O. K., Kerr, S. J., Lipshitz-Weister, R. and Borek, E. *Fed. Proc.*, **30,** 167 (1971).
183. Shatkin, A. J., and Sipe, J. D. *Proc. Nat. Acad. Sci.*, **61,** 1462 (1968).
184. Shatton, J. B., Donelly, A. J. and Weinhouse, S. *Cancer Res.*, **22,** 1372, (1962).
185. Shatton, J. B., Morris, H. P. and Weinhouse, S. *Cancer Res.*, **29,** 1161 (1969).
186. Shearer, R. W. and McCarthy, B. J. *Biochemistry*, **6,** 283 (1967).
187. Shonk, C. E., Morris, H. P. and Boxer, G. E. *Cancer Res.*, **25,** 671, (1965).
188. Shugart, L., Novelli, G. D., Stulberg, M. P. *Biochim. Biophys. Act.*, **157,** 83 (1968).
189. Sillero, A., Sillero, M. A. G. and Sols, A. *European J. Biochem.*, **10,** 351 (1969).
190. Sneider, T. W., Potter, V. R. and Morris, H. P. *Cancer Res.*, **29,** 40 (1969).
191. Snyder, S. P. and Theilen, G. H. *Nature*, Lond., **221,** 1074 (1969).
192. Spiegelman, S., Burny, A., Das, M. R., Keydar, J., Schlom, J., Travnicek, M. and Watson, K. *Nature*, Lond., **227,** 563 (1970).
193. Spiegelman, S., Burny, A., Das, M. R., Keydar, J. Schlom, J. Travnicek, M. and Watson, K. *Nature*, Lond., **228,** 430 (1970).
194. Spiegelman, S., Schlom, J. and Moore, D. H. *Nature* Lond., **231,** 97 (1970).
195. Stanislawski-Birencwajg, M., Uriel, J. and Grabar, P. *Cancer Res.*, **27,** 1990 (1967).
196. Stonehill, E. H. and Bendich, A. *Nature*, Lond., **228,** 371 (1970).
197. Sueoka, N. and Kano-Sueoka, T. *Prog. Nucl. Acid. Res. Mol. Biol.*, **10,** 23 (1970).
198. Sugimura, T. *Chemical Tumour Problems*, p. 261 Ed. Nakahara, W. *Jap. Soc. for the promotion of Science*, Tokyo (1970).
199. Sugimura, T., Matsushima, T., Kawachi, T., Kogure, K., Tanaka, N., Miyake, S., Hozumi, M., Sato, S. and Sato, H. *Gann Monograph No.* 13, **31,** Ed. Weinhouse, S. and Ono, T. Tokyo Univ. Press (1972).
200. Sweeney, M. J., Ashmore, J., Morris, H. P. and Weber, G. *Cancer Res.*, **23,** 995 (1963).
201. Sweeney, M. J., Hoffman, D. H. and Poore, G. A. *Proc. Am. Assoc. Cancer Res.*, **8,** 66 (1967).
202. Sweeney, M. J., Hoffman, D. H. and Poore, G. A. *Adv. Enz. Regln.*, **9,** 51 (1971).
203. Takeda, H., Sato, K., Saheki, R., Suzuki, R. and Tsuiki, S. *Gann*, **58,** 459 (1967).
204. Takeda, H. and Tsuiki, S. *Gann*, **58,** 221 (1967).
205. Taketa, K. and Pogell, B. *J. Biol. Chem.*, **240,** 651 (1965).
206. Tanaka, T., Harano, Y., Morimura, H. and Mori, R. *Biochem. Biophys. Res. Comm.*, **21,** 55 (1965).
207. Tanaka, T., Harano, Y., Sue, F. and Morimura, H. *J. Biochem.*, Tokyo, **62,** 71 (1967).
208. Tanaka, T., An, T. and Sakaue, Y. *J. Biochem*, Tokyo, **69,** 609 (1971).
209. Tanaka, T., Imamura, K., Ann. T. and Taniuchi, K. *Gann Monograph No.* 13, p. 219 (1972) Univ. of Tokyo Press Ed. Weinhouse, S. and Ono, T.
210. Taylor, C. B., Morris, H. P. and Weber, G. *Life Sci.*, **8,** 635 (1969).
211. Taylor, M. W., Buck, C. A., Granger, G. A. and Holland, J. *J. Mol. Biol.*, **33,** 809 (1968).
212. Temin, H. M. *Virology*, **20,** 577 (1963).

213. ———— *Virology*, **23,** 486 (1964).
214. ———— *Proc. Nat. Acad. Sci.,* **52,** 323 (1964).
215. ———— *Health Lab. Sci.*, **1,** 790 (1964).
216. ———— *J. Cell. Physiol.*, **69,** 53 (1967).
217. ———— *Cancer Res.*, **28,** 1835 (1968).
218. ———— and Baltimore, D. *Adv. Virus. Res.*, **17,** 129 (1972).
219. ———— and Mizutani, S. *Nature*, Lond., **226,** 1211 (1970).
220. Tocchini-Valentini, G. P. and Crippa, M. *Nature*, Lond., **228,** 995 (1970).
221. Todaro, G. J., Zeve, V., and Aaronson, S. A. *Nature*, Lond., **226,** 1049 (1970).
222. Todaro, G. J. and Gallo, R. C. *Nature*, Lond., **244,** 206 (1973).
223. Torelli, U. L., Torelli, G. M., Andreoli, A. and Mauri, C. *Nature*, Lond., **226,** 1163 (1970).
224. Tsuiki, S., Sato, K., Miyagi, T. and Kikuchi, H. *Gann Monograph No.* 13, p. 153 (1972). Ed. Weinhouse, S. and Ono, T. University of Tokyo Press.
225. Tsuiki, S. and Saheki, R. *Gann Monograph No.* 1, p. 117 (1966). Ed. Hayashi, O. and Morris, H. P. University of Tokyo Press.
226. Turkington, R. W. *J. Biol. Chem.,* **244,** 5140 (1969).
227. Turkington, R. W. *Biochim. Biophys. Acta*, **213,** 478 (1970).
228. Turkington, R. W. and Self, D. J. *Cancer Res.*, **30,** 1833 (1970).
229. van de Woude, G. F., Polatnik, J. and Ascione, R. *J. Virol.*, **5,** 458 (1970).
230. Vaughan, M. H., Soeiro, R., Warner, J. R. and Darnell, J. E. *Proc. Nat. Acad. Sci.*, U.S., **58.** 1527 (1967).
231. Verma, I. M., Meuth, N. L., Bromfeld, E., Manly, K. F. and Baltimore, D. *Nature New Biol.*, **233,** 131 (1971).
232. Vigier, P. and Goldé, A. *Virology*, **23,** 511 (1964).
233. Villar-Palasi, *Meth. Enzymol.*, **8,** 374 (1966).
234. Viñuela, E., Salas, M. and Sols, A. *J. Biol. Chem.*, **238,** 1175 (1963).
235. Viola, M. V. *J. Nat. Cancer Inst.*, **50,** 1175 (1973).
236. Volkers, S. A. S. and Taylor, M. W. *Biochemistry*, **10,** 488 (1971).
237. Wainwright, S. D. and Wainwright, L. K. *Can. J. Biochem.*, **45,** 255 (1967).
238. Walker, D. G. *Biochim. Biophys. Acta*, **77,** 209 (1963).
239. Walker, P. M. B. *Progr. Nucl. Acid. Res.*, **9,** 301 (1969).
240. Walker, P. R. and Potter, V. R. *Adv. Enz. Regln.*, **10,** 339 (1972).
241. Wallace, J. C. and Newsholme, E. A. *Biochem. J.*, **104,** 378 (1967).
242. Warburg, O. *The Metabolism of Tumours*, Constable, London (1930).
243. Warburg, O. *Science*, **123,** 309 (1956).
244. Weber, G. *Cancer Res.*, **23,** 1491 (1963).
245. ———— *Adv. Enz. Regln.*, **1,** 321 (1963).
246. ———— *Gann Monograph No.* 1, 151, Ed. Hayaishi, O. and Morris, H. P. Japanese Foundation for Cancer Research and The Japanese Cancer Association, (1966).
247. ———— *Naturwiss.*, **55,** 418 (1968).
248. ———— *Adv. Enz. Regln.*, **7,** 15 (1969).
249. ———— *Gann Monograph No.* 13, p. 47. Ed. Weinhouse, S. and Ono, T. Tokyo University Press (1972).
250. ———— *Adv. Enz. Reglu.*, **11,** 79 (1973).
251. ———— and Cantero, A. *Cancer Res.*, **17,** 995 (1957).
252. ———— and Cantero, A. *Cancer Res.*, **19,** 763 (1959).
253. ———— and Lea, M. A. *Adv. Enz. Regln.*, **4,** 115 (1966).
254. ———— and Lea, M. A. *Meth. Cancer Res.*, **2,** 523. Ed. Busch, Academic Press New York and London (1967).
255. ———— and Morris, H. P. *Cancer Res.*, **23,** 987 (1963).

256. ———— Banerjee, G. and Morris, H. P. *Cancer Res.*, **21,** 933 (1961).
257. ———— Lea, M. A. and Stamm, N. B. *Adv. Enz. Regln.*, **6,** 101 (1968).
258. ———— Queener, S. F. and Ferdinandus, J. A. *Adv. Enz. Regln.*, **9,** 63 (1971).
259. ———— Morris, H. P., Love, W. C. and Ashmore, J. *Cancer Res.*, **21,** 1406 (1961).
260. ———— Singhal, R. L., and Srivastava, S. K. *Adv. Enz. Reglu.*, **3,** 43 (1965).
261. ———— Singhal, R. L., Stamm, N. B. and Srivastava, S. K. *Fed. Proc.*, **24,** 745 (1965).
262. ———— Stamm, N. B. and Fisher, E. A. *Nature*, **149,** 67 (1965).
263. Weinhouse, S. *Adv. Cancer Res.*, **3,** 269 (1955).
264. ———— *Gann Monograph No.* 1, p. 99. Ed. Hayaishi, O. and Morris, H. P. Japanese Foundation for Cancer Research and the Japanese Cancer Association (1966).
265. ———— In: *Homologies in Enzymes and Metabolic Pathways, Metabolic Alterations in Cancer*, Miami Winter Symposia, **2,** Ed. Whelan, W. J. and Schultz, J. Amsterdam North Holland Publ. Co. (1970).
266. ———— *Cancer Res.*, **32,** 2007 (1972).
267. ————and Ono, T. Eds. *Isozymes and Enzyme Regulation in Cancer, Gann Monograph No.* 13. University of Tokyo Press (1972).
268. Whiteley, A. H., McCarthy, B. J. and Whiteley, H. R. *Proc. Nat. Acad. Sci.*, **55,** 519 (1966).
269. Winocour, E. *Adv. Cancer Res.*, **14,** 37 (1971).
270. Wood, T. *Biochem. Biophys. Res. Comm.*, **31,** 779 (1968).
271. Yang, W. *Cancer Res.*, **31,** 639 (1971).

Chapter 7

SYSTEMIC FACTORS PRODUCED BY HUMAN NEOPLASMS

A. MUNRO NEVILLE, Ph.D., M.D., M.R.C.Path.
Professor of Experimental Pathology, Institute of Cancer Research, London

and T. SYMINGTON, M.D., F.R.I.C., F.R.C.P.G., F.R.C.Path., F.R.S.E.
Professor of Pathology and Director in the Institute of Cancer Research, London

---

In recent years, the observation that many tumours can form and release various different factors which are inappropriate (ectopic) with respect to their time, site and amount of production, has received increasing attention (Azzopardi, 1966[1]; Liddle *et al.*, 1969[2]; Abelev, 1971[3]; Gold, 1971[4]; Laurence and Neville, 1972[5]). There are two broad categories of these inappropriate materials: hormones and foetal-associated macromolecules. This division into separate categories probably reflects the different methods of their detection rather than any basic difference in tumour behaviour; indeed, they almost certainly represent different manifestations of the same basic phenomenon—the abnormal tumour phenotype (Ellison and Neville, 1973[6]).

This review is concerned with some of these tumour products. We do not imply that they are the only factors released by tumours into the blood stream, but we believe that they illustrate important changes in gene expression—changes that have profound significance in clinical medicine and pathology and which may lead to a deeper understanding of the basic biology of neoplasia.

'Inappropriate' factors

HORMONES

The metabolic and systemic manifestations of 'non-endocrine' neoplasms include cutaneous, haematological, metabolic and endocrine, neurological, osseous and soft tissue changes (Azzopardi, 1966[1]). Many may be explained by hormone production but others, such as the nephrotic syndrome, seem to have an immunological basis (Grace and Dao, 1959[7]; Curtis *et al.*, 1961[8]; Landaw, 1964[9]; Lewis *et al.*, 1971[10]; Plager and Stultzman, 1971[11]). The range of hormones produced, the associated clinical syndromes, and the tumour sites most commonly involved are shown in Table 7.1.

Table 7.1. Inappropriate hormone production: the clinical syndromes and tumour sites

Clinical syndrome	*Hormonal products*	*Principal tumour sites*
Cushing's syndrome	ACTH (with MSH)	Bronchus Islets of Langerhans Thymus Carcinoid tumours
Inappropriate antidiuresis	ADH	Bronchus
Gynaecomastia Precocious puberty	Gonadotrophins	Liver Bronchus
Erythrocytosis	Erythropoietin	Kidney Cerebellum
Hypoglycaemia	Insulin-like	Retroperitoneal mesenchyme Liver
Hypertrophic osteoarthropathy	Growth hormone	Bronchus Uterus
Hypokalaemic alkalosis	Renin	Bronchus
Hyperthyroidism	TSH HCT	Gastro-intestinal Trophoblast
Zollinger–Ellison syndrome	Gastrin	Islets of Langerhans
Hypercalcaemia	Parathormone	Kidney Bronchus Breast

ACTH—adrenocorticotrophic hormone; MSH—melanocyte-stimulating hormone; ADH—antidiuretic hormone; TSH—thyroid-stimulating hormone; HCT—human chorionic thyrotrophin.

The demonstration of inappropriate hormone production by a neoplasm which arises from cells not considered to be a normal source of that hormone is required before the tumour can be considered responsible for the 'ectopic' hormone syndrome. This is achieved by assaying the tumour for its content of hormone, studying its *in vitro* biosynthetic ability, examining arteriovenous differences in hormone levels across the tumour vascular bed, or by observing that the excessive amounts of hormone production disappear following surgical removal of the tumour (Omenn, 1970[12]).

Various aspects of these functional aberrations may be illustrated by reference to the ectopic production of adrenocorticotrophic hormone (ACTH) which has been extensively documented. Inappropriate ACTH production has been recorded most frequently in association with oat cell carcinoma of the bronchus; other tumours include medullary carcinoma of the thyroid and phaeochromocytoma (Symington, 1969[13]) (Table 7.1). More recent evidence has indicated that ectopic ACTH production may be more widespread than was previously considered and some workers consider that most, if not all, bronchial tumours may secrete ACTH.

Other factors associated with tumours may cause Cushing's syndrome.

They include a corticotrophin releasing factor (CRF) which apparently releases ACTH from the pituitary and perhaps from the tumour itself (Upton and Amatruda, 1971[14]). It is also possible that a tumour product with adrenal weight maintaining properties but without steroidogenic function (Nichols and Gourley, 1965[15]) may be formed by various neoplasms, including those of bronchial origin; such a product would account for the very large adrenal glands found at autopsy of patients dying with bronchial carcinoma.

FOETAL MACROMOLECULES

The renewed interest in tumour immunology has been responsible for the delineation of a group of products (Table 7.2), often referred to as 'embryo-

Table 7.2. Human tumour-associated foetal macromolecules (antigens)

1. Present in tumours and body fluids
   - (a) without known metabolic effects
     - Carcinoembryonic antigen (CEA)
     - α_1–Foetoprotein (AFP)
     - α_2H–Foetoprotein
     - βS–Foetoprotein
     - Leukaemia associated antigens (LAA)
     - γ–Foetal proteins
     - Foetal sulphoglycoprotein antigen (FSA)
   - (b) with metabolic effects
     - Placental alkaline phosphatase
     - Placental-type hormones and related products
2. Present in tumours only

specific' or 'onco-foetal antigens': they are associated with both human (Gold and Freedman, 1965a[32]; Tee *et al.*, 1965[16]; Yashi *et al.*, 1968[17]; Häkkinen and Viikari, 1969[18]; Abelev, 1971[3]; Klavins *et al.*,[19] 1971; Trouillas, 1971[20]) and animal tumours (Pearson and Freeman, 1968[21]; Brawn, 1970[22]; Coggin *et al.*, 1970[23]; Duff and Rapp, 1970[24]; Stonehill and Bendich, 1970[25]). Their reappearance was first postulated in human neoplasms in 1929 (Hirzfeld, 1929[26]) and was noted by Stonehill and Bendich (1970[25]) in diverse animal tumours induced by physical, viral and chemical agents, as well as in those occurring spontaneously. Stonehill and Bendich (1970[25]) suggested that this was a universal oncological phenomenon which they termed 'retrogenetic expression'.

Human tumour-associated foetal macromolecules (antigens) fall into two principal categories depending upon whether or not they pass from the tumour cells into the plasma or other body fluids (Table 7.2). Those which occur outside the tumour may be further subdivided according to the presence or absence of demonstrable biological activity. Of the various principles, the carcinoembryonic antigen (CEA) and α_1-foetoprotein (AFP) are the two antigens whose structure, significance and role have been best elucidated.

Structure-function relationships

Bronchial carcinomas appear to be the tumours most commonly associated with hormone production at the present time (Table 7.1). ACTH and ADH are associated mainly with oat cell carcinomas (Table 7.3), squamous cell carcinoma of lung most often produces parathyroid hormone (PTH), and giant cell tumours synthesize gonadotrophins (Omenn and Wilkins, 1970[27]). But these structure-function relationships are not absolute: cases have been recorded where squamous cell carcinomas of the lung have produced ACTH, and oat cell carcinomas have produced gonadotrophins (Hauger-Klevene,

Table 7.3. Hormones produced by tumours of the lung

Hormone	*Typical tumour cell type*
ACTH	Oat cell
ADH	Oat cell
PTH	Squamous cell
Gonadotrophins	Giant cell
Growth hormone	
Renin	
Prolactin	
Glucagon	
Calcitonin	
TSH-like	

Table 7.4. Serum α_1-foetoprotein (AFP) Assay: results by gel diffusion methods*

Site	*Disorders*	*Incidence of Positive Serum AFP Assays*	
		Number	%
—	Normal controls	0/15, 730	(0)
Liver	Hepatocarcinoma	589/868	(68)
	Cholangiocarcinoma	1/73	(1.4)
	Non-neoplastic†	15/6484	(0.2)
Gonad	Teratocarcinoma	49/108	(45)
	Seminoma	0/39	(0)
	Choriocarcinoma	2/15	(13)
	Other tumours	0/13	(0)
Kidney	Nephroblastoma	0/59	(0)
—	Neuroblastoma	0/70	(0)
—	Non-hepatic primary malignant tumours‡	10/1169	(0.8)

*From the data reviewed by Laurence and Neville, 1972[5].
†Twelve of the positive assays had either viral hepatitis or cirrhosis.
‡All ten positive assays were in patients with hepatic metastases.

1968[28]; Cottrell *et al.*, 1969[29]). Too few examples of the other ectopic hormones in association with lung tumours have yet been reported to allow more detailed correlation of structure and function. Nonetheless, there appears to be a distinct non-random tendency within the ectopic hormone-producing syndromes. A clear-cut tumour structure-function relationship exists with regard to AFP, the α_1-globulin which is the major protein component of early foetal plasma and which is produced by the foetal liver, gastrointestinal tract and yolk sac. Approximately 70 per cent of patients with hepatomas and about 45 per cent with malignant teratomas have raised AFP levels as detected by gel diffusion in the plasma (Table 7.4). By contrast, raised levels of AFP are encountered only rarely in cholangiocarcinoma and apparently not at all in seminoma. If the so-called endodermal sinus tumour was truly of vitelline origin (Teilum, 1971[30]), Laurence and Neville (1972[5]) predicted that it, too, should be associated with raised AFP levels. This forecast has now been proved accurate (Ballas, 1972[31]).

When more sensitive methods of assay are employed, notably radioimmunoassay, AFP is detectable in the serum of healthy persons, and in the serum of greater numbers of patients with gastrointestinal, pancreatic and prostatic carcinomas, particularly if hepatic metastases are present. AFP is found also in the serum of subjects with inflammatory and/or regenerative diseases of the liver (see Table 7.4), partly vitiating the initial structure-functional relationship.

The carcinoembryonic antigen (CEA) is known to be a product of the foetal gastrointestinal tract, pancreas, and liver; it is a glycoprotein found in the cell glycocalyx (Gold and Freedman, 1965a[32], b[33]; Gold *et al.*, 1968[34], 1970[35]; von Kliest and Burtin, 1969a[36], b[37]). CEA was considered initially to be produced only by endodermally-derived neoplasms (Gold, 1971[4]) but, with increasing experience, this unique structure-function relationship has been brought into question and the antigen appears to be associated with a wide variety of tumours of differing histogenesis, including neuroblastomas (Reynoso *et al.*, 1972[38]): some important examples are shown in Table 7.5. Since urothelium is of endodermal origin (Hall *et al.*, 1972[39]) it is interesting that raised CEA levels have been found in the *urine* of patients with bladder carcinomas. However, raised levels are also associated with regenerative and inflammatory disorders of bladder.

Considerably less is known about other foetal proteins which may occur in the plasma of patients with neoplastic diseases (Table 7.2). α_2-H-Foetoprotein (Buffe *et al.*, 1970[40]; Martin *et al.*, 1971[41]; Wada *et al.*, 1971[42]), βS-foetoprotein (Takahashi *et al.*, 1967[43]; Wada *et al.*, 1971[42]) and γ-foetal proteins 1 and 2 (Edynak *et al.*, 1972[44]) do not occur with any particular type of tumour (Laurence and Neville, 1972[5]) and may be found in association with non-neoplastic disorders. On the other hand, the leukaemia-associated antigens (LAA) (Harris *et al.*, 1971[45]) are apparently localized to leukaemias and lymphomas and the foetal sulphoglycoprotein antigen of gastric juice has only been noted so far in patients with gastric carcinomas (Häkkinen and Viikari, 1969[18]).

Foetal-associated macromolecules with biological activity are related to normal placental products and are either hormonal or isozymic in nature

Table 7.5. Incidence of raised plasma carcinoembryonic antigen (CEA) levels in gastro-intestinal, bronchial and mammary disorders*

Site	*Disorder*	*(% incidence)*
	Healthy controls	1/335 (0.3%)
	Carcinoma of	
	Colon and Rectum	230/316 (73%)
	Pancreas	48/52 (92%)
	Liver	12/18 (67%)
	Other sites	51/85 (60%)
	Polyps of	
	Colon and Rectum	6/67 (9%)
Gastrointestinal tract	*Inflammatory/Reactive*	
	Ulcerative colitis and Crohn's disease	20/95 (21%)
	Diverticulitis, Peptic ulceration	7/33 (21%)
	Cirrhosis and alcoholic liver disease	28/66 (42%)
	Alcoholic pancreatitis	17/32 (53%)
	Other	2/43 (5%)
	Carcinoma	82/159 (52%)
Breast	*Benign tumour*	1/24 (4%)
	Reactive	
	Fibroadenosis	5/70 (7%)
	Carcinoma of	
	Bronchus	65/90 (72%)
	Upper respiratory tract	8/15 (53%)
Respiratory tract	*Inflammatory/Reactive*	
	Pulmonary tuberculosis	8/21 (38%)
	Chronic bronchitis and emphysema	16/63 (25%)

*From data of LoGerfo *et al.*, 1971[110], 1972[83]; Moore *et al.*, 1971[111]; Laurence *et al.*, 1972[55]; Reynoso *et al.*, 1972[38]; Zamchek *et al.*, 1972[56].

(Table 7.2). The synthesis of gonadotrophins, including human placental lactogen, by bronchial carcinomas and hepatomas has already been discussed. Both these tumours may also produce plasminogen activators (Davidson *et al.*, 1969[46]) which occur normally in the placenta. The embryonic (placental) origin of such substances serves to illustrate the similarity in the mechanisms which account for the tumour production of foetal macromolecules and hormones.

The induction of experimental neoplasms is frequently associated with the appearance in the tumours of isozymes typical of foetal or neonatal tissues. Usually, there is a quantitative change toward the foetal pattern in enzymes such as lactic dehydrogenase and aldolase (Leese, 1969[47]). While these observations have important basic connotations in the field of differentiation, only qualitative isozymic alterations found in body fluids will have potential clinical importance. To date, the only isozyme fitting the latter category is *placental alkaline phosphatase*—a heat stable variant, inhibited by L-phenylalanine (Fishman *et al.*, 1968[48]), and never found in the serum of normal *male* subjects though it is present in maternal serum during the third trimester of pregnancy.

The isozyme first detected in a patient named Regan with bronchial carcinoma—hence the eponym Regan isozyme—occurs in the serum of a minority of patients with various mammary, genito-urinary and gastro-intestinal neoplasms, and also in many inflammatory disorders. It thus fails to exhibit any unique structure-function relationship.

Polyfactor Production

The ability of a tumour to synthesize more than one inappropriate factor has been studied in detail only for hormones. Whereas certain tumours are capable of producing a variety of hormones, others occasionally elaborate several hormones at the same time (Table 7.6). Sometimes, a tumour arising in an endocrine organ produces the hormone appropriate to its site together with the ectopic production of another hormone: thus medullary carcinoma of the thyroid may produce calcitonin and ACTH (Melvin *et al.*, 1970[49]; Croughs *et al.*, 1972[50]). More rarely, a tumour synthesizes the hormone appropriate to its site of origin and also several ectopic hormones (O'Neal *et al.*, 1968[51]), or a tumour may produce more than one hormone, all of which are 'inappropriate'. However, it is not known if an ectopic hormone-producing tumour is also capable of releasing simultaneously one of the foetal macromolecules. Nor is it known if CEA and AFP are formed by the same gastro-intestinal or hepatic tumour, though some light is shed on this problem by the finding that a variant of the carcinoplacental alkaline phosphatase isozyme (Warnock and Reesman, 1969[52]) occurs in the serum of patients with hepatomas if they are also producing AFP.

Table 7.6. Polyhormonal potential of tumours

Tumour Site	*Hormones*	*Refs.**
A. Appropriate plus ectopic hormones		
Thyroid	Calcitonin—ACTH	1, 6
Islets of Langerhans	Insulin—ACTH	5
Kidney	Erythropoietin—PTH	8
Adrenal medulla	Noradrenaline—ACTH	7
B. Multiple ectopic hormones		
Islets of Langerhans	ACTH—MSH—Gastrin—Glucagon—?PTH, ?ADH	7
	ACTH—MSH—Gastrin	3
Lung	ACTH—MSH—PTH	4
	ACTH—ADH	2
	ACTH—MSH—Serotonin	7
	ACTH—MSH—Serotonin	7
	Insulin—Glucagon	9
Mediastinum	ACTH—ADH	7
Ileum	ACTH—Serotonin	7

**References*
1. Croughs *et al.*, 1972[50]
2. Cullen and Tomlinson 1968[112]
3. Law *et al.*, 1965[113]
4. Liddle *et al.*, 1965[60a]
5. Marks *et al.*, 1965[114]
6. Melvin *et al.*, 1970[49]
7. O'Neal *et al.*, 1968[51]
8. Salama *et al.*, 1971[115]
9. Unger *et al.*, 1964[116]

ACTH, MSH, ADH—See Table 7·1; PTH—parathormone.

Structure of the inappropriate materials compared to their normal counterparts

In trying to reach an understanding of the underlying cellular mechanisms responsible for the formation of inappropriate products, it is important to establish that such products are indeed synthesized and released by the tumours and are similar in structure to their normally formed counterparts.

There is now overwhelming evidence from *in vivo* and *in vitro* studies that hormones and foetal macromolecules such as AFP, CEA and the carcinoplacental alkaline phosphatase isozyme are biosynthetic products of the tumour cells. The decline of foetal antigens to normal levels in the serum after complete removal of the tumour and their increase in serum with recurrence of the disease argue strongly in favour of an active secretory function (Purves *et al.*, 1968[53]; Nathanson and Fishman, 1971[54]; Hall *et al.*, 1972[39]; Laurence *et al.*, 1972[55]; Zamchek *et al.*, 1972[56]). By measuring venovenous or arteriovenous gradients across the liver and kidney, parathormone-like materials have been shown to be produced by a cholangiocarcinoma (Buckle *et al.*, 1970[57]) and a renal carcinoma (Knill-Jones *et al.*, 1970[58]). Radioactively-labelled amino acids are incorporated into antidiuretic hormone (ADH) and growth hormone *in vitro* by bronchial carcinomas (George and Capen, 1972[59]; Greenberg *et al.*, 1972[60]), while ACTH (Liddle *et al.*, 1965[60a]; Tashjian, 1969[61]) and CEA (Todd, 1972[62]) can be formed by a variety of tumours in tissue culture. This evidence, together with ultrastructural observations of hormone-secreting-type granules in some tumours (Corrin and McMillan, 1970[63]; Kay and Willson, 1970[64]; Johnston and Waisman, 1971[65]) and immunofluorescent localization—of AFP in the hepatoma cell cytoplasm and CEA in the tumour cell glycocalyx (Gold *et al.*, 1968[34], 1970[35]; von Kliest and Burtin, 1969a[36]; Gusev *et al.*, 1971[66]; Nishioka *et al.*, 1972[67])—is further evidence of the active part tumour cells seem to play in the process.

All known inappropriate tumour products are polypeptides, proteins or glycoproteins; but none has yet been proved by amino acid sequence analysis to be identical with the normally produced counterpart. Nevertheless, much of the available evidence from hormone (Cameron *et al.*, 1969[68]; Knight *et al.*, 1971[69]; Roof *et al.*, 1971[70]; Shapiro *et al.*, 1971[71]; George and Capen, 1972[59]; Greenberg *et al.*, 1972[60]) and foetal macromolecule studies (Nishi, 1970[72]; Rüoslahti *et al.*, 1971[73]) has shown a reasonable correspondence between the normal and tumour materials. Future studies of the amino acid sequences of these ectopic materials will determine if the polypeptides formed are normal or abnormal in structure and could throw light on the molecular mechanisms underlying their production. From the clinical standpoint, structural differences may be used to design appropriate reagents and assay tests for detecting truly specific tumour products.

Pathological aspects

FOETAL ANTIGENS

The detection of inappropriate production of foetal macromolecules or hormones has contributed to our understanding of the structural and functional differentiation of tumours, their histogenesis and their prognosis. Tumours arising from tissues which in foetal life form AFP may also be associated with the production of this material. Most hepatocytes in the normal liver are involved initially in AFP synthesis by the sixth week of foetal life. As the serum level of the antigen falls during gestation, the numbers of cells stained by immunofluorescence also decline. Küpffer cells, bile duct epithelium and haematopoietic cells do not appear to synthesize AFP at any time (Englehardt *et al.*, 1969[74]). In regenerating liver (Englehardt *et al.*, 1969[74]) and in hepatomas (Gusev *et al.*, 1971[66]), only cells adjacent to tumour blood vessels or larger cells with more hyperchromatic nuclei contain AFP demonstrable by immunofluorescence. This suggests that the production of AFP is not entirely a random process (Nishioka *et al.*, 1972[67]).

The time course of AFP production is little understood. Hull *et al.*, (1969)[75] have shown that AFP production can precede the development of some diethylnitrosamine—induced hepatomas in monkeys: in others, where there is no apparent AFP production, the tumours possess a prominent lymphocytic infiltrate which disappears if and when these lesions start to form AFP. Kroes and Weisburger (1972)[76] observed a burst of AFP production in rats 3–5 weeks after administering 3-methyl-4-dimethylaminoazobenzene together with aflatoxin. The AFP level returned to normal until hepatomas redeveloped when a second increase in serum AFP concentration occurred.

While Abelev *et al.* (1967)[77] found a correlation between AFP levels and the time required for transplantable hepatomas to kill the host animal, no such association was found for humans with hepatocellular carcinoma, though Purves *et al.* (1970)[78] found lower serum levels in patients with the more differentiated tumours. This does not apply to teratocarcinomas (Mawas *et al.* (1971)[79]).

There is a wide range of AFP levels in patients with hepatomas. Although the total range between patients is 500,000-fold, the variation for a given patient is rarely more than 10-fold over the time of observation (Purves *et al.* 1970[78]). The outcome of the disease does not appear to depend on the AFP levels, suggesting that there is a homeostatic control mechanism in tumour cells for AFP production.

CARCINOEMBRYONIC ANTIGEN (CEA)

CEA seems to be retained by the glycocalyx of the plasma membrane of colonic carcinoma cells, localized particularly to their luminal aspect (Gold *et al.*, 1968[34], 1970[35]; von Kliest and Burtin, 1969a[36]; Martin *et al.*, 1972[80]). As the cell acquires CEA, it appears to lose normal cytoplasmic and membrane antigens (Nairn *et al.*, 1962[81]; Burtin *et al.*, 1971[82])—a finding that

Table 7.7. Correlation of histological type with CEA levels*

Site of Carcinoma	*Cell Type or Grade*	*Incidence of Positive Assays*
Colon and Rectum†	Well differentiated	9/16
	Moderately well differentiated	20/33
	Poorly differentiated	11/19
Breast†	I	2/5
	II	10/31
	III	5/18
Bronchus†	Oat-cell	12/14
	Squamous	10/17
	Adenocarcinoma	4/6
Bladder‡	Well differentiated	2/3
	Moderately well differentiated	6/9
	Poorly differentiated	7/10

*From data of Laurence and Neville, 1972[5]; Laurence *et al.*, 1972[55]; Hall *et al.*, 1972[39].
†Plasma or ‡urinary CEA assays.

Table 7.8. Influence of stage of tumour progression on the incidence of elevated plasma CEA levels*

Carcinoma of	*Stage*	*Total (%incidence)*
Colon and Rectum	Dukes' A†	20/48 (42%)
	Dukes' B	36/52 (69%)
	Dukes' C	27/38 (71%)
	Metastasized	66/74 (89%)
Bronchus	Local NO, MO‡	15/24 (63%)
	Local N+, MO	5/6 (83%)
	Metastases	6/7 (86%)
Breast	Local NO, MO‡ } Local N+, MO }	22/69 (32%)
	Metastases	21/32 (66%)
Prostate	Local	5/28 (18%)
	Metastases	7/13 (54%)
Bladder	Local	40/108 (37%)
	Metastases	13/24 (54%)
Cervix	Stage 0§	1/7 (14%)
	Stage 1	5/14 (36%)
	Stage 2	5/9 (55%)
	Stage 3	5/9 (55%)

*Data derived from Laurence and Neville (1972)[5].
†Dukes (1958)[117].
‡NO—no nodes involved with tumour.
N+—nodes contain metastatic tumour.
MO—no distant metastases.
§UICC classification.

suggests a precursor-product relationship. This is supported by immunofluorescent studies which revealed that the area of CEA 'acquisition' is the area of normal antigen 'loss' (Burtin *et al.*, 1971[82]).

Plasma CEA levels are seemingly uninfluenced by the degree of structural differentiation of tumours (Table 7.7), but seem to be more dependent on the extent of tumour spread (Table 7.8; Laurence *et al.*, 1972[55]). However, this is not invariably true as some apparently localized tumours are associated with raised CEA levels (Table 7.8).

Recent experimental studies suggest that glycoproteins in the glycocalyx from both normal and neoplastic cells pass into the blood stream. The glycoproteins of the normal cell glycocalyx have a half-life of about one day and pass from the cells into the blood stream. This time scale seems to be applicable to CEA. After complete resection of tumours, plasma CEA levels fall to normal between the second and eighteenth post-operative days (Laurence *et al.*, 1972[55]; LoGerfo *et al.*, 1972[83]). The different rates of decline may be related to the rate of CEA clearance (Laurence and Neville, 1972[5]).

Kim and Carruthers (1972)[84] examined two mammary carcinomas with differing metastasizing potential in rats and found an inverse relationship between the tumour content of a glycocalyx antigen (not necessarily CEA) and its concentration in the serum. As the surface glycoprotein declined in amount, it increased in the blood stream and the metastasizing potential of the tumour was more pronounced. Some preliminary data on humans (Zamchek *et al.*, 1972[56]) suggest that the prognosis in patients with primary colonic tumours and raised plasma CEA levels is worse than in patients with tumours similar in morphology and extent of spread but in whom plasma CEA is normal. However, more work is needed on the dynamics of CEA production and its metabolism to refute or substantiate this conclusion.

ECTOPIC HORMONES

Studies of foetal antigens and their relationship to tumour cell type, differentiation and prognosis are still at a preliminary stage compared with the extensive investigations which have been carried out on ectopic hormone production. Many ectopic hormone-secreting tumours arise from cells or organs normally associated with endocrine function (Table 7.1). Azzopardi and Williams (1968)[85] suggested that all acceptable examples of the ectopic ACTH syndrome were either tumours of endocrine origin or oat cell carcinomas of the bronchus, and they presented reasons for accepting that the oat cell carcinoma was an endocrine tumour. Subsequent work has shown that ACTH-secreting tumours may contain cytoplasmic secretory granules (Corrin and McMillan, 1970[63]; Kay and Willson, 1970[64]; Johnston and Waisman, 1971[65]) which resemble the granules of pancreatic islet cell tumours and carcinoid tumours (Bensch *et al.*, 1965a[86]; Goldenberg *et al.*, 1969[87]). These ultrastructural features should be viewed in conjunction with similarities in the light microscope of not only oat cell carcinomas, bronchial carcinoids, thymic and medullary thyroid carcinomas, but also islet cell and gastrointestinal carcinoid tumours. There is added support for their interrelationship when it is noted that each of the tumours may secrete ACTH and a wide range of other hormonal products Table 7.6). This evidence suggested that each of those tumours arose from a single progenitor cell-type normally associated with peptide production. Pearse (1966[88], 1969[89]) has described a group of peptide-hormone forming cells (APUD cells*) (Table 7.9) which

Table 7.9. Cells of the APUD Series—(cells capable of Amine Precursor Uptake and Decarboxylation)

Site	*Cell type*	*Product*
Pituitary	Corticotroph Melanotroph	ACTH MSH
Thyroid and extrathyroid	C-cell	Calcitonin
Islets of Langerhans	β-cell α_2-cell α_1-cell	Insulin Glucagon *
Stomach	Argyrophil cell Enterochromaffin cell	Gastrin *
Intestine	Argyrophil cell Enterochromaffin cell	Secretin Serotonin *
Adrenal	Phaeochromocyte	Catecholamines Calcitonin
Lung	Clear cell	*
Carotid body	Type I cell	*
Skin	Melanocyte	*

Data compiled from Kaplan *et al.*, 1970[118]; Pearse, 1969[89]; Polak *et al.*, 1971[91].
*Identification of definitive polypeptide still to be made.

seem to explain partially this phenomenon. It is proposed that the association goes further than the identifying characteristics, and that APUD cells are linked developmentally with a common origin from the neural crest (Pearse, 1969[89]). While the neural crest origin of the chromaffin cells of the adrenal medulla (Coupland, 1965[90]; Polak *et al.*, 1971[91]) and the C-cells of the ultimobranchial body or parafollicular cells of the thyroid (LeDouarin and Le-Lievre, 1970[92]) is now established, numerous attempts to confirm a similar source for other APUD cells have been less conclusive. Indeed, the work of Andrews (1963)[93], LeDouarin (1972)[94] and Ellison and Neville (1973)[6] suggests that they are endodermally derived. Consequently, the similar characteristics which led to the inclusion of phaeochromocytes, thyroid 'C' cells, some pituitary, gastrointestinal and pancreatic endocrine cells in the APUD cell systems may be more a reflection of their similar function than of a common embryonic origin.

The embryological origins for APUD cells—neuroectoderm for phaeochromocytes and 'C' cells of the thyroid, and endoderm for the islets of Langerhans and enterochromaffin cells—are paralleled by the existence of

*APUD cells—i.e. cells that are capable of Amine Precursor Uptake and Decarboxylation.

two separate groups of tumours within the framework of the APUD concept. Medullary carcinoma of the thyroid and phaeochromocytomas are neuro-ectodermal tumours, sometimes familial, which occur not infrequently in association with each other and with multiple neural tumours (Williams, 1965[94a]). Tumours of the carcinoid syndrome and pancreatic islet cell tumours causing the Zollinger-Ellison syndrome are considered to arise from the argyrophil and/or enterochromaffin cells of the gastrointestinal tract and pancreas and can be viewed as endocrine tumours which exhibit metaplastic function.

While the production of ACTH by the APUD tumours just mentioned may represent a change in the role of the APUD cell types, additional assumptions are necessary before thymic and oat cell carcinomas causing Cushing's syndrome can be viewed as arising from APUD cells. Using fluorescence and electron microscopy, various authors have recently described APUD cells in the foetal bronchial mucosa (Hage, 1972[95]), around bronchial glands in the adult (Bensch *et al.*, 1965b[96]) and in the neck (Pearse, 1968[97]), but there is still no direct evidence to confirm the origin of thymic or oat cell carcinoma from this cell type.

It is even more difficult to include, within the hypothesis of APUD cells, the ectopic production of parathormone (Knill–Jones *et al.*, 1970[58]; Melick *et al.*, 1972[98]), gonadotrophins (Rudnick and Odell, 1971[99]), renin (Hauger–Klevene, 1970[99a]), growth hormone (Sparagana *et al.*, 1971[100]; Greenberg, *et al.*, 1972[60]) or thyrotrophin-like substances (Hennen, 1967[101]). None of these hormones is produced normally by APUD cells, yet they can be secreted by a wide variety of tumours including oat cell carcinomas of the bronchus (Table 7.3). Moreover, the range of tumours which secrete hormones with parathormone-like properties include those of bronchial, renal, genito-urinary, gonadal, pancreatic, gastro-intestinal and hepatic origin. Yet such a wide distribution has not been proposed for APUD-type cells. Although tumours producing ectopic hormones may appear to have embryological and morphological affinities, the full extent of the para-endocrine syndrome probably can only be explained if their structural characteristics are a result of their functional attributes.

In a recent review, Ellison and Neville (1973)[6] critically reappraised the theoretical mechanisms which might result in the inappropriate formation of hormones. They concluded that it was due to a non-random change in the pattern of gene expression, and that the theory of gene regulation proposed by Britten and Davidson (1971)[102] provided a rational and satisfactory explanation in molecular terms. By analogy it would appear that the production of foetal macromolecules represents a similar change in gene expression.

Sensitive radioimmunoassays have shown that small amounts of substances, immunologically identical to the foetal-associated tumour macromolecules, are formed by normal adult tissues. This aspect of gene expression is not, therefore, completely suppressed in the adult. It will be extremely interesting to ascertain whether normal APUD-type cells can also form trace amounts of hormones other than the ones appropriate to their site—e.g. ACTH production by enterochromaffin cells.

Increasingly, current studies are suggesting that most human tumours are monoclonal in origin (Fialkow *et al.*, 1972[103]). This poses an interesting problem in cell differentiation. Does one tumour cell have poly-factorial productive ability or do different tumour cells each produce single different inappropriate materials? The theory of Britten and Davidson (1971)[102] certainly suggests that single extrinsic factors such as a carcinogenic agent, could have a diverse effect on the cell and result in the manifestation of different 'new' products. The relationship of these changes at cellular and subcellular levels to the degree of differentiation of the tumour, assessed morphologically or by the presence or absence of tissue isoantigens, is a topic of great potential interest.

Role in clinical medicine

The detection of ectopic hormones and foetal macromolecules in the body fluids may be valuable in the clinical diagnosis and management of patients with cancer.

Bagshawe (1969)[104] assayed human chorionic gonadotrophin (HCG) in the urine of patients with choriocarcinoma (this is not an example of ectopic production) and showed that HCG levels in urine could be used to monitor the dose and effectiveness of chemotherapy. Early recurrences of disease were detected by a rise in the urinary HCG titre.

Assay of plasma CEA may be useful in the management of carcinomas of the gastrointestinal tract and pancreas; also in carcinoma of the bronchus and neuroblastoma (Laurence *et al.*, 1972[55]: LoGerfo *et al.*, 1972[83]; Martin *et al.*, 1972[80]; Reynoso *et al.*, 1972[38]; Zamchek *et al.*, 1972[56]). Urinary CEA assays have a role to play in the investigation of urothelial carcinomas (Hall *et al.*, 1972[39]). The detection rate of early tumours by means of plasma CEA assays is unfortunately low, and the technique is of negligible value as a general tumour screening procedure. Instead, the estimation of CEA in plasma and urine is used mainly (i) as a monitor of effective treatment, providing a means of detecting residual tumour following surgery, and (ii) as a means of assessing local recurrences and/or distant metastases. Published results suggest that if the plasma CEA is raised pre-operatively, it declines to normal between the second and eighteenth post-operative day provided the tumour has been removed completely. Thus a high CEA level following surgery appears to indicate residual disease (Table 8; Laurence and Neville, 1972[5]). Whether this will affect the prognosis or long term survival remains to be determined.

The value of the AFP tests are related principally to the detection and therapeutic monitoring of patients with hepatomas and teratocarcinomas. Radioimmunoassays are now available (Ruoslahti *et al.*, 1971[73]) which should facilitate such studies, and may extend their usefulness—e.g. in obstetrics, as a means of assessing the well being of the foetus (see p. 19).

AFP tests could be better and safer than percutaneous liver biopsies in the investigtion of hepatic tumours (Houstek *et al.*, 1968[105]). There is evidence from the experimental production of hepatomas in monkeys that serum AFP levels may be elevated prior to the development of overt tumour. This may also be true in man (Hull *et al.*, 1969[75]): one patient with cirrhosis originally had normal AFP levels which were found by a gel diffusion method to be positive seven months before a hepatoma was discovered (Khasanov *et al.*, 1971[106]).

The actual levels of plasma AFP remain remarkably steady in any one patient with a hepatoma and appear to be independent of tumour sizes, stage or differentiation (Purves *et al.*, 1968[53]). Successful therapy, including chemotherapy, is associated with a decline in serum levels which rise again with relapse to reach the same or higher levels.

AFP assays are also valuable in the differential diagnosis of teratoma and seminoma (Table 7.4) and in following the response of teratomas to therapy. Mawas *et al.* (1971[79]) observed that teratomas in patients with raised AFP levels are more malignant; most examples of teratomas without detectable AFP in the plasma respond to therapy. Recent results of radioimmunoassays have shown that the AFP content of the sera of pregnant women is abnormal (Abelev *et al.*, 1971[107]; Seppälä and Ruoslahti, 1972a[108]). During the first, second and third trimesters the maternal serum levels are 18–119ng/ml, 96–302ng/ml and 103–550ng/ml respectively, dropping shortly before term to normal. Levels in excess of 1000ng/ml have been found before and after foetal death, and it has been postulated that increased amounts of AFP may be released because of foetal distress (Seppälä and Ruoslahti, 1972b[109]).

The use of these various radioimmunoassays to monitor therapy and to detect tumour recurrences is still relatively restricted. This may be due partly to the inaccessability of such techniques to the clinical oncologist. But a more fundamental problem is that with the exception of human placental lactogen (HPL), which does not occur in normal males, there is always a background level against which measurements have to be made. Small changes in concentration are thus difficult to detect and evaluate.

Conclusion

In this review, we have not discussed in biochemical, biological or pathological detail any of the inappropriate factors formed by tumours, nor the clinical syndromes which they produce. Instead, we have tried to illustrate and outline the general aspects of the subject. The main aim in the future will be to develop suitable radioimmunoassays for the various tumour-associated products which can be used to detect tumours and their recurrences, and to monitor therapy. This approach seems appropriate since earlier detection and treatment of cancer offers better prospects for survival. Furthermore, by characterizing these products more completely, we shall obtain a better understanding of differentiation and function in normal cells and—perhaps—some of the aberrations that occur in the corresponding neoplasms.

References

1. Azzopardi, J. G. *Recent Advances in Pathology*, *8th edition*, Ed. C. V. Harrison, London: Churchill, p. 98 (1966).
2. Liddle, G. W., Nicholson, W. E., Island, D. P., Orth, D. N., Abe, K. and Lowder, S. C. *Rec. Prog. Horm. Res.*, **25,** 283 (1969).
3. Abelev, G. I. *Adv. Cancer Res.*, **14,** 295 (1971).

4. Gold, P. *Ann. Rev. Med.,* **22,** 85 (1971).
5. Laurence, D. J. R. and Neville, A. M. *Br. J. Cancer*, **26,** 335 (1972).
6. Ellison, M. L. and Neville, A. M. In *Modern Trends in Oncology*. Part. I p. 163 (1973). Ed. R. W. Raven. London: Butterworth.
7. Grace, J. T. and Dao, T. L. *Cancer*, **12,** 648 (1959).
8. Curtis, A. C., Heckaman, J. H. and Wheeler, A. H. *J. Am. med. Assn.*, **178,** 571 (1961).
9. Landaw, S. A. *J. Mt. Sinai Hosp.*, **31,** 167 (1964).
10. Lewis, M. G., Loughridge, L. W. and Phillips, T. M. *Lancet*, **ii,** 134 (1971).
11. Plager, J. and Stultzman, L. *Am. J. Med.*, **50,** 56 (1971).
12. Omenn, G. S. *Ann Int. Med.*, **72,** 136 (1970).
13. Symington, T. *Functional Pathology of the Human Adrenal Gland.* Livingstone: Edinburgh, p. 128. (1969).
14. Upton, G. V. and Amatruda, T. T. *New Engl. J. Med.*, **285,** 420 (1971).
15. Nichols, J. and Gourley, W. *J. Am. med Assn.*, **185,** 696 (1965).
16. Tee, D. E. H., Wang, M. and Watkins, J. *Europ. J. Cancer,* **1,** 315 (1965).
17. Yashi, A., Matsumura, Y., Carpenter, C. M. and Hyde L. *J. Nat. Cancer Inst ,* **40,** 663 (1968).
18. Häkkinen, I. and Viikari, S. *Ann. Surg.*, **169,** 277 (1969).
19. Klavins, J. V., Mesa-Tejada, R. and Weiss, M. *Nature, New Biol.*, **234,** 153 (1971).
20. Trouillas, P. *Lancet*, **ii,** 552 (1971).
21. Pearson, G. and Freeman, G. *Cancer Res.*, **28,** 1665 (1968).
22. Brawn, R. J. *Int. J. Cancer*, **6,** 245 (1970).
23. Coggin, J. H., Ambrose, K. R. and Anderson, N. G. *J. Idmmnol.*, **105,** 524 (1970).
24. Duff, R. and Rapp, F. *J. Immunol.*, **105,** 521 (1970).
25. Stonehill, E. H. and Bendich, A. *Nature*, **228,** 370 (1970).
26. Hirzfeld, L. *Z. Immunitätsforsch.*, **64,** 81 (1929).
27. Omenn, G. S. and Wilkins, E. W. *J. Thorac. Cardiovas. Surg.*, **59,** 877 (1970).
28. Hauger-Klevene, J. H. *Cancer*, **22,** 1262 (1968).
29. Cottrell, J. C., Becker, K. L. Matthews, M. J. and Moore, C. *Am. J. clin. Path.*, **6,** 720 (1969).
30. Teilum, G. *Special Tumors of Ovary and Testis.* Copenhagen: Munksgaard. p. 33. (1971).
31. Ballas, M. *Am. J. clin. Path.*, **57,** 511 (1972).
32. Gold, P. and Freedman, S. O. *J. exp. Med.*, **121,** 439 (1965a).
33. Gold, P. and Freedman, S. O. *J. exp. Med.*, **122,** 467 (1965b).
34. Gold, P., Gold, M. and Freedman, S. O. *Cancer Res.*, **28,** 1331 (1968).
35. Gold, P., Krupey, J. and Ansari, H. *J. Nat. Cancer Inst.*, **45,** 219 (1970).
36. Von Kliest, S. and Burtin, P. *Cancer Res.*, **29,** 1961 (1969a).
37. Von Kliest, S. and Burtin, P. *Int. J. Cancer*, **4,** 874 (1969b).
38. Reynoso, G., Chu, T. M., Holyoke, D., Cohen, E., Nemoto, T., Wang, J-J., Chuang, J., Guinan, P. and Murphy, G. *J. Am. med. Assn.*, **220,** 361 (1972).
39. Hall, R. R., Laurence, D. J. R., Darcy, S., Stevens U., James, R., Roberts, S. and Neville, A. M. *Br. Med. J.*, **3,** 609 (1972).
40. Buffe, D., Rimbault, C., Lemerle, J., Schweisguth, O. and Burtin, P. *Int. J. Cancer*, **5,** 85 (1970).
41. Martin, J. P., Charlionet, R. and Ropartz, C. *Rev. Europ. Etudes Clin. et Biol.*, **26,** 266 (1971).
42. Wada, T., Anzai, T., Yachi, A., Takahashi, A. and Sakamoto, S. In *Protides*

of the Biological Fluids. Ed. H. Peeters. Oxford: Pergamon Press. p. 221. (1971).
43. Takahashi, A. Yashi, A., Anzai, T. and Wada, T. *Clin. Chim. Acta*, **17,** 5 (1967).
44. Edynak, E. M., Lardis, M. P. and Vrana, M. *Cancer*, **28,** 1457 (1972).
45. Harris, R., Viza, D., Todd, R., Phillips, J., Sugar, R., Jennison, R. F., Marriott, G. and Gleeson, M. H. *Nature*, **233,** 556.
46. Davidson, J. F., McNicol, G. P., Frank, G. L., Anderson, T. J. and Douglas, A. S. *Br. med. J.*, **1,** 88 (1969).
47. Leese, C. L. *Ciba Foundation Symposium on Homeostatic Regulators*. Ed. G. E. W. Wolstenholme and J. Knight. p. 144. (1969).
48. Fishman, W. H., Inglis, N. R., Green, S., Antiss, C. L., Gosh, N. K., Reif, A. E., Rustigan, R., Kraut, M. J. and Stolback, L. L. *Nature*, **219,** 697 (1968).
49. Melvin, K. E. W., Tashjian, A. H., Cassidy, C. E. and Givens, J. R. *Metabolism*, **19,** 831 (1970).
50. Croughs, R. J. M., Eastham, W. N., Hackeng, W. H. L., Schopman, W., Feltkamp-Vroom, T. M., Dolman, A. and Hennemann, G. *Clin. Endocrinol.*, **1,** 157.
51. O'Neal, L. W., Kipnis, D. M., Luse, S. A., Lacy, P. E. and Jarett, L. *Cancer*, **21,** 1219 (1968).
52. Warnock, M. and Reesman, R. *Clin. Chim. Acta*, **24,** 5 (1969).
53. Purves, L. R., MacHab, M. and Bersohn, I. *S. Afr. J. Med.,* **42,** 1138 (1968).
54. Nathanson, L. and Fishman, W. H. *Cancer*, **27,** 1388 (1971).
55. Laurence, D. J. R., Stevens, U., Bettelheim, R., Darcy, D., Leese, C., Turberville, C., Alexander, P., Johns, E. W. and Neville, A. M. *Br. med. J.*, **3,** 605 (1972).
56. Zamchek, N., Moore, T. L., Dhar, P. and Kupchik, H. *New Engl. J. Med.*, **286,** 83 (1972).
57. Buckle, R. M., McMillan, M. and Mallinson, C. *Br. med. J.*, **4,** 724 (1970).
58. Knill-Jones, R. P., Buckle, R. M. and Parsons, V. *New Engl. J. Med.*, **282,** 704 (1970).
59. George, J. M. and Capen, C. C. *J. clin. Invest.*, **51,** 141 (1972).
60. Greenberg, P. B., Martin, T. J., Beck, C. and Burger, H. G. *Lancet*, **i,** 350 (1972).
60a. Liddle, G. W., Givens, J. R., Nicholson, W. E. and Island, D. P. *Cancer Res.*, **25,** 1057 (1965).
61. Tashjian, A. H. Jnr. *Biotechnol. Bioeng.*, **11,** 109 (1969).
62. Todd, C. W. Personal communication (1972).
63. Corrin, B. and McMillan, M. *Br. J. Cancer*, **24,** 755 (1970).
64. Kay, S. and Willson, M. A. *Cancer*, **26,** 445 (1970).
65. Johnston, W. H. and Waisman, J. *Cancer*, **27,** 681 (1971).
66. Gusev, A. I. Engelhardt, N. V., Masseyeff, R., Camain, R. and Basteris, S. *Int. J. Cancer*, **7,** 207 (1971).
67. Nishioka, M., Ibata, T., Okita, K., Harada, T. and Fujita, T. *Cancer Res.*, **32,** 162 (1972).
68. Cameron, D. P., Burger, H. G., DeKretzer, D. M., Catt, K. J. and Best, J. B. *Australas. Ann. Med.*, **18,** 143 (1969).
69. Knight, R. A., Ratcliffe, J. G. and Besser, G. M. *Proc. Roy. Soc. Med.*, **64,** 52 (1971).
70. Roof, B. S., Carpenter, B., Fink, D. J. and Gordan, G. S. *Am. J. Med.*, **50,** 636 (1971).

71. Shapiro, M., Nicholson, W. E., Orth, D. N., Mitchell, W. M. and Liddle, G. W. *J. Clin. Endocr.*, **33,** 377 (1971).
72. Nishi, S. *Cancer Res.*, **30,** 2507 (1970).
73. Rüoslahti, E., Seppälä, M., Pihko, H. and Vuopio, P. *Int. J. Cancer*, **8,** 283 (1971).
74. Engelhardt, N. V., Shipova, L. Ya., Gusev, A. I., Yazova, A. K. and Ter-Grigorova, E. N. *Byull. Eksp. Biol. Med.,* **68,** 62 (1969).
75. Hull, E., Carbone, P., Gitlin, D., O'Gara, R. and Kelly, M. *J. Nat. Cancer Inst.*, **42,** 1035 (1969).
76. Kroes, R. and Weisburger, J. H. *Proc. Am. Ass. Cancer Res.*, **13,** 53 (1972).
77. Abelev, G. I., Perova, S. D., Bakirov, R. D. and Irlin, I. S. In *Specific Tumor Antigens.* Ed. R. J. C. Harris. UICC Monograph Series. Copenhagen: Munksgaard. Vol. **2,** p. 32. (1967).
78. Purves, L. R., Bersohn, I. and Geddes, E. W. *Cancer*, **25,** 1261 (1970).
79. Mawas, C., Buffe, D., Schweisguth, O. and Burtin, P. (1971). quoted by Abelev (1971).
80. Martin, F., Martin, M. S., Bordes, M. and Bourgeaux, C. *Europ. J. Cancer*, **8,** 315.
81. Nairn, R. C., Fothergill, J. E., McEntegart, M. G. and Richmond, H. G. *Br. med. J.*, **1,** 1791 (1962).
82. Burtin, P., Von Kliest, S. and Sabine, C. *Cancer Res.*, **31,** 1038 (1971).
83. LoGerfo, P., LoGerfo, F., Herter, F., Barker, H. G. and Hansen, H. J. *Am. J. Surg.*, **123,** 127 (1972).
84. Kim, U. and Carruthers, C. *Proc. Am. Assoc. Cancer Res.*, **13,** 69 (1972).
85. Azzopardi, J. G. and Williams, E. D. *Cancer*, **22,** 274 (1968).
86. Bensch, K. G., Gordon, G. B. and Miller, L. R. *Cancer*, **18,** 592 (1965a).
87. Goldenberg, V. E., Goldenberg, N. S. and Benditt, E. P. *Cancer*, **24,** 236 (1969).
88. Pearse, A. G. E. *Vet. Rec.*, **79,** 587 (1966).
89. Pearse, A. G. E. *J. Histochem. Cytochem.*, **17,** 303 (1969).
90. Coupland, R. E. *The Natural History of the Chromaffin Cell.* London: Longmans. (1965).
91. Polak, J. M., Rost, F U. D. and Pearse, A. G. E. *Gen. Comp. Endocr.*, **16,** 132 (1971).
92. LeDouarin, N. and LeLievre, C. *Compte. rendus.*, **270,** Serie D., 2857 (1970).
93. Andrews, A. *J. Embryol. exp. Morph.*, **11,** 307 (1963).
94. LeDouarin, N. Personal communication (1972).
94a. Williams, E. D. *J. clin. Path.*, **18,** 288 (1965).
95. Hage, E. *Acta path. microb. scand.* 80*A*, 225.
96. Bensch, K. G., Gordon, G. B. and Miller, L. R. *J. Ultrastruct. Res.*, **12,** 668 (1965b).
97. Pearse, A. G. E. *Advances Pharmacol.*, **6,** 156 (1968).
98. Melick, R. A., Martin, T. J. and Hicks, J. D. *Br. med. J.*, **2,** 204 (1972).
99. Rudnick, P. and Odell, W. D. *New Engl. J. Med.*, **284,** 405 (1971).
99a. Hauger-Klevene, J. H. *Cancer*, **26,** 1112 (1970).
100. Sparagana, M., Phillips, G., Hoffman, C. and Kucera, L. *Metabolism*, **20,** 730 (1971).
101. Hennen, G. *J. Clin. Endocr.*, **27,** 610 (1967).
102. Britten, R. J. and Davidson, E. H. *Quart. Rev. Biol.*, **46,** 111 (1971).
103. Fialkow, P. J., Martin, G. M., Klein, G., Clifford, P. and Singh, S. *Int. J. Cancer,* **9,** 133 (1972).

104. Bagshawe, K. D. *Choriocarcinoma: The Clinical Biology of the Trophoblast and its Tumour*. London: Arnold. (1969).
105. Houstek, J., Masopust, J., Kithier, K. and Radi, J. *J. Ped.*, **72,** 186 (1968).
106. Khasanov, A. I., Abelev, G. I., Perova, S. D., Polenko, V. K., Ryapsova, U. K. and Shirenkova, O. (1971) quoted by Abelev, G. I. (1971).
107. Abelev, G. I., Tsvetkov, V. S., Biryulina, T. I., Elgort, D. A. Olovnikov, A. M., Gusev, A. I., Yazova, A. K., Perova, S. D. Rubtsov, I. V., Kantorovich, B. A., Tur, V., Khasanov, A. I. and Levina, D. M. *Byull. Eksp. Biol. Med.*, **71,** 75 (1971).
108. Seppälä, M. and Ruoslahti, E. *Am. J. Obstet. Gynec.*, **112,** 208 (1972a).
109. Seppälä, M. and Ruoslahti, E. *Lancet*, **i,** 375 (1972b).
110. LoGerfo, P., Krupey, J. and Hansen, H. J. *New Engl. J. Med.*, **285,** 138 (1971).
111. Moore, T. L., Kupchik, H. Z., Marcon, N. and Zamchek, N. *Am. J. Dig. Dis.*, **16,** 1 (1971).
112. Cullen, D. R. and Tomlinson, B. E. *Postgrad, med. J.*, **44,** 472 (1968).
113. Law, D. H., Liddle, G. W., Scott, H. W. and Tauber, S. D. *New Engl. J. Med.*, **273,** 292 (1965).
114. Marks, V., Samols, E. and Bolton, R. *Br. med. J.*, **1,** 1419 (1965).
115. Salama, F., Luke, R. G. and Hellebusch, A. A. *J. Urol.*, **106,** 820 (1971).
116. Unger, R. H., Lochner, J. and Eisentraut, A. M. *J. Clin. Endocr.*, **24,** 823 (1964).
117. Dukes, C. In *Cancer*. Ed. R. W. Raven. London: Butterworth, Vol. **2,** p. 136 (1958).
118. Kaplan, E. L., Arnaud, C. D., Hill, B. J. and Peskin, G. W. *Surgery*, **68,** 146 (1970).

Chapter **8**

THE EPIDEMIOLOGY OF CANCER

C. A. LINSELL, M.B., B.S., D.C.P., F.R.C.Path.
Chief, Nairobi Research Centre, International Agency for Research on Cancer, Kenya

---

'*Prodigies are always seen in proportion as they are expected.*' Samuel Johnson.

Although the first systematic collection of cancer statistics dates from a census in London in 1728 and Pott gave his classic description of the occupational hazard of chimney sweeps to contract scrotal cancer in 1775[1], it is surprising that the general application of epidemiology to the study of cancer was delayed so long. For many years, epidemiology was limited to consideration of epidemics but the subject subsequently grew to include more general studies of non-infectious diseases in populations or communities; of these, cancer is now a notable example.

It has been suggested that the majority of human cancers are initiated by potentially removable environmental agents (Higginson, 1968[2]—see also Chapters 1 and 9) and prevention of at least some forms of cancer is now feasible. The demonstration of any extrinsic factor as 'the cause' of a particular human cancer is, however, difficult as a direct experimental approach cannot be adopted in man. Much stress has to be attached to fortunately rare events such as whole body irradiation from atomic bombs, the iatrogenic radiological exposure of the foetus during treatment of the mother, or the use of immuno-suppressive drugs. One must therefore rely—and this can serve as a general definition of epidemiology— on the interpretation of 'natural experiments' to identify risk factors, or on analogies derived from laboratory animal experimentation. The former will be the main subject of this chapter.

The use of experimental data and its extrapolation to man has been the subject of much discussion. Man may appear to have many similarities—anatomical, physiological and immunological—to other animals and, even at the subcellular level, molecular structure and enzyme function may be paralleled; yet the suitability of animal models for problems of human carcinogenesis must be questioned. The utility of animal experiments where, for example, genetic or dietary factors can be controlled, is undoubted, for in man the variations and combinations of these two factors alone may make it difficult to standardize a human risk factor. As the number of variables in the uncontrolled human experiment is large, the difficulties in extrapolating from an experiment of, say, 300–500 animals (a large laboratory experiment by current standards) to many millions of human subjects may be almost overwhelming, particularly when it is recalled that the animals used in such experiments are as homogeneous as modern science can make them.

Although it can be said that almost all agents carcinogenic in man are also active in appropriate animal models—the classic exception is arsenic—the reverse situation cannot be assumed to exist. The number of agents first shown to be carcinogenic in animals which have subsequently been demonstrated to cause cancer in man is small. This may seem surprising, but many of the carcinogens tested were devised in the laboratory and primarily studied to demonstrate biological correlations; the overall risk to man from such artificial agents was naturally minimal. Furthermore, the compounds tested were often very potent or were used in unnaturally high doses. Any possibility that exposure of man will take place is obviously prevented by the personal intervention of the scientists involved and by legislation. An example is afforded by 2-acetylaminofluorene which in 1940 was shown to be a potentially useful insecticide; it was later found to be a potent and versatile carcinogen (Weisberger, 1958[3]). If its dangerous potential had not been recognized and its widespread use in the environment forbidden, an exceptional hazard might have been created. Such situations must reinforce the necessity for animal testing of chemicals used in public health campaigns, in medicine generally and in food production (see also Chapter 9). Risk-benefit assessments are often necessary in deciding whether agents suspected of carcinogenic activity on the basis of animal tests should continue to be allowed for human use, and these may pose complex problems.

It is inappropriate to discuss theories of causation of cancer here but, to illustrate the utility of epidemiology, a comment from Sir Macfarlane Burnet (1969)[4] may be quoted—'Cancer arises as an accidental by-product of the very essence of life and evolution'. Epidemiology can assist in the measurement of the circumstances surrounding this accident, and it can be used to assess the possibilities of chance being responsible for the 'prodigies' scorned by Dr. Johnson in the eighteenth century. The aetiology of cancer is recognized as the complex interplay of a number of factors which are ultimately responsible for the escape of cells from normal control mechanisms, their abnormal replication, and their excessive growth. Epidemiology can be employed to separate some of these factors into measurable entities, and it remains the most effective means of identifying environmental carcinogens. Except in the field of industrial hazards, prevention unfortunately tends to depend on the reversal of social or personal customs and we are only just beginning to appreciate the difficulties that such changes entail.

The theoretical basis of cancer epidemiology

Epidemiology is used in the investigation of disease to establish a relationship between initial biological events and subsequent disease. It produces the basis for a hypothesis primarily by describing a clinical problem in terms of its incidence in a community. After a study of the variation of incidence of a given disease between individuals, communities or populations of different geographical regions, and of the influence of age distribution and time trends, formulation of a hypothesis may be justified. The next phase will be the evaluation of this hypothesis which will call for all the resources of analytical epidemiology and the assessment of specific hazards of the environment, internal or external, which are inherent in the hypothesis. There may be selection of cases and comparison with controls to assess the significance or otherwise of the presence of the suspect factor; or investigations can be designed to measure directly the risk of developing the disease in a population, some members of which will be exposed while others will be free from the influence of the aetiological agent or mechanism. The first type of study is commonly termed 'retrospective' and mainly uses comparative studies of past experience of individual cases; the second considers 'prospectively' whether selected individuals have or have not the characteristics to be investigated and follows them for a period of time to determine the morbidity or mortality of the disease. Investigation of a problem usually begins with a retrospective consideration of available data, a procedure that is less expensive in time and money than a prospective study. When the evidence favouring a particular factor is strong, derived either from a retrospective survey or from other data, then more detailed and reliable information can be sought by a prospective investigation. The expectations from prospective studies of cancer will be influenced by the large numbers of subjects required to attain statistical significance (cases may be few) and by the long latent period of induction. Retrospective studies have the disadvantages that they must rely on the often uncertain memory of past events, and it is difficult to avoid bias in the design of questions and in the methods of eliciting answers. Prospective studies designate the individuals with the factor, and personal bias is avoided since data are recorded before the result is known. The principles and detailed methods of such studies are dealt with in 'Methods of Epidemiology' (MacMahon *et al.*, 1961[5]) and, particularly for cancer in 'Cancer Epidemiology: Methods of Study'. (Lilienfeld *et al.*, 1967[6]).

The practice of epidemiology in cancer research

DEFINITION OF A CANCER CASE

Cancer is not a single disease but a collection of many different clinico-pathological entities. Even a broad definition may be difficult; as Virchow remarked, 'No man can say, even under torture, what exactly a tumour is' (Ewing, 1916[7]). In view of the problems of precise biological definition reliance has to be placed on the accumulated experience of clinicians and pathologists to supply the current concept of an individual neoplasm. It is particularly important, therefore, to decide on diagnostic criteria and classification before applying statistical methods.

CLASSIFICATION OF NEOPLASMS

An aetiological classification would be the most informative but, as this is the aspect of neoplasia most in question, the following more prosaic groupings are used:

1. anatomical site of the primary tumour
2. histological type
3. stage of the disease.

The type of classification chosen will depend on the particular tumour and the type of study. In the study of oesophageal cancer, for example, anatomical location is important: although the histopathology of oesophageal cancers may be reasonably uniform, aetiology and clinical progress depend on precisely where they arise in the oesophagus—the upper, middle or lower thirds. In contrast, for primary liver tumours in adults (which can develop from either hepatic parenchyma or bile duct epithelium) a histological classification is useful: cancers of the intrahepatic biliary tract may be associated with liver flukes as opposed to those of the hepatic parenchyma where toxic agents (viral or chemical) are suspect.

ANATOMICAL CLASSIFICATION

The most widely used classification of anatomical site is detailed in the International Classification of Diseases, Injuries and Causes (I.C.D.) provided by the World Health Organization. It is not, however, possible to classify all neoplasms solely by site—for example, malignancies of the reticuloendothelial system—and, for such neoplasms, the I.C.D. merges into an histological classification. There are many difficulties associated with classifications of cancer, principally because of the differences in diagnostic criteria sometimes used by clinicians, pathologists, and radiologists in defining a specific disease entity. These problems are discussed in the introduction to 'Cancer Incidence in Five Continents (Doll *et al.*, 1970[8]), a collection of material from a number of cancer registries throughout the world. The authors of this important study emphasize that difficulties of classification, coding and other registration technicalities are often preventable and that future registries could be much more valuable once international agreement was reached on nomenclature and classification.

HISTOLOGICAL CLASSIFICATION

Neoplasms from the same anatomical site may show a wide range of histological appearances. Not only has it been shown that aetiology may vary markedly in different histological types—notably in cancers of the lung, liver and bladder and in the leukaemias—but it is also clear that accurate histological classification may be of prognostic value. Classifications designed by the American Cancer Society and the Union Internationale Contre le Cancer (U.I.C.C.) are widely used and, to demonstrate the need for international agreement, the World Health Organization has established reference centres to assess and publicize standard nomenclature and histological classifications. But even when agreement on classification has been reached, there is still the problem of individual interpretation of histological material. In any analytical study, close liaison must be established between clinicians and pathologists and among the researchers themselves to ensure that error between observers is minimized, and that by blind review the diagnoses of individual pathologists are consistent. The difficulties associated with the definition and classification of Burkitt's lymphoma illustrate the problem. Aetiological research on Burkitt's lymphoma depended on whether or not this tumour was unique to particular areas in Africa (as originally suggested) and whether it could be separated from other reticuloendothelial malignancies. A group of pathologists experienced in the diagnosis of Burkitt lymphoma were able to establish that this tumour was, indeed, occasionally seen in other areas of the world and that a working definition of diagnostic criteria could be established (Bulletin of the W.H.O.[9]).

CLASSIFICATION BY STAGE OF DISEASE

This form of classification is mainly used by those interested in clinical trials and the assessment of therapy. It may be based on clinical assessment alone or together with information from other investigative procedures (e.g. radiology) and from subsequent surgery and histopathology. This method of staging is clearly subject to individual bias since those using it are themselves intimately involved in the study and its success.

A standard scheme is provided by the TNM System (T—Primary Tumour, N—Regional Lymph Node, M—Distant Metastases), first described by Denoix (1940)[10] and later developed by the Classification Committee of the U.I.C.C. Whereas the classification of cancers of accessible sites presents few difficulties, those of deeper origin pose special problems which have been reviewed by Sellars (1971)[11].

Although in summary it must be recognized that the definition, nomenclature and classification of cancers is complex, the present lack of uniformity perhaps owes as much to the tenacity of individual prejudice as to any inherent problems.

Descriptive epidemiology

Fully appreciating the difficulties of the definition and classification of a 'case', the methods of computing measurements of cancer in populations are now reviewed. These are usually expressed as rates.

RATES

The construction of a rate requires a numerator—the number of persons with cancer; a denominator—the population in which the cancer cases are observed; and a time factor. Incidence rates which provide a direct measurement of the probability of developing cancer are particularly important in the study of aetiology. An incidence rate for lung cancer per 100,000 per year is expressed as—

$$\frac{\text{number of new cases developing lung cancer in the year } \mathbf{X}}{\text{the number of persons exposed to the risk of developing lung cancer in that year}} \times 100{,}000$$

It is necessary for the numerator and denominator to be restricted to the same terms. For example, if the denominator in the above fraction is the population of a defined area, then every precaution must be taken to ensure that the numerator consists only of cases from that area. When assessing the validity of such rates one has to consider not only the question of case definition but the sociological background of the populations from which the data are derived. Factors influencing the numerator will be the type and quality of available medical services (both diagnostic and therapeutic), and the ability and willingness of the population to present themselves for medical care. The definition of the population or denominator may be difficult as it need not be a 'population' in the strict demographic sense. It may be a group with a special characteristic such as an occupation which, nevertheless, can be considered the related population at risk. Demography is a complex subject which cannot be discussed here and specialized text-books (Cox (1959)[12], Yeats (1953)[13] and Lilienfeld *et al.* (1967)[64]—also the demographic year-book of the United Nations Organization) should be consulted.

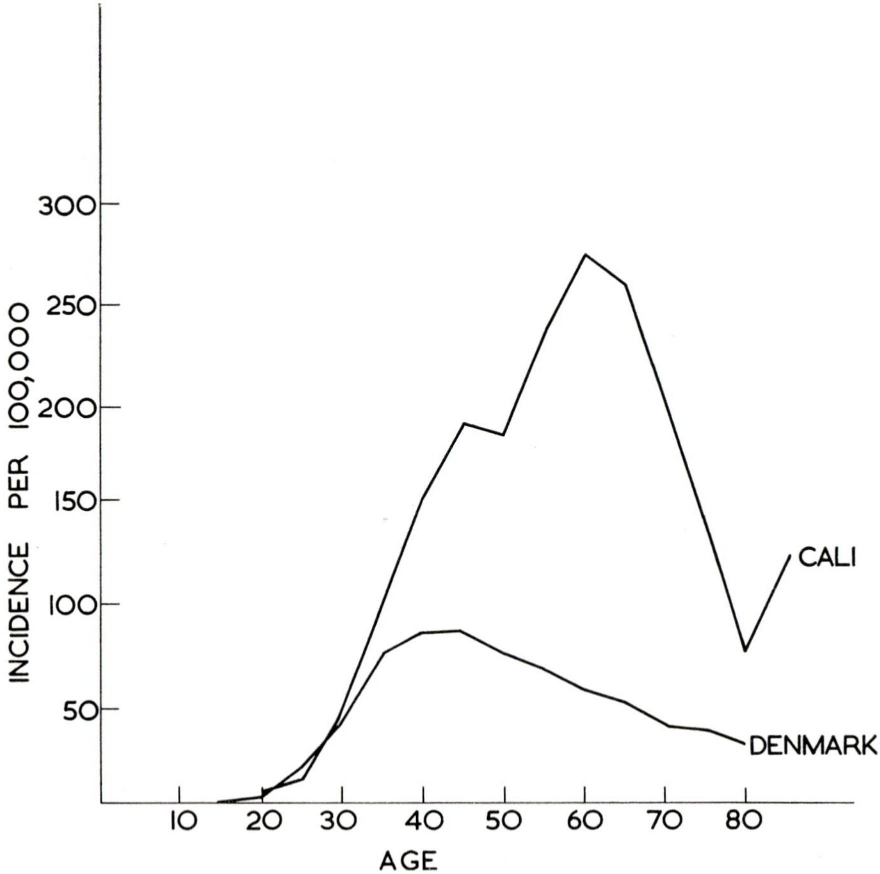

Fig. 8.1. Age incidence of cancer of cervix uteri in Cali (Columbia) and Denmark: source—Cancer in Five Continents (8).

AGE

Age is an important variable in evaluating statistics of cancer and the study of its effects have formed the basis for theoretical models of carcinogenesis (Doll 1971[14]). The influence of age distribution within a population on crude rates is so strong that other variables cannot be assessed unless this is eliminated. This is done by the use of age-specific rates or 'standardization' to adjust for the differences of age structure of the populations to be computed. Bio-statistical text-books (Hill, 1970[15]; Bailey, 1959[16]) should be consulted for details of methods. Birth registration is not obligatory in some countries and age assessment is often inaccurate. Calendars of events familiar to the population and which can be related to the birth of a child have been found useful for checking age in such circumstances.

The age incidence pattern of a cancer can be examined for aetiological clues. *Figure 8.1* shows the incidence of cancer of the cervix in Cali, Columbia and Denmark. As the curve falls sharply in the latter years it would appear that either the tumour is not the consequence of uniform exposure to some carcinogenic stimulus throughout adult life, or that those over forty-five in Denmark or over sixty in Columbia are less susceptible to the effects of such a stimulus. It is also reasonable to suggest that a continuous hazard starting in the teens is maintained in Denmark up to forty-five years and to sixty in Columbia, after which it is less effective. The decline after forty-five in Denmark may parallel the menopause but speculation that this is the sole factor in both Denmark and Columbia is hardly tenable as this physiological condition would have to be grossly disturbed to explain the age trend in Columbia. If an initiating event some twenty years before the development of the cancer is postulated to account for the peak, then we must explain why it is fifteen years later in Columbian women—or else suggest an entirely different aetiology. *Figure 8.2,* showing the age distribution of cancer of the penis, illustrates the typical increase with age which is found with many cancers. Cook *et al.* (1969)[17] examined the shape of age incidence curves for a number of cancers using information from various sources and suggested that the genesis of tumours of the alimentary tract, skin and penis was related at least in part to continuous exposure to environmental agents. There have been studies linking these two cancers—cervix and penis—Martinez (1969)[18] reporting eight wives of 889 men with cancer of the penis having cancer of the cervix compared with none in a control population. If there are some common factors of aetiology then there must indeed be other profound differences.

It has been suggested that the shape of the age curve is determined largely by:

(i) the length of the latent period
(ii) the age at which exposure first takes place
(iii) the intensity of the initiating event.

Hueper (1952)[19] considered that the long latent period found in most cancers make it inevitable that most neoplasms should occur in the older age groups, even if exposure was first effective at birth.

The events that take place during the latent period of neoplasia are ill understood and difficult to interpret. It seems likely that host factors are important in cancer where many may be exposed yet a limited number exhibit the disease, an aspect that has been emphasized by Burnet (1970)[20] and by Doll (1970)[21]. Many patients with advanced cancer are immunologically incompetent, perhaps as a consequence of a premature failure of immune surveillance (Levin *et al.*, 1964[22]), though direct evidence for this attractive

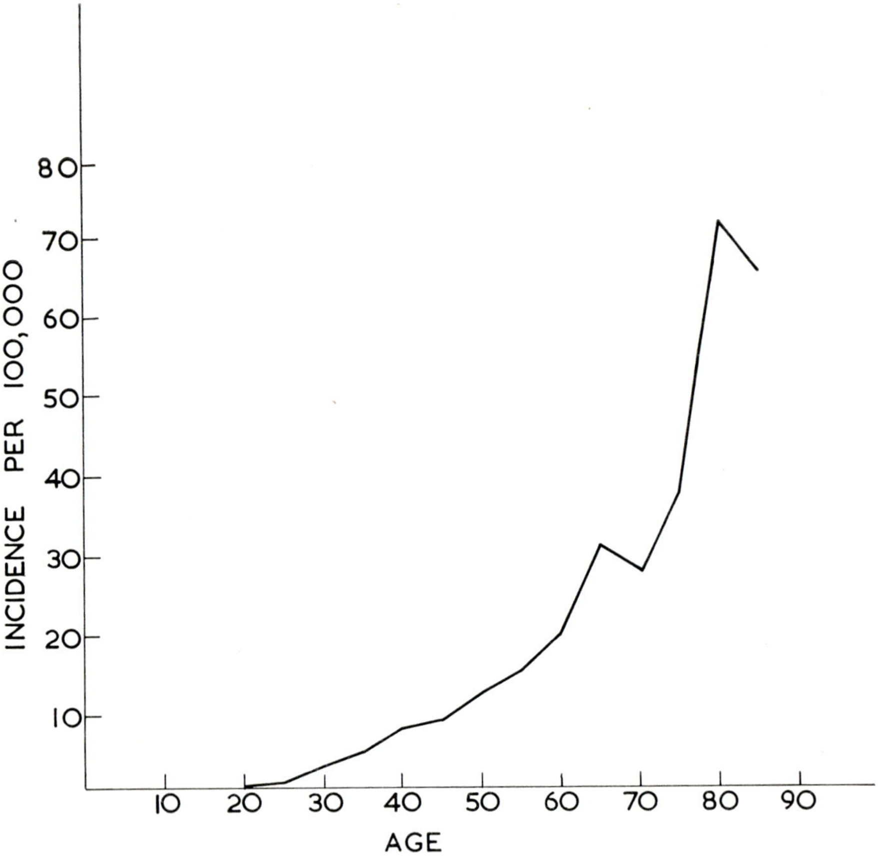

Fig. 8.2. Age incidence of cancer of the penis in Puerto Rico: source— Martinez (18).

view is scanty. But if one postulates a physiological exhaustion of immune surveillance with ageing, this itself may be one factor regulating clinical emergence of a cancer and responsible for the increased incidence of cancer at the end of the life span. The latent period which is broadly equivalent to the incubation period of an infection, is characteristically prolonged in malignant disease. From studies on the relationship of cigarette smoking and lung cancer, the latent period for bronchogenic carcinoma is thought to be approximately 20–40 years; and the association between sideropenic dysphagia and cancer of the hypopharynx indicates that a disease manifested at puberty may lay the foundation for the development of cancer in the fifth and sixth decade. The tumours of children, of course, show shorter latent periods. Studies on identical twins developing acute leukaemia during the first year of life suggest that, following the first case, the twin is at a high risk to develop leukaemia within months. This risk seems to be associated with the body's initial (ill-understood) defence against the reponsible aetiological agent(s); the risk fades rapidly with age, and disappears entirely after the age of six (Miller, 1971[23]). The evaluation of frequency curves of acute leukaemia, neuroblastoma and Wilm's tumour (nephroblastoma) indicates that many of these childhood malignancies are likely to have been initiated during intra-uterine life. Increase in cancer risk as a result of prenatal influences is indicated by the observation of Herbst *et al.* (1971)[24], of a high risk of adenocarcinoma of the vagina following exposure of the mother to large doses of stilboestrol during early pregnancy (see also I.A.R.C. monograph on transplacental carcinogenesis, 1973)[25].

MORBIDITY AND MORTALITY STATISTICS

There are two main sources of information on the occurrence of cancer—morbidity studies and mortality statistics. Although one would expect mortality statistics to be the method of choice for the examination of an invariably fatal disease, progress in treatment makes mortality statistics increasingly inadequate as a measure of cancer incidence and emphasis is increasingly being transferred to morbidity studies. Information from mortality statistics must be limited to that provided by official death certification, a procedure that varies widely in content and accuracy. A valuable extension of the study of morbidity has been the etablishment of cancer registries to assess incidence. However, mortality statistics remain indispensable for international comparisons and they may be the final arbiters of whether a particular regimen of diagnosis or treatment has been effective. Steinitz and Costin (1971)[26] compared the mortality of cancer from vital statistics of the Central Bureau of Statistics with those of the Israel Cancer Registry and found marked discrepancies, illustrating the care which must be exercised in interpretation.

MORBIDITY STUDIES

Information on the occurrence of cancer to give the numerator of a rate is available from various sources.

Hospital studies

Case histories can be collected from hospital records and, although the value of this information is limited, it may be the only source available—particularly in developing countries where epidemiological studies are of increasing importance in cancer research. Such record retrieval is simple to operate but it is not a reliable index of cancer frequency because the population served by a given hospital is seldom well-defined. Socioeconomic factors may influence attendance, and special facilities and skills of the hospital may further bias the numbers or pattern of cancer cases detected. If figures for head and neck cancer are compared in Bombay between the Tata Memorial Hospital specializing in cancer treatment (Paymaster, 1967[27]) and the Bombay Cancer Registry, the hospital data show these tumours to represent 44 per cent of all cancers as opposed to 28 per cent in the local cancer registry. When mouth and tongue cancers are compared the frequency of cancer in the hospital material is twice as high as that of the registry. And, as mentioned earlier, the initial diagnosis of cancer may be inaccurate (see Bauer & Robbins, 1972[28]).

Pathological material—biopsy and autopsy studies

Although diagnoses from pathological material have one major advantage—that they can be readily reassessed—the interpretation of data from biopsy collections must be cautious as there may be an artificially high proportion of tumours from readily accessible sites. In addition, factors such as age, sex, and nearness of residence to hospital will determine which patients present themselves for biopsy. Even in countries with well-developed health services, the proportion of all recognized cancers submitted to biopsy varies widely. (McMahan (1963)[29], reviewing the bias of selection associated with autopsy series, considered that as such data could not be referred to a definite population, no estimate of cancer frequency could be made. The examination of biopsy and autopsy material can, however, give important extra information on the occurrence of occult cancers and of suspicious 'precancerous lesions'. Despite inherent biases, the examination of pathological and hospital series has yielded much interesting information—particularly proportional frequencies illustrating regional variations of cancer patterns. Although many reviews of cancer data are presented as relative or proportional frequencies, caution must be emphasized in their interpretation as unqualified estimates of the risk of developing cancer. An extreme case is illustrated in Table 8.1.

Table 8.1. The difference in meaning of relative frequencies and rates

	Population A			Population B		
Primary site	*Incidence rate per 100,000 population*	*Computed number of cases*	*Per cent of total*	*Incidence rate per 100,000 population*	*Computed number of cases*	*Per cent of total*
	1	2	3	4	5	6
Lung	20	16	10.0	20	30	6.7
Breast	60	48	30.0	60	90	20.9
Uterus	50	40	25.0	50	75	16.7
All other	70	56	35.0	170	255	56.6
Total	200	160	100.0	300	450	100.0

Source: Dorn, H. F. 1955. J.Chron.Dis., 1, 638.

Despite the fact that the three cancers are more frequent relative to all cancers in population A as compared with B, their incidence is the same in both populations. The difficulty with proportional rates is that the proportion of one type of cancer is affected by an increase or decrease of other types. Methods of assessing these anomalies by a restriction of the age groups studied and, when there is an extremely high incidence of a particular type of cancer, of expressing this as a proportion of all other cancers rather than as a proportion of the total cancers is discussed by Doll (1968)[30].

Cancer registries

To overcome difficulties in interpreting data obtained solely from hospital or laboratory records, population-based cancer registries have been established in a number of countries. The cancer registry collects information on all cancer detected in a selected population from hospital and laboratory records, from general practitioners, from social services, and from the examination of death certificates. As it is essentially prospective in nature, attempts can be made to provide information which would not be available from either medical records or death certification. For example, information of a social or ethnic nature can be recorded, the significance of which is often vaguely recognized when the registry is first set up. It is true that population-based cancer registries are both complex and expensive but they should not be limited to developed countries with comprehensive health and social services and effective demography. In developing countries, registries can indicate opportunities for vital environmental studies and provide essential data for field work which can often only be established in these societies remote from industrialization. Indeed the position of developing countries is one of crucial importance. The patterns of cancer in such regions must be 'established as soon as possible, since the close contacts with the environment have already began to be broken and local cultural differences are fast disappearing. It is, however, not too late to grasp the present unique opportunities, since much cancer would seem to result from a lifetime of exposure to some environmental stimulus and, in the study of tumours developing today, the way of life twenty or thirty years ago is perhaps more relevant than are present conditions' (Cook and Burkitt, 1971[31]) Short term surveys of various kinds may be valuable in examining specific problems and they are particularly useful when there is little cancer data, where medical services are rudimentary, and demographic information is virtually non-existent. *Ad hoc* surveys in the United States have shown good correlation with cancer registries, except that registries tend to lose cases by under-reporting and surveys may overestimate by including cases diagnosed before the start of the survey. Mass examination of populations to assess the prevalence of all cancers, or cancers from a specific site, requires considerable administrative effort and expense but it may be the only feasible method of obtaining information.

MORTALITY STUDIES

These are mainly derived from the official death certificates which are obligatory in many countries. Although there have been international attempts to standardize the diagnoses recorded, great variation of detail is encountered. In addition to the cause of death, there is usually information about sex, date and place of death, residence, occupation and marital state. If an adequate census is available, death rates from the various types of cancer can be computed, and a pattern of cancer mortality delineated. The use of mortality statistics to illustrate geographical or regional patterns of cancer presents many difficulties. Although official statistics are collected within defined political boundaries, it is clear that disease will not be so confined. The broad patterns obtained by comparison of mortality statistics have proved valuable but only when the rates can be assumed to indicate incidence. Whereas the death rate computed from mortality statistics for a rapidly fatal cancer such as bronchial carcinoma may closely reflect incidence, the relationship between mortality and incidence rates of carcinoma of the skin will be poor. Mortality statistics are available regularly from the World Health Organization Epidemiological and Vital Statistics Reports. The collection of mortality statistics from twenty-four countries by Segi *et al.* (1969)[32] and from urban areas of fifteen Soviet Republics by Merkov *et al.* (1963)[33] are particularly useful. The problem of the choice of standard populations for age adjustment has been greatly aided by the acceptance of Segi's standard population and the standard African population as devised by Knowelden (1962)[32]. The usefulness of mortality patterns as clues to aetiology is proportional to the order of magnitude of the differences in age-adjusted rates. The finding that age-adjusted rates of stomach cancer among males in Japan is 67·5 per 100,000 compared with 16·3 for U.S. Whites (Haenszel, 1958[35]), cannot fail to excite interest in spite of the problems which are inherent in the registration of deaths from this type of cancer. However, reliable mortality rates are often not available in situations which may offer the most intriguing contrasts. This deficiency dictates that information from all sources—cancer registries, special surveys and hospital or pathological records—should be collected for assessment.

DISTRIBUTION BY OCCUPATION

The evaluation of occupation and its relation to cancer is usually only possible when vital and health statistics are of a high standard. Occupation is a major element of the definition of social class or socio-economic status which may be a general aetiological factor or can be associated directly with exposure to a specific carcinogenic hazard. Asbestos and mesothelioma, β-naphthylamine and bladder cancer, nickel and haematite with lung cancer, wood-working and air sinus cancer, are all associations which have emerged from examination of specific occupational groups. Studies on industrial workers using their spouse as controls may assist in deciding whether the increased incidence is related to a specific occupational hazard. The exact definition of an occupation may be difficult and official records often use very broad categories of registration. It is necessary to examine the industrial process in detail as in Case's studies, in the dye industry[36,37] to discover whether all or only some of the registered workers come into contact with the suspect carcinogen. In all such investigations it is essential to ensure that the occupation recorded is the one in which the subject spent most of his working life, as changes of work may often be dictated by illness.

DISTRIBUTION IN TIME

Where mortality statistics are available over a number of years the time trends can be assessed. The difficulties associated with the influence of age are dealt with elsewhere, and the use of age specific rates and a standardized cancer population is again stressed. Apart from real changes in incidence, improved diagnosis or registration may suggest an apparent increase in the disease. As distribution in time is often related to observation over a considerable period, the effects of the quality and availability of both diagnosis and therapy and even of observation itself may be considerable. A complete evaluation of the procedures of death certification including classification of neoplastic disease is also necessary before the trends can be interpreted. In 1915, Hoffman stated—'When every reasonable allowance is made for the want of accuracy and completeness in the available returns for the African continent it would seem safe to assume that cancer is of a relatively very low degree of frequency in African countries. Even among the white population, as a general rule, malignant disease is extremely rare'.[38] Just how unwise it is to make assumptions of this kind, particularly in developing countries, has been proved beyond doubt by modern epidemiological surveys in many parts of Africa.

In some countries, for example Norway, the death rates from gastric cancer has halved in twenty-five years. It is possible, though unlikely, that the original diagnoses inadvertently included cancers of other organs in close relation to the stomach. As the decline is more pronounced in younger age groups and is seen in rural as well as urban areas it is unlikely to be solely related to diagnostic changes. Treatment has not improved to such an extent to be responsible for this marked decrease, and a review of the Norwegian evidence seems to warrant the conclusion that the decrease in incidence is real (Pederson and Magnus, 1961[39]).

Studies of mortality in lung cancer suggest the reverse situation; here, there seems to have been an absolute increase of this cancer in the recent past (Clemmensen, 1965[40];—see also *Smoking and Health*, World Health Organization, 1971[41]). This trend has been confirmed by many statistical analyses, and when it is recognized that the greater part of the increase is restricted to certain readily identifiable histological types, squamous and the anaplastic 'oat-cell' tumours, it becomes difficult to conclude that the increase is other than real. Changes in cancer frequency in defined geographical regions may be very striking and the rise in oesophageal cancer in the Transkei of South Africa first reported by Burrell (1767[42]) appears to be real and almost epidemic in its proportions (Rose, 1965[43]; Burrell, 1969[44]).

Cancer incidence can clearly vary both in space as well as time and valuable information can be obtained by techniques to test space-time clustering. In the West Nile district of Uganda, Pike *et al.* (1967)[45] considered that variation of incidence in time and space might confirm that an infectious agent was a factor in the aetiology of Burkitt's tumour. Clustering of cases has also been reported in Hodgkin's Disease. Davies and his colleagues in Albany, New York, have found that 'on occasion Hodgkin's disease can occur in the pattern of a long lasting epidemic with a period of high incidence followed by one of low incidence; the disease can spread in a slowly contagious pattern, with a long incubation period, both by case-to-case and case-to-contact-to-case transmission; and the direction of transmission may be from young to young or young to old persons with contacts remaining in good health, and on occasion apparently giving rise to multiple cases' (Davies, 1972)[46].

Analytical epidemiology

Retrospective or case history studies

Such studies compare the influence of a suspect factor in a group of cancer patients with a group of controls or persons known to be free of the disease in question. Evaluation of the history of cases with or without the factor is made by interview or questionnaire. The finding of a greater frequency of the factor in cancer patients compared with controls indicates a degree of association which is expressed usually as a 'relative risk'. The computation of this risk and the assessment of the effects of other variables on it are described in detail by Mantel and Haenszel (1959)[47].

Although the fundamental issue is whether this statistical association is a biological one, a major problem with the assessment of such studies is the elimination of bias in the selection of either case or control. Most investigators are obliged to use cancer cases seen in hospital but these may not be representative of the behaviour of the cancer in the general population. Nearly 20 per cent of patients included in the comprehensive cancer registry of the state of Connecticut were found to have had no hospital care—(Griswold *et al.* (1955)[48]). Advanced cases which attract little medical or surgical interest may be neglected in favour of those with an early disgnosis which are more likely to respond favourably to treatment. If such sources of bias are not appreciated, the association demonstrated may only represent the selection of patients for hospital admission and this effect may be particularly marked in retrospective studies in developing countries. The selection of controls must give rise to an even more anxious search for bias. The controls or comparison groups should ideally not differ from the affected groups except in the one factor being investigated, but the chances of achieving this are remote. Although matching of cases and controls by age or sex is desirable, one immediately introduces the tacit assumption that age or sex has no influence on the association. Matching a factor rejects it as an independent variable and the controls can only be used for assessment of additional factors. Often other patients attending the same hospital are used as the general population from whom controls are to be chosen to minimize the factors of selection associated with hospital attendance. Relatives whose socio-economic environment is similar to the affected cases may form a control group, but they are obviously limited in number and matching here may be difficult.

Sampling of the control group may be undertaken if it is too large to be used for comparison. This sampling may be random or systematic by choosing every second or tenth individual. However, it is not always possible to enumerate the whole population to effect such a method of sampling so a system of pairing based on some relationship to the affected person such as the next hospital admission or nearest neighbour is often used. The details of techniques for sampling populations and for the examination for differences between groups are fully presented in text-books of bio-statistics[6, 15, 16, 49]. Even if statistical significance is suggested, it is advisable to confirm this by studies using differing methods and control groups.

Prospective or cohort studies

If evidence for an association is strong *prima facie* or following a retrospective investigation, then a study can be mounted to collect information prospectively on a 'cohort'—a group of individuals identified by a demographic characteristic such as an age group or occupation. These longitudinal studies have the advantage of making a direct measurement of the suspect factor. Biased associations are less likely than in retrospective studies and reliance on the fraility of memory is eliminated. A sample of a population is selected, examined for the suspect factor, and then followed for a number of years to see whether cancer develops. Basic data, often retrospective in nature, may be used but the main part of the study is prospective in that the selected cohort is followed in anticipation of the biological event. Such studies may be on general population samples or on readily identified groups such as industrial workers, insured persons or self-selected groups of volunteers. An important population are those who are suspected of being at a high risk of developing a particular cancer. Prospective studies are expensive in time and money for, if the disease is rare, large numbers will be required for study and in any case a long period of observation is necessary. Furthermore, the interest generated in the disease process within the population during the investigation may itself create bias and lead to a falsely high incidence. This effect is not marked in cancer research, but loss to follow-up which may give a false low incidence is of great concern and comprehensive coverage throughout the study must be maintained. British doctors involved in the study by Doll and Hill (1964)[50] to define the risk of cigarette smoking and lung cancer were followed not only by death certification in the Registrar General's Office but by the administrative organizations of the profession and only a few cases were recorded as lost to follow-up when the doctor population was requestioned after some years.

The evaluation of statistical data—biological deductions

Tests of significance are designed to check the biases of chance Johnson had in mind, and it must be conceded that although there has been increasing appreciation of this necessity, we still need to beware of sampling biases in the collection of data and of the misconceptions often associated with statistical significance. Statistical significance may indicate that the difference is (within limits) a real one, but it certainly does not prove that the difference is causal.

In the absence of experimental proof, a number of factors must be evaluated before considering the causality of a relationship. It must be noted that, by definition, statistical significance can be applied only to groups. Individual events cannot be related causally except by experimental proof. The strength and the specificity of the association of the factor with the incidence of cancer are of great importance. The ratio of the death rate from lung cancer of heavy smokers to that of non-smokers is 10:73, whereas the ratio of smokers to non-smokers in bladder cancer is 2:17—(Hammond and Horn, 1958, 1966[51, 52]).

Although there is statistical significance to support association of both cancers with smoking, the evidence of the former relationship being causal is much stronger than the second. A statistical association can also be deceptively indirect or related to a third factor known or not appreciated in the light of present biological knowledge. It may be proved that lung cancer develops more commonly in those who have had coronary thrombosis, whereas the relationship may arise because both diseases are related to cigarette smoking. A graduation between incidence and degree of exposure, a dose-response relationship, is useful supporting evidence but often environmental factors are difficult to define and measure quantitatively. As it is not feasible to expect experimental proof to be the final arbiter in cancer epidemiology, it is important to consider whether a hypothesis which has statistical significance fits other evidence. This may be provided by further analyses to test geographical or sex differences and time trends.

Finally, the question must be asked as to whether a given hypothesis is biologically reasonable or plausible. Particularly when dealing with cancer, this requirement should not be obligatory as our judgment will depend on current biological knowledge; we certainly should not reject a hypothesis because we cannot envisage the precise biological mechanism. It was difficult to appreciate immediately how altitude alone would affect the incidence of the tumour entity reported by Burkitt (1958)[53, 48]; nevertheless, it initiated an exciting new series of investigations into the viral aetiology of childhood tumours. To quote Bradford Hill[15]—'There was no biological knowledge to support (or to refute) Pott's observation in the eighteenth century of the excess of cancer in chimney sweeps. It was lack of biological knowledge in the nineteenth century that led a prize essayist writing on the value and the fallacy of statistics to conclude, amongst other "absurd" associations, that "it could be no more ridiculous for the stranger who passed the night in the steerage of an emigrant ship to ascribe the typhus, which he there contracted, to the vermin with which bodies of the sick might be infected"'. The logic of some investigations is dictated by lay commonsense. The association of cigarette smoking and lung cancer was not difficult to conceive but it was the excellent statistical design of the investigations to test this association which makes it such a frequently quoted model. 'Armchair' epidemiological speculation always has to be fully supported by what Burnet calls 'shoeleather' epidemiology before a hypothesis can be put forward in any reasonable form. How rarely we are able to do this illustrates the complexity of the problems posed by cancer, yet it must be conceded that the majority of known risk factors for man have been defined by observations on human data using epidemiological methods.

References

1. Pott, P. *The Chirurgical Works of Percival Pott*, London. (1775).
2. Higginson, J. From Canadian Cancer Conference, Proceedings of the Eighth Canadian Cancer Conference, Honey Harbour, Ontario (1968).
3. Weisberger, E. K. and Weisberger, J. H. *Advances in Cancer Research*. J. P. Greenstein and A. Haddow, Eds. New York, New York Academic Press Inc. Vol. **5,** 331 (1958).
4. Burnet, M. *Changing Patterns*, American Elsevier Publishing Co. Inc., New York (1969).
5. MacMahon, B., Pugh, T. F., Ipsen, J. *Epidemiologic Methods,* Little, Brown & Co. Boston, Mass. (1960).
6. Lilienfeld, A. M., Pedersen, E. and Dowd, J. E. Cancer Epidemiology—Methods of Study, John S. Hopkins Press, Baltimore, U.S.A. (1967).
7. Ewing, J. *J. Cancer Res.*, **1,** 71 (1916).
8. Doll. R., Muir, C. S. and Waterhouse, J. *Cancer in Five Continents*, Vol. **II.** Springer-Verlag, Berlin, Heidelberg, New York (1970).
9. *Bulletin of W.H.O.*, **40,** 601 (1969).
10. Denoix, P. F. *Bull. Int. Nat. Hys.*, Paris., **1,** 69 (1944).
11. Sellars, A. H. *Canad. med. J.*, **105,** 836 (1971).
12. Cox, P. R. *Demography,* 3rd Edition. University Press, Cambridge (1959).
13. Yates, F. *Sampling Methods for Census and Survey.* 2nd Edition. Griffin, London (1953).
14. Doll, R. *J. Roy. Stat. Soc.*, **134,** 133 (1971).
15. Hill, A. B. *Principles of Medical Statistics.* 8th Edition. London (1970).
16. Bailey, N. T. J. *Statistical Methods in Biology*, English University Press, London (1959).
17. Cook, P. J., Doll, R. and Fellingham, S. A. *Int. J. Cancer*, **4,** 93 (1969).
18. Martinez, I. *Cancer, Philad.*, **24,** 777 (1969).
19. Hueper, W. C. *Archs. Path.*, **58,** 360 (1952).
20. Burnet, F. M. *Lancet*, **ii,** 358 (1970).
21. Doll, R. *Br. med. J.*, **4,** 420 (1970).
22. Levin, A. G., McDonough, E. F. Jnr., Miller, D. G. and Southam, C. M. *Ann. N.Y. Acad. Sci.*, **120,** 400 (1964).
23. Miller, R. W. *J. Nat. Cancer Inst.*, **46,** 203 (1971).
24. Herbst, A. L., Ulfelder, H. and Pozkarer, D. C. *New Engl. J. Med.*, **284,** 878 (1971).
25. I.A.R.C. *Monograph on Transplacental Carcinogenesis.* L. Tomatis, U. Mohr and W. Davis, Eds. Lyon (1973).
26. Steinitz, R. and Costin, C. *Israel. J. med. sci.*, **7,** 1405 (1971).
27. Paymaster, J. C. Oral and Pharyngeal Cancer in India. Washington, Butterworths, 308 (1967).
28. Bauer, F. W. and Robbins, S. L. *J. Am. med. Assn.*, **221,** 1471 (1972).
29. McMahan, C. A. *Archs. Path.*, **73,** 40 (1962).
30. Doll, R. *Cancer in Africa*, p. 108. Ed. Clifford Linsell Timms, East-African Publishing House, Nairobi. 108 (1968).
31. Cook, P. J. and Burkitt, D. P. *Br. med. Bull.*, **27,** 14 (1971).
32. Segi, M., Kurihara, M. and Matsuyama, T. Cancer mortality for selected sites in twenty-four countries. Department of Public Health, Tohoka Uni-

versity, Japan and Japan Cancer Society. 1950–57, 1958–59, 1960–61, 1962–63, 1964–65, 1966–67.
33. Merkov, A. M., Tserkovnogo, G. F. and Kaufman, B. D. Morbidity and Mortality from Malignant Neoplasms in the U.S.S.R. English Edition, J. G. Dean (1963).
34. Knowelden, E. L. *Lancet*, **ii**, 328 (1952).
35. Haenszel, W. *J. Nat. Cancer Inst.*, **21,** 213 (1958).
36. Case, R. A. M. and Hosker, M. E. *Br. J. prev. and soc. Med.*, **8,** 39 (1954).
37. Case, R. A. M. *Annls. Roy. Coll. Surg.*, Eng., **39,** 213 (1966).
38. Hoffman, F. L. Mortality from Cancer Throughout the World. New Jersey, 1915. Quoted by Linsell, C. A. and Martyn, E. *E. Afr. med. J.*, **39,** 642 (1962).
39. Pedersen E. and Magnus, K. *Acta. Un. Int. Cancer*, **17,** 373 (1961).
40. Clemmensen, J. *Statistical Studies in the Aetiology of Malignant Neoplasms*, Part I. Review and Results. Munksgaard, Copenhagen (1965).
41. *Smoking and Health*, W.H.O. (1971).
42. Burrell, R. J. W. *S. Afr. med. J.*, **31,** 401 (1957)—see also *J. Nat. Cancer Inst.*, **28,** 495 (1962).
43. Rose, E. F. *S. Afr. med. J.*, **39,** 1098 (1965).
44. Burrell, R. J. W. *J. Nat. Cancer Inst.*, **43,** 877 (1969).
45. Pike, M. C., Williams, E. H. and Wright, B. *Br. med. J.*, **1,** 395 (1967).
46. Davies, J. N. P. *Human Pathol.*, **3,** 297 (1972).
47. Mantel, N. and Haenszel, W. *J. Nat. Cancer Inst.*, **22,** 719 (1959).
48. Griswold, M. H., Wilder, C. S., Cutler, S. J. and Pollack, E. S. *Cancer in Connecticut*, 1935–1951. Connecticut Department of Health, Harlford, Conn. (1955).
49. Snedecor, G. W. *Statistical Methods.* 5th Edition, Iowa State College Press, Ames, Iowa (1962).
50. Doll, R. and Hill, A. B. *Br. med. J.*, **1,** 1399 and 1460 (1964).
51. Hammond, E. C. and Horn, D. *J. Am. med. Assn.*, **166,** 1159 and 1204 (1958).
52. Hammond, E. C. *N.C.I. Monogr.*, **19,** 127 (1966).
53. Burkitt, D. *Br. J. Surg.*, **46,** 218 (1958).

Chapter **9**

THE CHEMICAL INDUCTION OF CANCER

D. B. CLAYSON, Ph.D.

Professor of Cancer Research, Department of Experimental Pathology and Cancer Research, University of Leeds

Since the first edition of this book was published, major progress has been made in obtaining evidence to support the unifying concept of the metabolic activation of carcinogens to reactive ions (Miller, 1970)[1], and in studies of the interaction of carcinogens with tissue components—exemplified by the alkylation hypothesis put forward by Magee (1969)[2] as a result of his work on nitrosamines.

Despite this progress, stemming largely from biochemical studies of carcinogenesis, underlying fundamental and practical questions remain unanswered. We are little further towards understanding how chemicals alter the behaviour of cells and organisms to induce cancer, and we are still unable to translate results obtained in animals to man with any degree of certainty.

The molecular structure of chemical carcinogens

OCCUPATIONAL CARCINOGENS

The majority of chemicals known to be carcinogenic in man have been discovered because attention was drawn to them, or to related chemicals, by investigations into occupational cancer (Table 9.1). The recognition of a particular cancer hazard has tended to follow a predictable pattern. First, astute clinical observation has drawn attention to an excessive number of cases of a particular form of cancer in men working in a given employment. For example, Pott (1775)[3] noticed an abnormal number of cases of cancer of scrotal skin among chimney sweeps; Rehn (1895)[4] reported an unusual clustering of cases of bladder cancer in a factory making the dyestuff fuchsin. The clinicians' suspicions were shown to be well founded when epidemiological methods were subsequently used to confirm the earlier observations (Henry 1947[5]; Case *et al.*, 1954[6];—see also Chapter 8). Finally it has usually proved possible to demonstrate the carcinogenicity for laboratory animals of some contaminants of the industrial environment, and then, by the use of further tests, to identify the actual chemicals responsible. Occupational skin cancer led to the discovery of the carcinogenicity of certain polycyclic hydrocarbons, bladder cancer to that of a number of aromatic amines, some forms of lung

Table 9.1. Extrinsic carcinogenic chemicals discovered by their action in man

Tissue of election of human cancer or related condition	*People affected*	*Class of Carcinogen*	*Example*
Skin	Chimney sweeps Pitch and tar workers Mule-spinners	Hydrocarbons	3:4-Benzpyrene
Bladder	Chemical workers Rubber workers Dyestuffs workers	Aromatic amines	2-Naphthylamine
Lung (Nose)	Metal refiners (nickel processors)	Metals	Chromium Nickel
Liver	Chemical workers (liver cirrhosis)	Dialkylnitrosamines	
Bone and Leukaemia	Dial Painters Radiochemical workers	Radiochemicals	Radium

and (in the case of nickel) nasal cancer to the knowledge that certain metals have carcinogenic potential bone cancer and certain leukaemias to the carcinogenicity of radiochemicals.

NATURALLY OCCURRING CARCINOGENS

Naturally occurring carcinogens are now attracting more attention (Table 9.2). The fortuitous discovery of metabolites of the mould *Aspergillus flavus*,

Table 9.2. Examples of naturally-occurring carcinogens

Source	*Species*	*Carcinogen*
Mould	*Aspergillus flavus*	Aflatoxin
	Aspergillus versicolor	Sterigmatocystin
Plant	*Pteris aquilana*	Compound $C_7H_8O_4$
	Senecio, Crotolaria Heliotropium, etc.	Pyrrolizidium alkaloids, e.g. retrorsine
	Cycas circinalis	Cycasin

known as aflatoxins, as a result of the poisoning of some 100,000 turkey poults, led to the demonstration of the considerable hepatotoxicity and later hepatocarcinogenicity of aflatoxin B_1(I) and G_1(II). It was thought that,

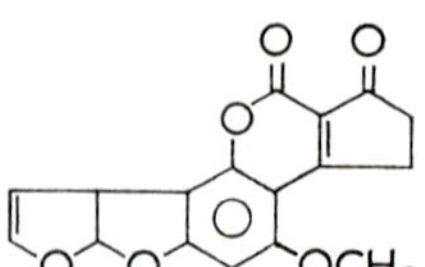

(I)

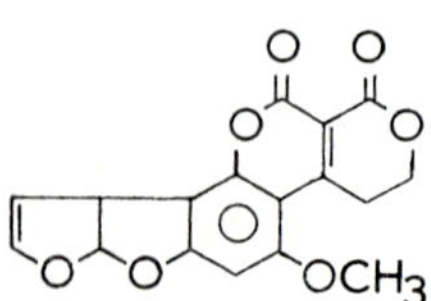

(II)

because mould contamination was more likely in hot, moist countries than in temperate climates, aflatoxin or other mould metabolites might be responsible for the relatively high incidence of human liver cancer in some parts of the tropics. Attempts have been made to substantiate this view by comparing the concentration of aflatoxins in foodstuffs purchased by people in areas with high and low incidences of liver cancer (Shank *et al.*, 1972a[7], b[8], c[9]). Although the results support the hypothesis that aflatoxins may be implicated, the small differences in incidence of liver cancer between the areas under study, a lack of knowledge of the effects of different ways of preparing food for consumption, and the possible presence of other carcinogenic mould metabolites (e.g. sterigmatocystin) still leaves the significance of the association in doubt.

Other natural products which may induce cancer and which have been found as contaminants in human foodstuffs include cycasin—the glucoside of methylazoxymethanol (III) (IARC Monographs, 1972[10])—and a toxic

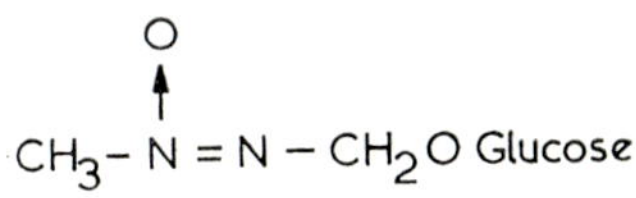

(III)

principle, so far unidentified, in bracken fern, *Pteris aquilana* (Evans, 1968)[11]. The study of such naturally occurring carcinogens may be of the utmost importance in determining the causation of human and animal cancers hitherto regarded as spontaneous in origin.

ENDOGENOUS CARCINOGENS

Endogenous carcinogens (i.e. carcinogens produced within the body) have attracted attention as possible causes of naturally occurring tumours (Table 9.3). Physiological levels of circulating hormones are normally maintained

Table 9.3. Endogenous chemical carcinogens

Type of Compound	*Tissues affected*	*Species*	*Example*
Hormones	Endocrine (e.g. pituitary, ovary, . . .) Endocrine dependent (e.g. breast, uterus, . . .)	Various	Oestrogens
Cholesterol	Subcutaneous tissues	Mouse, rat	Cholesterol
Tryptophan metabolites	Bladder	Mouse	3-Hydroxy-anthranilic acid

within the body by homeostatic regulatory mechanisms, most of which involve the pituitary gland and other endocrine tissues. Disruption of homeostasis may lead to excessive stimulation of certain endocrine or endocrine-responsive tissues and ultimately, if the stimulus is sufficiently prolonged, to cancer. Breakdown of homeostasis has been brought about by the administration of excessive amounts of oestrogenic substances, or by surgical or chemical procedures which lead one or more endocrine tissues to over-secrete certain hormones (see Clayson, 1962[12]).

Cholesterol (Hieger, 1958[13]) and certain *metabolites of tryptophan* (Price, 1966[14]) have been put forward as possible endogenous carcinogens. The evidence in the case of the former substance is unconvincing. Cholesterol was claimed to be carcinogenic because it gave rise to subcutaneous sarcomas on injection in rats and mice. The induction of these tumours was dependent on the vehicle used: oily solutions were effective whereas aqueous solutions were not. Bischoff (1963)[15] suggested that the carcinogenic effect might be due to oxidation products present in the cholesterol, or that the tumours arose in response to a thin film of cholesterol being deposited in the tissues. Thin films or sponges of sufficient area made from a wide variety of materials of different chemical compositions, are able to induce sarcomas in the subcutaneous tissues of rats and mice (references: see Clayson, 1962[12]; Bischoff, 1972[15a]).

The status of tryptophan metabolites as endogenous carcinogens is more difficult to evaluate. Price (1966)[14] found that all the aromatic amines normally present in human urine were metabolites of the essential amino acid, tryptophan. Patients with bladder cancer, not exposed to occupational bladder carcinogens, excreted more of these substances in their urine than subjects without bladder cancer; the difference was especially marked after a loading dose of L-tryptophan. The metabolites were shown to possess carcinogenic activity by the bladder implantation technique (Allen *et al.,* 1957[16]; Bryan *et al.,* 1964[17]) but not by more conventional methods. Bladder implantation is not, however, a satisfactory method of carcinogenic testing (Clayson, 1973[18]). More recent investigations of patients with bladder cancer failed to demonstrate as high a proportion of individuals with abnormal tryptophan metabolism as in the former series (Brown *et al.,* 1969[19]). This discrepancy may reflect the fact that the earlier group of patients was drawn from a largely rural population while the later group came from the greater Boston conurbation where exposure to industrial bladder carcinogens is, perhaps, more likely. Radomski *et al.* (1971)[20] found that feeding seven times the normal intake of L-tryptophan to dogs induced hyperplasia of the bladder epithelium. This was apparent as early as three months after the start of feeding and persisted until the experiment was terminated seven years later; nevertheless, no tumours were found. The present author's opinion is that the status of tryptophan metabolites as endogenous carcinogens has not been satisfactorily established.

OTHER CHEMICAL CARCINOGENS

These have been discovered as a result of animal tests which are now required before regulating bodies license the use of proposed food additives, pesticides, drugs and certain other chemicals that may become environmental contaminants. The compounds which have been shown to be carcinogenic as a result of obligatory routine tests do not always fall into any category of known chemical carcinogen (Table 9.4): they have sometimes been useful in demonstrating how apparently non-specific factors may affect the course of carcinogenesis in animals (p. 175).

Table 9.4. Principal chemical groups that are associated with carcinogenic activity (possession of one of these structural characteristics does not mean that a chemical is carcinogenic, but increases the probability that it is)

Substances that do not require metabolic activation	
1. Biological Alkylating Agents	(i) S-mustards
	(ii) N-mustards
	(iii) Epoxides
	(iv) Arizidines
	(v) Alkyl alkane sulphonates
	(vi) Strained ring lactones
	(vii) Nitrosamides
2. Inorganic chemicals	(i) Certain metals and metalloids
	(ii) Asbestos
3. Radiochemicals	
Substances requiring metabolic activation	
4. Polycyclic hydrocarbons	(i) Carbocyclic compounds
	(ii) Heterocyclic analogues
5. Aromatic amines	(i) Carbocyclic compounds
	(ii) Heterocyclic amino and nitrocompounds
	(iii) Aminoazo compounds
6. Nitrosamines	
7. Hydrazines	(i) Hydrazine
	(ii) Alkyl hydrazines
	(iii) Alkyl azocompounds
	(iv) Alkyl azoxycompounds
8. Hormones and related substances	(i) Oestrogens
	(ii) Goitrogens
9. Miscellaneous	(i) Urethane
	(ii) Carbontetrachloride, DDT, dieldrin

Metabolic activation of carcinogens

It was observed at a relatively early stage in the study of chemical carcinogenesis that different species of experimental animals varied in their susceptibility to particular chemical carcinogens. This is most clearly illustrated in the case of the aromatic amines (Table 9.5). The analysis of the factors underlying

Table 9.5. The site of election of tumours induced by three aromatic amines

Species	*2-Naphthylamine*	*2-Acetamidofluorene*	*4-Aminodiphenyl*
Man	Bladder	Not known	Bladder
Dog	Bladder	Bladder, liver	Bladder
Cat	None	Lung, liver, kidney	Not known
Rat	Bladder (pre-cancer)	Various	Intestine, breast
Rabbit	None	Bladder, ureter	Bladder

these species differences in susceptibility has played a major role in showing how chemical carcinogens react with the tissues.

It was found that many of the tumours induced by aromatic amines occurred at sites of metabolism or excretion of the test compound—kidneys, bladder, intestine or liver—rather than at sites such as the mouth or stomach, where orally administered carcinogens would be expected to reach the highest concentrations. This led to the suggestion that the aromatic amines need to be metabolized before they become active carcinogens. The first substantial information concerning the nature of metabolic activation followed from the demonstration of a novel metabolic pathway in which the aromatic amine derivative, 2-acetylaminofluorene (AAF-IV), was converted to N-hydroxy-2-acetylaminofluorene (N-hydroxy-AAF-V) (Miller *et al.*, 1960[21]). The N-

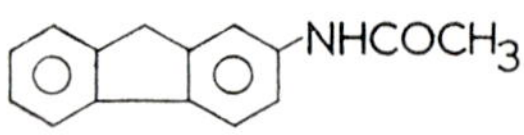

(IV)

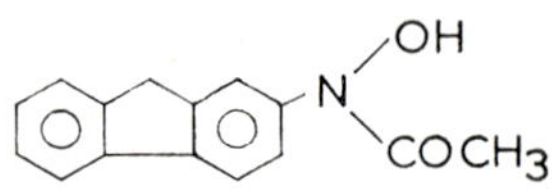

(V)

hydroxy compound was shown to be a more active carcinogen than the compound from which it was derived; in equimolar doses it induced more tumours in some, but not all, tissues than the parent acetamide. It was carcinogenic to the subcutaneous tissues of the rat on injection and induced tumours in the stomach on feeding; AAF itself was inactive under the same conditions. The N-hydroxy compound induced tumours in the guinea pig whereas the acetamide was apparently without carcinogenic activity in this species. It was also shown that the guinea pig lacks the ability to N-hydroxylate aromatic amines. The importance of N-hydroxylation in carcinogenesis is further demonstrated by the fact that concomitant feeding of 3-methylcholanthrene (as an enzyme-inducing agent rather than as a carcinogen) and AAF, or N-hydroxy AAF, inhibited hepatocarcinogenesis in the rat induced by the former but not by the latter acetamide. It was shown that the overall effect of 3-methylcholanthrene was to inhibit N-hydroxylation of AAF (Lotlikar *et al.*, 1967[22]).

The evidence available leaves little doubt that N-hydroxylation is important in the activation of AAF. It is not by itself sufficient because if 9-^{14}C-AAF is fed to rats, it is possible to demonstrate that the carcinogen has reacted chemically with the DNA, RNA and protein of the liver and it is believed (Miller *et al.*, 1966[23]) that this interaction plays an essential role in the induction of tumours. Such binding is not found if N-hydroxy-AAF is incubated with these tissue macromolecules *in vitro*. The demonstration that certain synthetic esters of N-hydroxy AAF were potent local carcinogens and able to interact with tissue macromolecules *in vitro* indicated that esterification is probably the second activation step (Miller *et al.*, 1966[24]). The identity of the ester formed *in vivo* has been established in only one system, the rat liver. It was thought that the sulphate or phosphate esters were the most likely to be involved. Using a microsomal fraction to supply the enzyme, sulphotransferase, phosphoadenosine-phosphosulphate as a source of active sulphate, magnesium or manganese ions to activate the enzyme, and methionine as a trapping agent, De Baune *et al.* (1970)[25] found that it was possible to react N-hydroxy-AAF with methionine to give products identical to those obtained by hydrolyzing the proteins from the liver of rats fed with AAF. Furthermore, the sulphotransferase levels in liver microsomes correlated well with the ability of AAF to induce liver tumours in the species from which the microsomes were prepared (De Baune *et al.*, 1970[25]). Indirect evidence in support of this hypothesis has been obtained by demonstrating that the inhibition of N-hydroxy AAF carcinogenesis induced by a large excess of acetanilide is due to the metabolism of acetanilide to *p*-hydroxyacetanilide ester sulphate which depletes the animal of sulphate. The carcinogenicity may be restored by feeding excess sulphate in the diet (Weisburger *et al.*, 1972[26]).

Although there is much evidence to support the importance of N-hydroxylation in the metabolic activation of aromatic amines, it is only in the induction of tumours by AAF in the rat liver that there is evidence that the sulphate ester is involved. In the rat, tumour formation in the mammary gland and acoustic duct results from different forms of metabolic activation (Irving *et al.*, 1971[27]). It appears that there is more than one way of activating an N-hydroxy compound. Bartsch *et al.* (1972)[27a] have discussed the possibility that one electron oxidation of N-hydroxy-AAF *in vivo* may play a part in carcinogenesis. *In vitro*, it was shown that one electron oxidation of N-hydroxy-AAF led to 2-nitrosofluorene and N-acetoxy-AAF. In reacting with the tissues, it is thought that N-hydroxy esters of aromatic amines decompose with the loss of the negatively-charged ester ion leaving a highly reactive positively-charged intermediate

$$\begin{matrix} CH_3CO \\ Ar \end{matrix}\!\!\!\!\!>\!N-OX \longrightarrow \begin{matrix} CH_3CO \\ Ar \end{matrix}\!\!\!\!\!>\!N^+ + OX^-$$

This positively-charged intermediate reacts with nucleophilic groups in the tissues, some of which are shown in *Fig. 9.1.*

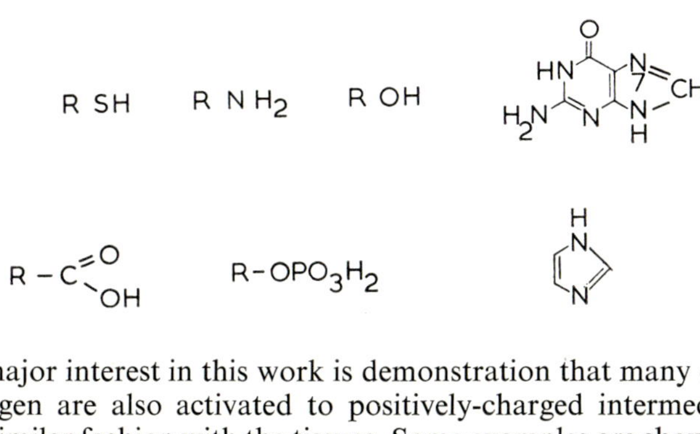

The major interest in this work is demonstration that many other classes of carcinogen are also activated to positively-charged intermediates which react in a similar fashion with the tissues. Some examples are shown in *Fig.9.2.* The majority of the very diverse types of chemical carcinogens (Table 9.4,)

Nitrosamines

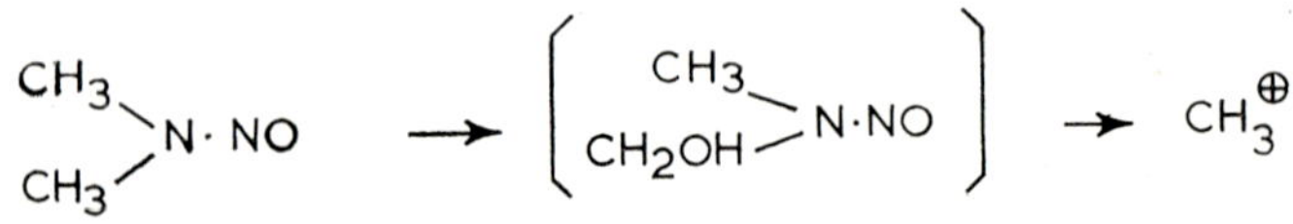

Aromatic Amines

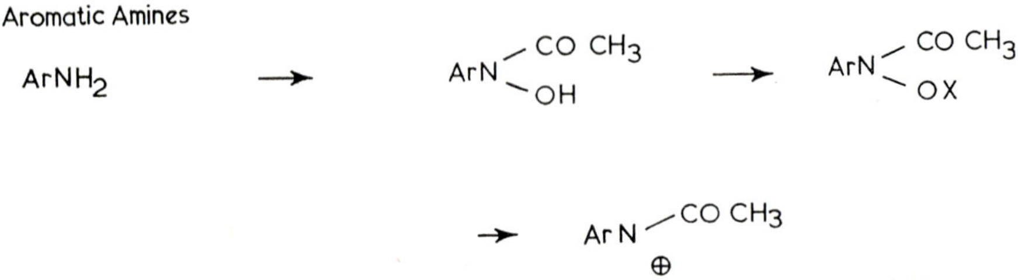

Polycyclic Hydrocarbons

(i)

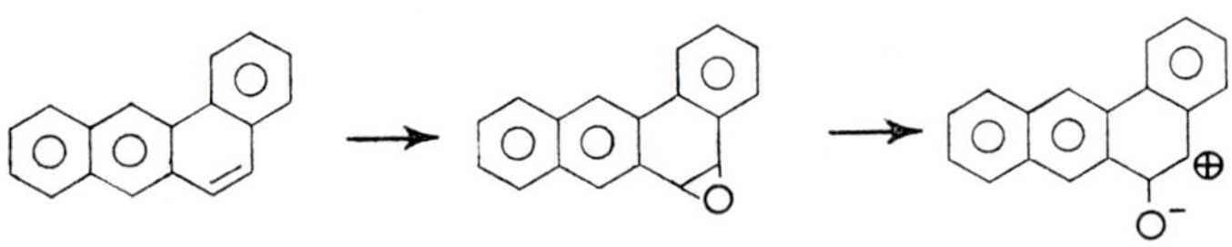

(ii)

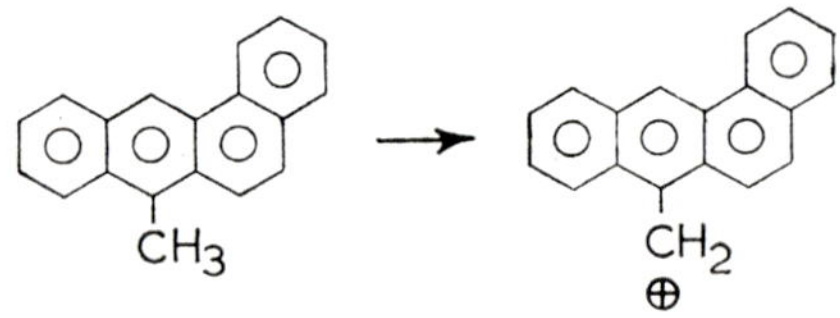

Aflatoxin

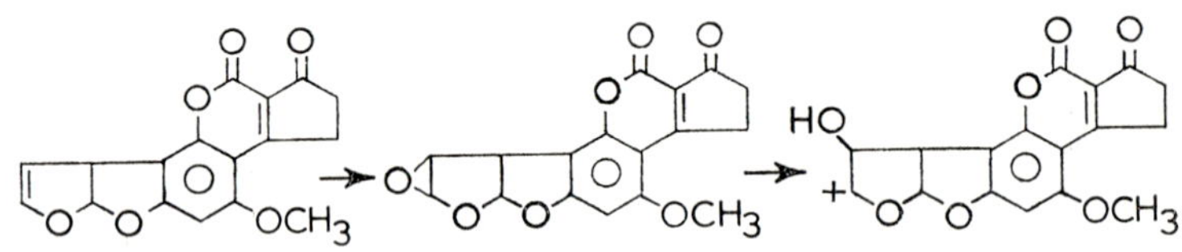

which at one time seemed so bewilderingly different, now appear to have a common path of action.

Interaction of carcinogens with tissue components

The presence of covalently bound carcinogen residues on many cellular macromolecules is the consequence of the interaction of the metabolically activated carcinogens with nucleophilic groups in the tissues. Since the earliest demonstration of carcinogen-protein binding (Miller *et al.*, 1947[28]) there have been many attempts to link such binding with the ultimate appearance of tumours. Speculation is at present centred around three types of interaction—(*a*) carcinogen to DNA; (*b*) carcinogen to protein, and (*c*) carcinogen to transfer RNA: all three of them are discussed in more detail in Chapter 10.

BINDING TO DNA

The idea that cancer might be the result of one or more interactions in the genome of somatic cells has had many adherents since Boveri (1929)[29] reported that the chromatin of cancer cells stained irregularly compared to that of normal cells (See also Chapter 2). The somatic mutation hypothesis is particularly apposite for speculation because, by assuming that mutation occurs in genes with specified actions and that a suitable selection process operates, it is possible to account for the majority of biological phenomena. Substantial evidence is much more difficult to obtain. Earlier objections to the somatic mutation hypothesis were based on the observation that several important classes of carcinogen, including the polycyclic hydrocarbons and aromatic amines, were inefficient at inducing mutations in the monocellular organisms used in the classical work on chemical mutagenesis (Burdette, 1955[30]). The realization that chemical carcinogens require metabolic activation and that the monocellular organisms lack the necessary metabolizing enzymes has been followed by experiments which show that the active metabolites are potently mutagenic and can, for example, mutate isolated phage (Maher *et al.,* 1968[31]). A mutational hypothesis for the induction of cancer by chemicals as well as by radiation is therefore a real possibility.

It should not be thought, however, that every molecule of carcinogen which reacts with DNA necessarily induces a mutation; damage to DNA in most mammalian systems can be repaired by enzymes present in the cells affected (Chapter 10). Furthermore, particularly with carcinogens of low molecular weight (for example, the methylating agents such as dimethylnitrosamine), it has been shown that the position in the DNA molecule at which binding occurs is vitally important in the induction of mutations (Chapter 10).

The extent of binding to DNA *in vivo* varies according to the agent, the dose and its susceptibility to metabolic activation. Brookes (1966)[32] in a review of the literature, reported that six moles of sulphur mustard bound to 10^5 nucleotide pairs in DNA in mouse ascites cells whereas only 0·75 moles of benzo(a)pyrene bound to the same number of nucleotide pairs in mouse skin. If this binding is random and leads to simple point mutations, the chance of obtaining the series of specific mutations postulated to be necessary for the induction of cancer would appear to be remote. Yet results obtained in *in vitro* studies suggest that malignant as well as morphological transformation is not uncommon. For example, Chen and Heidelberger (1969)[33] induced many morphological transformations by adding 3-methylcholanthrene (1μg/ml) to adult C3H mouse ventral prostate cells in culture. Implantation of only 100 of these transformed cells into each of three isologous hosts led to tumours in two mice. This suggests that a mechanism other than specific somatic mutation may operate in cancer induction. These observations could however be artefactual in view of the finding that the addition of a chemical carcinogen, diethylnitrosamine, to rat embryo cells infected with Rauscher virus led to morphological transformation, whereas neither virus nor chemical alone had this effect (Freeman *et al.*, 1970[34]). Before accepting that certain results contra-indicate a somatic mutation mechanism for cancer induction, it is necessary to establish that the cells used in transformation experiments with chemicals do not contain incomplete cancer-inducing viruses.

Huebner has postulated that all cancers have a viral origin and that chemicals act as carcinogens by activating an intrinsic cancer virus (Huebner and Todaro, 1969[35]). The truth of this suggestion is difficult to determine. On semantic grounds, it demands strict definition of the term 'virus' and on a more practical level, actual techniques to differentiate oncogenic viruses from other nucleic acid sequences of the cell genome.

BINDING TO PROTEIN

The demonstration that in certain systems carcinogen to protein binding could be correlated with the degree of activity of the carcinogen led to attempts to explain the mechanism of cancer induction. The enzyme deletion hypothesis (Miller and Miller, 1952[36]) represented the first of such attempts. It was suggested that binding to cell protein led to the deletion of enzymes controlling growth and thus to cancer. The mechanism by which interaction with a protein could lead to its elimination was not at that time explained.

Further work showed that certain proteins had a greater affinity for activated carcinogens than others. Sorof *et al.* (1960)[37], for example, showed that a group of proteins characterized by their electrophoretic mobility (the h_2 proteins) had the highest affinity for 4-dimethylaminoazobenzene metabolites of all proteins in the soluble fraction of rat liver; and a similar group of polycyclic hydrocarbon-binding proteins was demonstrated in mouse skin (Abell and Heidelberger, 1962[38]). More recently Litwack *et al.* (1972)[39] have characterized the binding protein in rat liver, ligandin, they have shown that it has a high binding affinity for a number of foreign compounds not all of which are carcinogens and many of which bind physically rather than chemically. Pitot and Heidelberger (1963)[40] suggested that the proteins bound to carcinogens were activators or repressors of gene action. Basing their arguments on the mechanism for the genetic control of bacteria by Jacob and Monod (1961)[41], they suggested that the binding of a repressor by a carcinogen could lead to a permanent alteration in gene expression.

BINDING TO TRANSFER-RNA

Transfer-RNA, as its name implies, is responsible for aligning the correct amino acid with messenger RNA in the ribosome during protein synthesis. Aberrations in transfer-RNA could lead to the production of abnormal proteins and thus interfere with the internal economy of the cell. The significance of transfer-RNA in carcinogenesis has recently been discussed (Zamecnik, 1971[42]). The degree of methylation of transfer-RNA is higher in foetal and in cancer tissues than in normal adults and it was believed that one action of methylating carcinogens, such as dimethylnitrosamine, might be to increase the level of methylation of transfer-RNA. The methylating carcinogens act on different bases in transfer-RNA than the methyl transferases naturally present in the tissue.

The practical implications of metabolic activation

It is current practice to test many compounds intended for use as food additives, growth promoters for livestock, pesticides, or pharmaceutical agents for possible carcinogenicity in animals before they are permitted to be used in the human environment. These investigations are extremely costly to carry out and, if the substance is carcinogenic in experimental animals but not in man, there is the additional expense of finding an adequate replacement for the proscribed substance. Difference in capacity for metabolic activation is a major reason why species differ in their response to carcinogens. It is neither ethical nor practical to contemplate studies on the metabolic activation of potential carcinogens in man. *In vitro* assays using human tissues are therefore being developed for the interpretation of animal carcinogenicity tests in relation to man. Ethical problems still remain in obtaining tissues unless fresh *post mortem* material proves adequate for these tests.

As metabolically activated carcinogens are usually highly reactive, they may be detected and quantified by the use of trapping agents. For example, the use of methionine or guanosine to trap the intermediate produced by the sulphation of N-hydroxy AAF has already been discussed. More recently the use of bacteria in combination with microsomal activating systems has been advocated (Ames, 1971[43]): the end point may be the toxicity of the activated carcinogen to the bacteria, measured by the reduction in the number of viable colonies found on subculture.

Alternatively, the induction of mutations by the activated carcinogen may provide a more appropriate parameter. In experimental animals, host mediated assays *in vivo* may offer certain advantages over the *in vitro* technique. In this approach bacteria are injected into the peritoneal cavity, the carcinogen administered by mouth or subcutaneous injection and, after an interval, the bacteria recovered and mutants quantified. Although these tests measure toxicity or mutagenicity, the present concensus of knowledge on the action of chemical carcinogens suggests that they may provide a useful guide to the likely response of different species to a carcinogen, whose activity has been confirmed in one species by a conventional test. Strains of *S. typhimurium* developed by Ames (1971)[43] are generally used. They have proved especially valuable in demonstrating that dimethylnitrosamine (Gabridge and Legator, 1969)[44] and aflatoxin (Garner *et al.*, 1972)[45] require metabolic activation for mutagenicity.

Other mechanisms of carcinogenesis

A carcinogen is commonly defined as an agent which will induce cancer. The carcinogens which have so far been considered share a group of common properties. They, or their active metabolites, generally interact chemically with nucleic acids and proteins and induce cell death, mutation and/or DNA repair (unscheduled DNA synthesis). Like radiation they can be described as genotoxic. If it is accepted that cancer is the result of a mutation-like event, it follows that the dose-response curve for these carcinogens will not show a threshold or no-effect level: even in the case of a single molecule of a mutagen there is a finite probability of its reacting with a receptor and ultimately giving rise to cancer. Too little is known from experimental studies about the shape of dose-response curves for carcinogens, especially at levels which the agent induces tumours in less than 5 per cent of animals exposed to it, to enable the calculation of even an approximation to the probable incidence of cancer in apopulation exposed to a defined but low dose of a carcinogenic agent. This uncertainty leads to the conclusion that, for example, all traces of carcinogens in foodstuffs must be proscribed, a dogma embodied in the Delaney clause of the U.S. Federal Food, Drug and Cosmetics Act. The rigid application of this dogma leads to great practical problems.

For certain substances a direct genotoxic mechanism of cancer induction appears inappropriate. The induction of thyroid tumours by the administration of goitrogens to rats, and of tumours of the endocrine tissues by natural or synthetic oestrogens has already been mentioned. Tumorigenesis by these agents appears to be the end-product of the excessive stimulation of the target tissue by the abnormal levels of these substances or by endogenous hormones released by the endocrine tissues to counteract the primary action. It is not known whether the induction of cancer results from 'spontaneous transformation' or whether the growth of foci of tumour cells induced by traces of other carcinogenic agents is involved.

The normal homeostatic mechanisms of the body may be able to protect against possible harm from low doses of exogenous goitrogens and oestrogens. However, it is possible that in the case of agents of this kind, threshold values could be derived. Some regulatory authorities consider that the hormonal activity of these compounds may conceal a direct genotoxic action and insist that no detectable level of synthetic material with hormonal activities should be present in food. Naturally occurring hormones present a more difficult problem to such authorities.

There is evidence (Chapter 12) that the development of tumours may be generally influenced by immunological factors. Many immunosuppressants are biological alkylating agents (e.g. cyclophosphamide) which have a genotoxic effect and are carcinogenic in their own right. The aromatic nitro group in azathioprine may account for its carcinogenic activity (Frankel *et al.*, 1970[46]) but biological agents such as anti-lymphocyte serum or anti-lymphocyte globulin which are not thought to be carcinogens on the basis of their chemical structures, may also potentiate the growth and development of tumours. For example, the development of leukaemia in response to Moloney Leukaemia Virus injected into *adult* Balb/C mice, which are normally resistant to this virus, may be brought about by anti-lymphocyte serum (Law, 1970)[47]. The incidence of reticulum-cell sarcoma and a variety of other cancers is much higher in patients bearing renal transplants than in the general population (Starzl *et al.*, 1970[48]; Yadav *et al.*, 1972[49]; Hoover and Fraumeni, 1973[49a]). Such patients are kept perpetually in a state of immuno-suppression.

It is not certain whether the increased incidence is secondary to immuno-suppression or in some way a result of the prolonged presence of foreign protein in a host in a partially immune-suppressed state. The fact that tumours often arise very soon after transplantation makes it highly improbable that they result from any direct carcinogenic action of the immuno-suppressive agents themselves.

A partial or complete failure of DNA repair mechanisms is observed in two skin conditions: xeroderma pigmentosa and the De Sanctis-Cacchione syndrome (De Weerd-Kastelein *et al.*, 1972[50]). These syndromes lead to the inability of the skin to make good the damage induced by exposure to sunlight (u.v. radiation) and thence to multiple skin tumours. It has been suggested that arsenic, which appears to be carcinogenic in man but not in experimental animals, inhibits DNA polymerase and thus DNA repair mechanisms in human cells but not those of other species (Jung and Traschsel, 1971[51]). Concentrations of arsenic as low as 10^{-5} to 10^{-6} molar were shown to be effective in inhibiting radiation-induced DNA repair in human fibroblasts *in vitro*: if these observations can be confirmed it may be possible to define threshold values for arsenic and other drugs which enhance the incidence of cancer by similar means (Annotation, Food and Cosmetic Toxicology, 1972[52]).

A classical example of enhancement of tumour production by a non-carcinogen is the effect of croton oil (or the derived phorbol esters (Hecker, 1968[53])) in promoting the development of tumours in mouse skin previously exposed to subcarcinogenic doses of a polycyclic hydrocarbon (Berenblum and Shubik, 1957[54]). Although croton oil has been shown to be carcinogenic by itself (Roe, 1956[55]), it is uncertain whether its active tumour-promoting constituents, the phorbol esters, have this property. In the case of croton oil itself it is impossible to be sure whether the tumours that appear are induced by the agent itself or are the result of initiation by background exposure to a carcinogen and promotion by the agent. Boutwell and Bosch (1958)[56] showed that tumours apparently induced by croton oil were in fact initiated through the exposure of the infant mice to creosote used in the impregnation of their breeding boxes. The mechanism by which croton oil or the phorbol esters induce hyperplasia and promote tumour formation in mouse skin has yet to be elucidated. Teebor *et al.* (1972[56a]) have, however, demonstrated that a phorbol ester inhibits DNA repair and this may help to explain why the phorbol esters behave differently to other irritants such as turpentine.

INDIRECT MECHANISMS

There are a few instances where a chemical may induce a biological disturbance in the animal, which in turn leads to cancer. This may be illustrated by the effects of feeding 4 per cent diethyleneglycol in the diet to rats (Weil *et al.*, 1965[57]). Stones of calcium oxalate, formed by the metabolism of the glycol are precipitated in male but not in female rats.

$$\begin{array}{l} CH_2OH \\ | \\ CH_2OH \end{array} \longrightarrow \begin{array}{l} CO_2H \\ | \\ CO_2H \end{array} \longrightarrow \begin{array}{l} COO^- \\ | \\ COO^- \end{array} \qquad Ca^{++}$$

This sex difference in response may be due to the anatomy of the male urethra favouring the retention of stones in the bladder: bladder epithelial tumours arise in male but not in female rats. That the stones and not the chemical give rise to the tumours has been demonstrated by transplanting the stones to the bladder lumen of other rats and showing that without further chemical treatment, these stones, and others of different composition, led to the formation of bladder tumours in both male and female animals. Stilboestrol is one of several chemicals which increase the risk of development of bladder tumours in rats by inducing vesical calculi.

The logical conclusion from these observations is that when bladder tumours and stones are found together in response to test chemicals, the agent may not be carcinogenic in the full sense of the term. This should, however, be interpreted cautiously. For example, 4-ethylsulphonylnaphthalene-1-sulphonamide (ENS-VI) is a carbonic anhydrase inhibitor. It raises the pH of the urine, leading to the deposition of stones of calcium phosphate and oxalate in the bladder lumen in mice; tumours are induced in the presence of these stones (Clayson and Bonser, 1965[58]). But it is unwise to assume that the stones are solely responsible for tumour formation because, in the acute phase of its action. ENS has a specific effect on the bladder epithelium leading to DNA synthesis and cellular proliferation, cell loss by desquamation into the bladder lumen, and an inflammatory response (Clayson *et al.*, 1967[59]; Levi *et al.*, 1969[60]; Lawson *et al.*, 1970[61]). This acute response to ENS suggests that it has other actions than precipitating stones, and these may play a role in carcinogenesis.

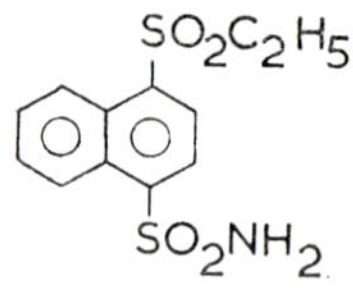

(VI)

These indirect actions on specific tissues have not been intensively explored in many instances. There is evidence that surface active agents and agents with other physical properties induce sarcomas local to the site of injection in rats (Grasso and Golberg, 1966[62]; Grasso *et al.*, 1969[63]; 1971[64]; Hooson *et al.*, 1973[65]; Carter, 1970[66]; Carter *et al.*, 1970[67]) and that in many rodent species the subcutaneous or intraperitoneal implantation of discs and films of a wide variety of materials lead to local sarcomas (for references, see Clayson, 1962[12]; Bischoff, 1972[15a]; Carter, 1970[66]).

In this brief review I have tried to touch upon the main growing points of knowledge in the field of chemical carcinogenesis. Facts and knowledge of mechanisms are accumulating rapidly, nevertheless precise information about chemical causes of human cancers remains scarce. Thus we know that smoking plays an important role in the causation of nearly 40 per cent of cancers in males, but despite much research we still know little of the precise mechanisms involved.

References

1. Miller, J. A. *Cancer Res.*, **30,** 559 (1970).
2. Magee, P. N. *Ann. N.Y. acad. Sci.*, **163,** 717 (1969).
3. Pott, P. *Chirurgical Observations*, (1775).
4. Rehn. L. *Arch. klin. Chir. Langenbecks*, **51,** 588 (1895).
5. Henry, S. A. Cancer of the Scrotum in Relation to Occupation, Oxford Univ. Press, London. (1946).
6. Case, R. A. M., Hosker, M. E., McDonald, D. B. and Pearson, J. T. *Br. J. Industr. Med.*, **11,** 75 (1954).
7. Shank, R. C., Wogan, G. N. and Gibson, J. B. *Fd. Cosmet. Toxicol.*, **10,** 51 (1972).
8. Shank, R. C., Wogan, G. N., Gibson, J. B. and Nondasuta, A. *Fd. Cosmet. Toxicol.*, **10,** 61 (1972).
9. Shank, R. C., Gordon, J. E., Wogan, G. N., Nondasuta, A. and Subhamani, B. *Fd. Cosmet. Toxicol.*, **10,** 71 (1972).
10. IARC Monographs on the Evaluation of Carcinogenic Risk of Chemicals to Man. Vol. **1,** pp. 157 (1972).
11. Evans, I. A. *Cancer Res.*, **28,** 2252 (1968).
12. Clayson, D. B. *Chemical Carcinogenesis*, Churchill, London (1962).
13. Hieger, I. *Br. Med. Bull.*, **14,** 159 (1958).
14. Price, J. M. *Canad. Cancer Conf.*, **6,** 224 (1966).
15. Bischoff, F. *Prog. Exp. Tumor Res.*, **3,** 412 (1963).

15a. Bischoff, F. *Clin. Chem.*, **18,** 869 (1972).

16. Allen, M. J., Boyland, E., Dukes, C. E., Horning, E. S. and Watson, J. G. *Br. J. Cancer*, **11,** 212 (1957).
17. Bryan, G. T., Brown, R. R., Morris, C. R., and Price, J. M. *Cancer Res.*, **24,** 586 (1964).
18. Clayson, D. B. In: *The Biology and Clinical Management of Bladder Cancer* ed. E. H. Cooper and R. E. Williams. Blackwell, Oxford (in press).
19. Brown, R. R., Price, J. M., Friedell, G. H. and Burney, S. W *J. Nat. Cancer Inst.*, **43,** 295 (1969).
20. Radomski, J. L., Glass, E. M. and Deichmann, W. B. *Cancer Res.*, **31,** 1690 (1971).
21. Miller, J. A., Cramer, J. W. and Miller, E. C. *Cancer Res.*, **20,** 950 (1960).
22. Lotlikar, P. D., Enomoto, M., Miller, J. A. and Miller, E. C. *Proc. Soc. Exp. Biol. Med.*, **125,** 341 (1967).
23. Miller, E. C. and Miller, J. A. *Pharmalogical Reviews*, **18,** 805 (1966).
24. Miller, E. C., Juhl, U. and Miller, J. A. *Science*, **153,** 1125 (1966).
25. De Baune, J. R., Miller, E. C. and Miller, J. A. *Cancer Res.*, **30,** 577 (1970).
26. Weisburger, J. H., Yamamoto, R. S., Williams, G. M., Grantham, P. H. and Matsushima, T. *Cancer Res.*, **32,** 491 (1972).
27. Irving, C. C., Janss, D. H. and Russell, L. T. *Cancer Res.*, **31,** 387 (1971).

27a. Bartsch, H., Miller, J. A. and Miller, E. C., *Biochem. Biophys. Acta*, **273,** 40 (1972).

28. Miller, E. C. and Miller, J. A. *Cancer Res.*, **7,** 468 (1947).
29. Boveri, T. *The Origin of Malignant Tumours*, Williams and Wilkins, Baltimore (1929).
30. Burdette, W. J. *Cancer Res.*, **15,** 201 (1955).

31. Maher, V. M., Miller, E. C., Miller, J. A. and Szybalski, W. *Mol. Pharmacol.*, **4,** 411 (1968).
32. Brookes, P. *Cancer Res.*, **26,** 1994 (1966).
33. Chen, T. T. and Heidelberger, C. *Int. J. Cancer*, **4,** 166 (1969).
34. Freeman, A. E., Price, P. J., Igel, H. J., Young, J. C., Maryak, J. M. and Huebner, R. J. *J. Nat. Cancer Inst.*, **44,** 65 (1970).
35. Huebner, R. J. and Todaro, G. J. *Proc. nat. Acad. Sci. U.S.A.*, **64,** 1087 (1969).
36. Miller, E. C. and Miller, J. A. *Cancer Res.*, **12,** 547 (1952).
37. Sorof, S., Young, E. M., Spence, M. M. and Fetterman, P. L. *Biochem. Biophys. Acta*, **38,** 559– (1960).
38. Abell, C. W. and Heidelberger, C. *Cancer Res.*, **22,** 931 (1962).
39. Litwack, G., Ketterer, B. and Arias, I. M. *Nature*, **234,** 466 (1971).
40. Pitot, H. C. and Heidelberger, C. *Cancer Res.*, **23,** 1694 (1963).
41. Jacob, F. and Monod, J. *J. Mol. Biol.*, **3,** 318 (1961).
42. Zamecnik, P. C. *Cancer Res.*, **31,** 716 (1971).
43. Ames, B. N. In Hollaender, A. (ed.) *Chemical Mutagens Principles and Methods for their Detection*, Vol. **1,** pp. 267–282, Plenum Press, New York (1971).
44. Gabridge, M. G. and Legator, M. S. *Proc. Soc. Exp. Biol. Med.*, **130,** 831 (1969).
45. Garner, R. C., Miller, E. C. and Miller, J. A. *Cancer Res.*, **32,** 2058 (1972).
46. Frankel, H. H., Yamamoto, R. S., Weisburger, E. K. and Weisburger, J. H. *Toxicol. appl. Pharmacol.*, **17,** 462 (1970).
47. Law, L. W. *Fed. Proc.*, **29,** 171 (1970).
48. Starzl, T. E., Porter, K. A., Andres, G., Halgrimson, C. G., Hurwitz, R., Giles, C., Teraski, P. I., Penn, I., Lilly, J., Starkie, S. J. and Putman, C. W. *Ann. Surg.,* **172,** 437 (1970).
49. Yadav, R. V. S., Marshall, V. C., Johnson, W., Matthew, T. H. and Kincaid-Smith, P. *Med. J. Austral.*, **i,** 729 (1972).
49a. Hoover, R. and Fraumeni, J. *F. Lancet*, **ii,** 55 (1973).
50. Weerd-Kastelein, E. A. De, Keijzer, W. and Bootsma, D. *Nature*, New Biol., **238,** 80 (1972).
51. Jung, E. G. and Traschsel, F. *Arch. klin. exp. Derm.*, **237,** 819 (1971).
52. Annotation. *Fd. Cosmet. Toxicol.*, **10,** 100 (1972).
53. Hecker, E. *Cancer Res.*, **28,** 2338 (1968).
54. Berenblum, I. and Shubik, P. *Br. J. Cancer*, **1,** 379 (1947).
55. Roe, F. J. C. *Br. J. Cancer*, **10,** 72 (1956).
56. Boutwell, R. K. and Bosch, D. *Cancer Res.*, **18,** 1171 (1958).
56a. Teebor, G. W., Duker, N. U., Ruacan, S. A. and Zachary, K. Y. *Biochem. Biophys. Res. Comm.*, **50,** 70 (1973).
57. Weil, C. S., Carpenter, C. P. and Smyth, H. F. *Arch. Environ. Hlth.*, **11,** 569 (1965).
58. Clayson, D. B. and Bonser, G. M. *Br. J. Cancer*, **19,** 311 (1965).
59. Pringle, J. A. S., Clayson, D. B. and Bonser, G. M. *Biochem. Pharmacol.*, **16,** 619 (1967).
60. Levi, P. E., Cowen, D. M. and Cooper, E. H. *Cell Tissue Kinet.*, **2,** 249 (1969).
61. Lawson, T. A., Dawson, K. M. and Clayson, D. B. *Cancer Res.*, **30,** 1586 (1970).
62. Grasso, P. and Golberg, L. *Fd. Cosmet. Toxicol.*, **4,** 297 (1966).
63. Grasso, P., Gangolli, S. D. and Hooson, J. *Br. J. Cancer*, **23,** 787 (1969).

64. Grasso, P., Gangolli, S. D., Golberg, L. and Hooson, J. *Fd. Cosmet. Toxicol.*, **9**, 463 (1971).
65. Hooson, J. Grasso, P. and Gangolli, S. D. *Br. J. Cancer*, **27**, 230 (1973).
66. Carter, R. L. 'Induced Subcutaneous Sarcomata: their development and critical appraisal.' In: *Metabolic Aspects of Food Safety*, Ed. F. J. C. Roe. p. 569. Blackwell Scientific Publications, Oxford.
67. Carter, R. L., Birbeck, M. S. C. and Roberts, J. D. B. *Br. J. Cancer*, **24**, 300 (1970).

Chapter **10**

NUCLEIC ACID MODIFICATIONS AND CANCER

J. J. ROBERTS, Ph.D., D.Sc.

Senior Lecturer, Division of Chemical Carcinogenesis, Chester Beatty Research Institute, Institute of Cancer Research, London

---

It is the ability of a single malignant cell to produce a tumour in animals (Furth and Kahn, 1937[1]; Ishibashi, 1950[2]) that clearly establishes the cellular nature of this disease. While host factors will obviously play a role in the induction process and in the subsequent development of a tumour (Furth (1963)[3]), there can be little doubt that the cancer cell is derived by modification of a normal cell in such a way as to produce a permanent heritable change in its properties, expressed phenotypically by a partial or complete loss of control of multiplication. Moreover, cytological and biochemical studies which indicate the clonal origin of tumours suggest that tumours can arise from a single chromosomally abnormal cell. A consistent finding from cytological observations is the similarity of the karyotype derived from any one single tumour tissue in contrast to the variability from tumour to tumour (Atkin (1969)[4]). Other evidence that the initial change in the development of neoplasia occurs in one cell, leading to a clone of similar cells, has come from studies on isoenzymic patterns in Burkitt's tumour (Fialkow *et al.*, 1970[5]) and in a variety of head and neck tumours (Fialkow *et al.*, 1972[6]).

From the time that nucleic acids and particularly deoxyribonucleic acid (DNA) were recognized as the source of genetic information within the cell, investigators have looked in this direction for a clue as to the nature of the cellular modification associated with neoplastic change. During the past few years, studies on the role of nucleic acids in cancer have followed essentially two courses. They have either sought differences in the levels, structure and function of nucleic acid molecules in the normal and malignant cell, or alternatively have been concerned with how these macromolecules may be modified by interaction with known chemical carcinogenic agents. While these efforts have not provided incontrovertible proof of the somatic mutation theory of cancer, most of the findings have been consistent with this possibility.

In the early days following the enunciation of the central dogma and the elucidation of the genetic code, it appeared that only a modification to DNA would produce a mutational event leading to the emergence of a cancer cell. But the discovery that some RNA molecules could act as a template for the synthesis of DNA indicated that DNA was not the only possible site of attack of chemical carcinogens which could produce mutational events. It is by no means axiomatic that a definite chemical modification of DNA is required in order to effect a change of gene expression. Thus, carcinogenesis can be likened to the changes of gene expression which are associated with cellular differentiation when (presumably) no permanent chemical changes in the DNA sequence occur. Much recent work has pointed to the possible role of various RNA molecules in controlling and regulating this epigenetic process by mechanisms which may involve various methylating enzymes (see Tsutsui *et al.*, 1966[7]; and Baliga *et al.*, 1969[8] for reviews). Again, reactions with proteins have been considered by Jacob and Monod (1961)[9] to result in alteration in gene expression, and a model which could convert such alteration to heritable or quasi-irreversible changes was subsequently proposed by Pitot and Heidelberger (1963)[10].

In this chapter I shall consider three questions concerning the role of nucleic acids in the development of neoplasia. (1) What chemical modifications occur to DNA when exposed to known chemical carcinogens which might induce a somatic mutation leading to cancer? (2) What chemical changes occur in molecules other than DNA that could modify gene expression leading to tumour induction? (3) What information is transcribed from DNA in malignant as compared with normal cells, and how is this controlled and regulated? A further aspect that should be borne in mind is the role of DNA and RNA tumour viruses in neoplastic transformation. Clearly the information contained in a virus can produce a hereditary change whether or not the viral genome eventually becomes integrated into the somatic cell: this aspect of cancer is discussed in Chapter 11.

Reactions of carcinogens with cellular macromolecules

BIOLOGICAL FACTORS

The last decade has seen the resolution of several outstanding problems in chemical carcinogenesis. The remarkable species- or organ-specificity of a number of chemical carcinogens can now be interpreted in terms of the availability at the appropriate receptor site of a reactive carcinogenic chemical species. Studies in this field are now at the stage of establishing (*a*) that reactions have occurred with nucleic acids, (*b*) the chemical nature of such reactions, and, when feasible, (*c*) the correlation of quantitative aspects of these reactions with the carcinogenic process. However, this last approach must necessarily be somewhat unsophisticated since it is recognized that many stages are involved in the course of development from a transformed cell to the appearance of a tumour (see review by Farber, 1968[11]). Thus a cell is constantly changing its properties by a process of progression (Foulds, 1969[12]) whereby some cells acquire growth advantages over their neighbours in the process of clonal selection. The formation of clones of abnormal cells, or clones within clones, presumably accounts for the fact that chemically-induced neoplasms each contain cell antigens which are unique to that tumour—in contrast to virus-induced neoplasms which contain antigens characteristic of the viruses and not of the transformed cell. Further aspects of oncogenesis which complicate the study of structure-activity relationships are the variable and often long latent interval that separates exposure to a carcinogen and the appearance of identifiable cancer cells, and the fact that this interval can be shortened by exposure to other chemical compounds that have been called 'promoters' or 'co-carcinogens'. Such compounds are usually not themselves carcinogenic or are only weakly so; hormones may sometimes occupy the role of endogenous promoting agents (Furth, 1963[3]). The need for cell proliferation to occur before the initial response to a carcinogen is apparent has been discussed by a number of authors (see Farber (1968)[11] for review) and introduces further complexity into the temporal events controlling carcinogenesis. Recently, much interest has been focused on the ability of a cell to recognize damage to its DNA. Depending on the nature of the lesion and the genetic constitution of the cell, the damage may either be eliminated or circumvented by means of appropriate enzyme systems. These processes are most clearly understood in relation to lethal damage to DNA in micro-organisms, and it is now clear that they have their counterpart in the eukaryotic cell. If reactions with DNA are indeed relevant to carcinogenesis, then the role of DNA repair mechanisms must be considered. Reactions of chemicals with cellular constituents other than DNA, such as proteins and RNA, would be expected to influence these secondary factors of promotion, cell division and DNA repair. In view of the above factors it is not surprising that quantitative evidence in support of a causative role for reaction with DNA in the carcinogenic process is limited.

The early work of Earle (Earle and Nettleship, 1943)[13] and Gey (Gey *et al.*, 1959)[14] indicated that normal cells, cultured serially for a long time,

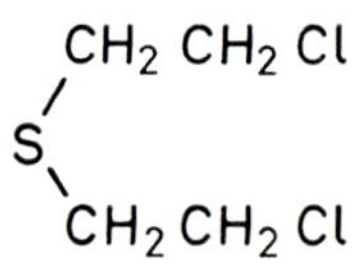

SULPHUR MUSTARD
MUSTARD GAS
(H)

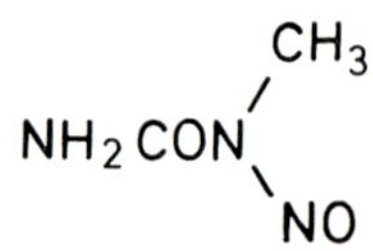

N-METHYL-N-NITROSOUREA
(MNU)

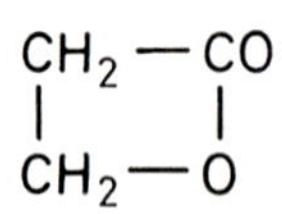

β-PROPIOLACTONE (BPL)

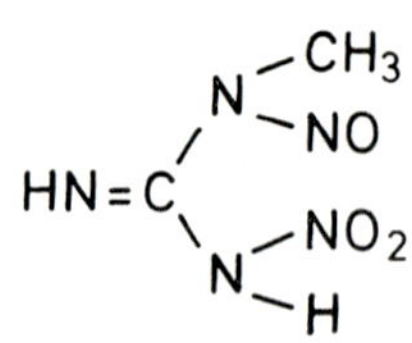

N-METHYL-N'-NITRO-N-NITROSOGUANIDINE (MNNG)

$CH_3SO_2O\ C_2H_5$

ETHYL METHANESULPHONATE
(EMS)

$CH_3SO_2OCH_3$

METHYL METHANESULPHONATE
(MMS)

Fig. 10.1. Reactive alkylating agents.

may undergo malignant transformation and give rise to tumours when injected into an appropriate host. Considerable efforts have subsequently been spent in developing *in vitro* systems for analysing this transformation process, notably by Sachs, Heidelberger and DiPaolo and their co-workers (Berwald and Sachs, 1963[15]; Huberman and Sachs, 1966[16]; Chen and Heidelberger, 1969a, b, c[17–19]; Mondal and Heidelberger, 1970[20]; Grover *et al.*, 1971[21]; Dipaolo, Donovan and Nelson, 1969, 1971[22, 23]). Macpherson (1970)[24] has discussed the criteria proposed for the detection of viral or chemically-transformed cells *in vitro*. Use of these various systems should help to elucidate the role of reactions with nucleic acids in the carcinogenic process.

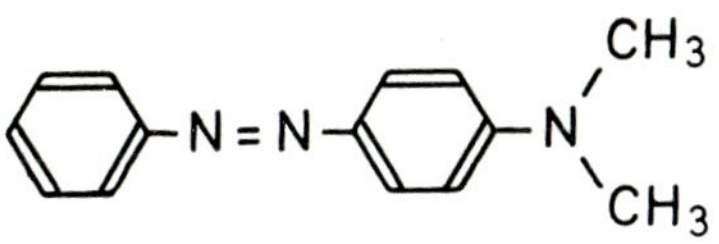

4-DIMETHYLAMINOAZOBENZENE
BUTTER YELLOW
(DAB)

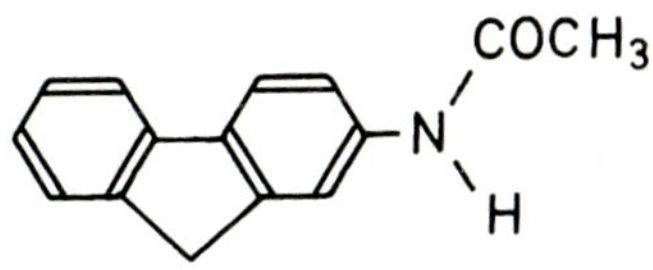

ACETYLAMINOFLUORENE (AAF)

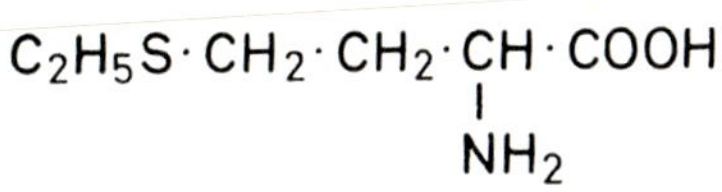

ETHIONINE

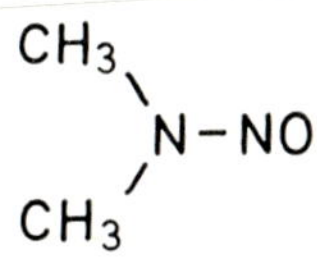

DIMETHYLNITROSAMINE (DMN)

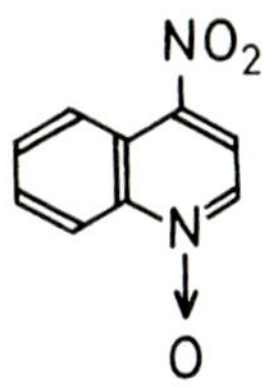

4-NITROQUINOLINE-1-OXIDE
(4NQO)

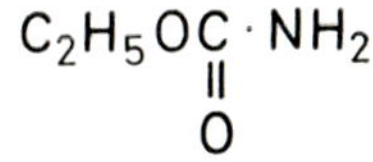

ETHYL CARBAMATE
URETHANE

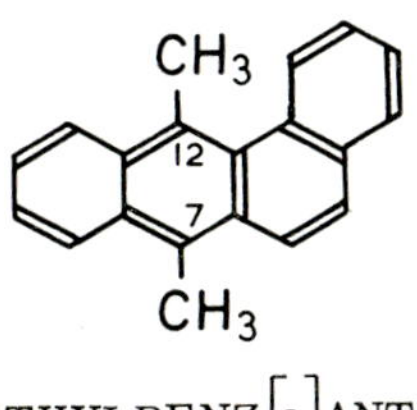

7:12-DIMETHYLBENZ[a]ANTHRACENE

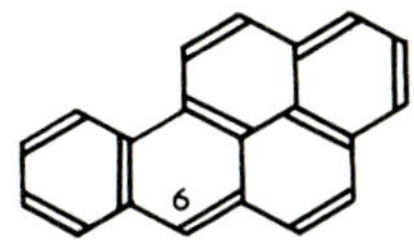

BENZO(a)PYRENE

Fig. 10.2. Synthetic carcinogenic chemicals which are probably metabolized to reactive electrophiles *in vivo*.

It now appears that most chemical carcinogens fall into two distinct categories: (*a*) compounds that can react directly with cell constituents and which are active *per se* in initiating the carcinogenic process, and (*b*) compounds that require preliminary metabolic conversion to an active metabolite which then initiates the neoplastic transformation. Biological alkylating agents such as β-propiolactone, the sulphur and nitrogen mustards, the alkyl sulphonates and alkyl nitrosamides and alkyl nitrosamidines are examples of the first group of agents (*Fig. 10.1*). In the second category are a number of synthetic chemical carcinogens (*Fig. 10.2*) as well as several natural carcinogenic products thought to cause cancer in man. Of the synthetic chemicals requiring intermediate metabolism, polycyclic hydrocarbons, aromatic amines, azo dyes, nitrosamines, 4-nitroquinoline-l-oxide, urethane and ethionine (*Fig. 10.2*) have been most extensively investigated and the chemistry of their enzymic activation has been comprehensively reviewed (Miller and Miller 1966, 1971[25, 26]; and Miller (1970)[27].

BINDING OF CARCINOGENS TO NUCLEIC ACIDS; SUBSEQUENT TUMOUR INCIDENCE

Covalent binding of residues of these various chemical carcinogens or their metabolites to macromolecules *in vivo* has now been demonstrated but attempts to correlate such binding to either DNA or RNA with the ultimate incidence of tumours from a series of closely related compounds of varying potency, or by a particular agent in susceptible and nonsusceptible tissues, have met with mixed success. A positive correlation between binding to DNA (but not RNA or protein) for a series of aromatic hydrocarbons was found by Brookes and Lawley (1964)[28] and by Colburn and Boutwell for β-propiolactone and related compounds (for review see Boutwell *et al.* (1969)[29]. A limited correlation between DNA binding and tumour initiation with azo dyes was suggested by the work of Dingman and Sporn (1967)[30] but this was not apparent from the previous results of Roberts and Warwick (1966)[31] who investigated binding with similar compounds in a variety of species and in susceptible and non-susceptible tissues. In these studies, azo-dye binding to DNA was initially determined following a single injection of drug whereas chronic feeding of rats for three months is required for tumour initiation. Subsequent comparison of binding of 4-dimethylaminoazobenzene and an inactive analogue — 2-methyl-4-dimethylaminoazobenzene—showed that under such chronic feeding conditions binding to DNA was eventually appreciably higher than that following a single injection; but major differences in the binding of each of these compounds to liver DNA were not revealed (Roberts, 1969[32]). Possibly the lack of tumour formation by the 2-methyl derivative was related to its greater toxicity which may have been a function of the relatively higher protein binding. Neither Swann and Magee (1968)[33] nor Den Engelse *et al.* (1969–70)[34] were able to correlate methylation of nucleic acids with the subsequent incidence of tumours. Matsushima and Weisburger (1969–70)[35] did, however, find that only with respect to DNA was there a relationship between depressed binding of radioisotope from N-hydroxy-acetylaminofluorene, after prefeeding selected agents, and the inhibitory effect of these agents on tumour induction in the liver of rats. In retrospect, and particularly in view of recent advances in our knowledge of DNA repair (see later), the lack of any close correlation in these studies on the overall binding to DNA is hardly surprising. The different alkylating agents or electrophiles will react at various nucleophilic sites in DNA (see later) only some of which (and not necessarily those formed in a major amount) will elicit biological events such as mutations leading to cancer.

BIOLOGICALLY ACTIVE ALKYLATING AGENTS

Sites of alkylation in DNA

This group of substances has been shown to alkylate a variety of macromolecules including DNA, RNA and protein in numerous biological systems. Extensive studies, notably by Brookes and Lawley (for review see Lawley, 1966[36]), have revealed several damaging effects following alkylation of DNA. These can be summarized as follows: (1) single base substitution; (2) depurination reaction; (3) single strand breaks; (4) double strand breaks; (5) inter- or intrastrand cross-links; (6) esterification of phosphate groups.

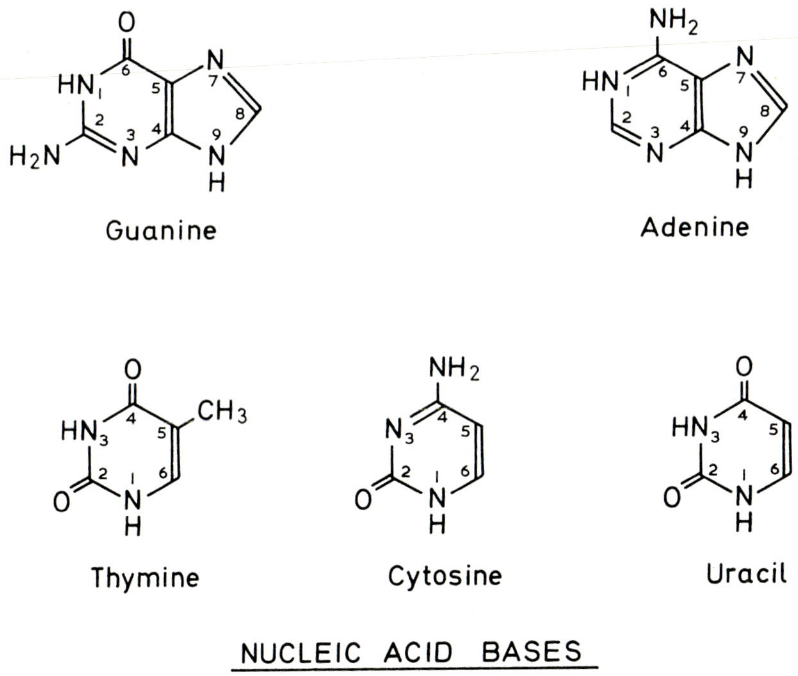

Fig. 10.3. Nucleic acid bases.

There are clearly numerous sites of reaction in DNA for monofunctional agents, but the 7-position of guanine usually accounts for up to 90 per cent of the total alkylation (see *Fig. 10.3*). Sites of monofunctional alkylation of purine and pyrimidine residues in nucleic acids *in vivo* and *in vitro* are now known to include in adenine residues, N–1, N–3 and N–7; in guanine N–3,

N–7 and 0–6; in cytosine N–3 and in uracil N–3 (Lawley, 1966[36]; Ross, 1962[77]; Loveless, 1969[38]; Lawley, Shah and Orr 1972[39]; and Lawley and Shah 1972[40]).

Ability to alkylate at the extranuclear 0–6 atom of guanine seems to be confined to agents such as the *N*-nitrosamines and *N*-nitrosamides and ethyl methanesulphonate which can react by an S_N1 mechanism. Lawley *et al.* (1972)[39] analysed the reactions of different alkylating agents with RNA and polynucleotides and suggested that these same agents—unlike those acting by an S_N2 mechanism such as mustard gas and dimethyl sulphate—could also react with phosphodiester groups and cause degradation of RNA. Whether or not phosphotriester formation occurs in DNA and contributes to its subsequent degradation is still a matter for conjecture, though it has been demonstrated in model systems (Ludlum, 1967[41]; Rhaese and Freese 1969[42]).

It should be noted that reactions at sites other than those listed, such as the C–8 position of guanine and the amino groups of guanine, adenine and cytosine have been described for certain other carcinogenic agents (to be discussed in a later section); some of these possibly react through formation of an intermediate electrophile.

Biological effect of alkylation

It is uncertain which type of damage in DNA is responsible for a particular effect. Swann and Magee (1968)[33] compared the tumorigenic capabilities of *N*-methyl-*N*-nitrosourea, methyl methanesulphonate, dimethylnitrosamine and dimethyl sulphate (*Fig. 10.1*) and found no correlation between the level of 7-methylguanine and the yield of tumours in certain organs of the rat. Colburn and Boutwell (Boutwell *et al.*, 1969[29]) have observed alkylation of DNA from mouse skin as a consequence of topical application of β-propiolactone. The amount of 7-(2-carboxyethyl)guanine in skin DNA could be correlated with the initiation of skin tumours when either the dose of alkylating agent or the susceptibility of the mice was varied. Recently, attention has focussed on the minor products of DNA alkylation. Loveless (1969)[38] has suggested that the greater extent of 0–6 alkylation by *N*-methyl-*N*-nitrosourea as compared with methyl methanesulphonate may not only account for its greater mutagenicity towards T2 bacteriophage (Loveless and Hampton (1969)[43]) but may also be related to its carcinogenic properties. On the other hand, cytosine substitution in the 3 position has been thought to be responsible for some of the mutagenic effects of *N*-methyl-*N'*-nitro-*N*-nitrosoguanidine in tobacco mosaic virus (Singer and Fraenkel-Conrat, 1969[44]). Depurination resulting from alkylation of the 7 position of guanine and 3 position of adenine has been suggested by Lawley *et al.* (1969)[45] to be a predominant cause of the inactivation of T7 phage.

The presence of an alkylated base in DNA could result in mispairing during DNA replication and this is presumably the basis for many of the mutagenic effects caused by alkylating agents. Alkylation of a base causes labilization of the purine glycoside link which leads to depurination. The gap so produced could then be filled by a variety of bases again leading to mispairing. The consequences of such mispairing can be elucidated by a variety of techniques including a study of point mutations, the frequency of mutation and reversion, or analyses of amino acid substitutions in the gene product. These methods have been discussed in detail by Loveless (1966)[46]. Evidence for mispairing, obtained in a number of systems (for review see Loveless (1966)[46]), suggests that a GC pair is changed to an AT pair but that other changes can also occur. Malling and de Serres (1969)[47], for example found that ethyl methanesulphonate (EMS) and *N*-methyl-*N'*-nitro-*N*-nitrosoguanidine (MNNG) gave mostly AT→GC transitions. Detailed *in vitro* studies on the consequences of particular base substitutions have been carried out by Ludlum[48–51, 53] in an attempt to define more precisely how damage to DNA is expressed during replication and transcription. Wilhelm and Ludlum (1966)[48] first showed that polyribonucleotides containing 7-methylguanine did not cause the theoretical misincorporation of an amino acid which would result if 7-methylguanine resembled adenine in its base pairing properties. These studies were extended to determine the mispairing which occurs when RNA polymerase acts on either a DNA or RNA strand to direct the synthesis of a daughter strand. It is interesting that while 7-methylguanine in a polynucleotide template retained the base-pairing properties of guanine (Ludlum, 1970a)[49], 3-methyl and 3-ethylcytosine, which are produced in much smaller amounts when DNA is alkylated, caused marked misincorporation of uridylic and adenylic acid into daughter polynucleotides (Ludlum and Wilhelm, 1968[50]; Ludlum, 1970b[51]; Singer and Fraenkel-Conrat, 1970)[52]. Polydeoxyribonucleotide templates behaved similarly in this respect (Ludlum (1971)[53]). Troll (Troll *et al.,* 1969[54]) investigated the effect of modifying DNA with various agents on its Tm, buoyant density and RNA polymerase priming activity. β-Propiolactone (BPL) and *N*-acetoxy-2-acetylaminofluorene (acetoxy-AAF) reduced the priming ability of DNA with bacterial RNA polymerase to a measurable extent with as little as I per cent substitution. Furthermore BPL, unlike acetoxy-AAF, caused more than double the incorporation of uridine than cytosine into the resulting RNA, thus supporting the notion that substituted guanine was ambiguous in its selection of cytosine and/or uridine. This ambiguity was confirmed in another system by showing that whereas poly G formed a double helix only with poly C, poly G reacted with BPL formed such a complex with poly C and poly U.

Difunctional alkylating agents are markedly more cytotoxic than monofunctional ones, and this enhanced activity is thought to be a consequence of their ability to introduce either inter- or intrastrand cross-links into DNA. Reversible denaturation experiments were used by Guiduschek (1965)[55] and subsequently by Kohn *et al.* (1966)[56] to demonstrate these cross-links in DNA. Kohn *et al.*[56] further demonstrated the removal of interstrand cross-links in the DNA of *E.coli* B/r but not B_{s-1} and this was elegantly confirmed by Venitt (1968)[57] by direct physical measurement. More recently, Ball and Roberts (1971)[58] demonstrated cross-links directly in mammalian cells by showing that 'heavy' and 'light' opposite strands of DNA (formed by growing cells in BUdR-containing medium) could not be separated in an alkaline caesium chloride gradient following treatment of the cells with mustard gas as they could when isolated from untreated control cells. Yamamoto *et al.* (1966)[59] compared the cytotoxicity of mono- and difunctional mustards on single- and double-stranded bacteriophages and concluded that intrastrand as well as interstrand cross-links could be important in killing cells. A similar conclusion as to the importance of intrastrand cross-linking was reached by Lawley *et al.* (1969)[43] in studies of the inactivation of bacteriophage T7 by mustard gas.

Experiments using synchronized populations of cells in culture have established that the cell killing action of a number of alkylating agents may be correlated with a depression in the rate of DNA synthesis consequent upon reaction with the DNA template (Roberts *et al.* (1971)[60]). With difunctional alkylating agents like mustard gas, this inhibition of DNA synthesis is detected in the cycle during which treatment is carried out if this is during the G_1 or S phase of the cell cycle. Treatment after the S phase is complete—i.e. during the G_2 phase of the cell cycle—results in a depression of DNA synthesis in the following cell cycle. Monofunctional alkylation of cellular DNA with methylating agents such as MNU or MMS does not depress DNA synthesis until the alkylated DNA has undergone one round of replication (Plant and Roberts (1971a, b[61, 62]). Following a depression in the rate of DNA synthesis, cells exhibit a mitotic delay. Since RNA and protein synthesis is only inhibited by much higher concentrations of these agents than those required to produce cell death, these mitotically inhibited cells grow into giant cells.

CHEMICAL CARCINOGENS METABOLIZED TO ELECTROPHILIC REACTANTS

Intensive investigations during the past few years have clearly established the mechanisms by which various carcinogens can be converted *in vivo* by enzymic or non-enzymic means to reactive alkylating agents or electrophilic reactants

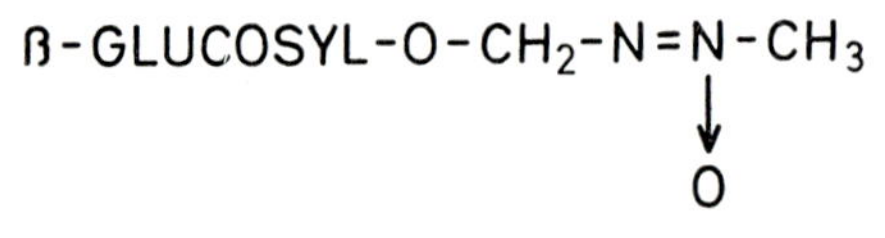

Cycasin

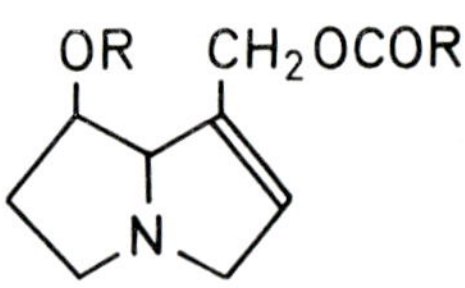

Pyrrolizidine alkaloids

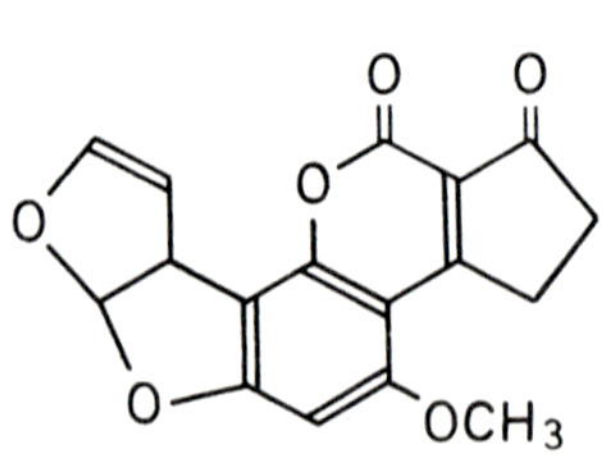

Aflatoxin B_1

Fig. 10.4. Some carcinogenic natural products which are probably metabolized to reactive electrophiles.

(see Miller, 1970[27] for review). Such potential alkylating agents include nitrosamines and nitrosamides (Magee and Barnes, 1967[63]) (see Fig. 10.2), naturally occurring compounds such as cycasin [the glycoside of methylazoxymethanol found in cycad nut meal, Matsumoto and Higa, 1966[64]; Nagata and Matsumoto 1969[65])], the pyrrolizidine alkaloids found in the genera *Senecio Crotalaria* and *Heliotropium* (Mattocks, 1968[66]; Culvenor *et al.* 1969[67]) and aflatoxin, the toxin produced by a strain of *Aspergillus flavus Fig. 10.4*): see Miller (1970[27] for review.) The amino acid analogue ethionines is converted to the ehylating agent S-adenosylethionine *in vivo* but Ortwerth and Novelli (1969)[68] have proposed that another, as yet unidentified, alkylating agent is responsible for the ethylation of transfer RNA in rat liver.

Aromatic amines

Metabolic activation and the properties of the derived active forms are most clearly understood in the case of aromatic amines such as acetylaminofluorene (AAF). The first step in the activation of AAF is the formation of an *N*-hydroxy derivative; the compound itself has little ability to react with nucleic acids *in vitro* but it is subsequently esterified to form a strong electrophilic reactant (*Fig. 10.5*). It is the ability of certain species or organs to perform these metabolic transformations that accounts in large measure for the observed specificity in tumour production of this and related compounds. The synthetic esters of *N*-hydroxyacetylaminofluorene react readily with guanine residues in nucleosides and nucleic acids and only to a limited extent with adenine residues (Kriek *et al.* (1967)[69]). Unlike the classical alkylating agents (see earlier), these esters react at the C-8 position to give, in the case of *N*-acetoxyacetylaminofluorene and guanosine, *N*-(guanosin-8-yl)-acetylaminofluorene (*Fig. 10.5*). When liver ribosomal RNA was isolated from rats given acetylaminofluorene or *N*-hydroxyacetylaminofluorene and then degraded by enzymes to the nucleoside level, a product was obtained which was indistinguisable chromatographically from the above guanine derivative (Kriek, 1969a, b[70, 71]). Debaun, Miller and Miller (1970)[72] have adduced considerable evidence that the *N*-hydroxy AAF is converted by a sulphotransferase to a sulphate ester *in vivo* and that this is the final proximate carcinogen. Other studies indicate that the carcinogenic azo dyes are also converted via *N*-hydroxylation to reactive esters which probably also react at the C-8 position of guanine moieties in DNA (Miller (1970[27]). Substitution at the C-8 of a purine residue with a bulky moiety such as a fluorenyl group would, according to the studies of Kapuler and Michelson (1971)[73] on 8-substituted guanines, require nucleotides to exist in the *syn* configuration rather than the *anti* form present in native DNA. Since the *syn* form could only exist in a denatured region of DNA, such reactions must inevitably lead to a permanent distortion of the helical configuration. Conversely, it would follow that reaction would be more likely to occur at denatured regions of DNA. Similar conformational changes have been elegantly demonstrated to occur in tRNA following reaction with *N*-acetoxyacetylaminofluorene (see later, Weinstein, 1969[74]).

The potent carcinogen 4-nitroquinoline-l-oxide (4NQO) is reduced enzymically to 4-hydroxy-aminoquinoline-l-oxide (Matsushima *et al.,* 1968[75])

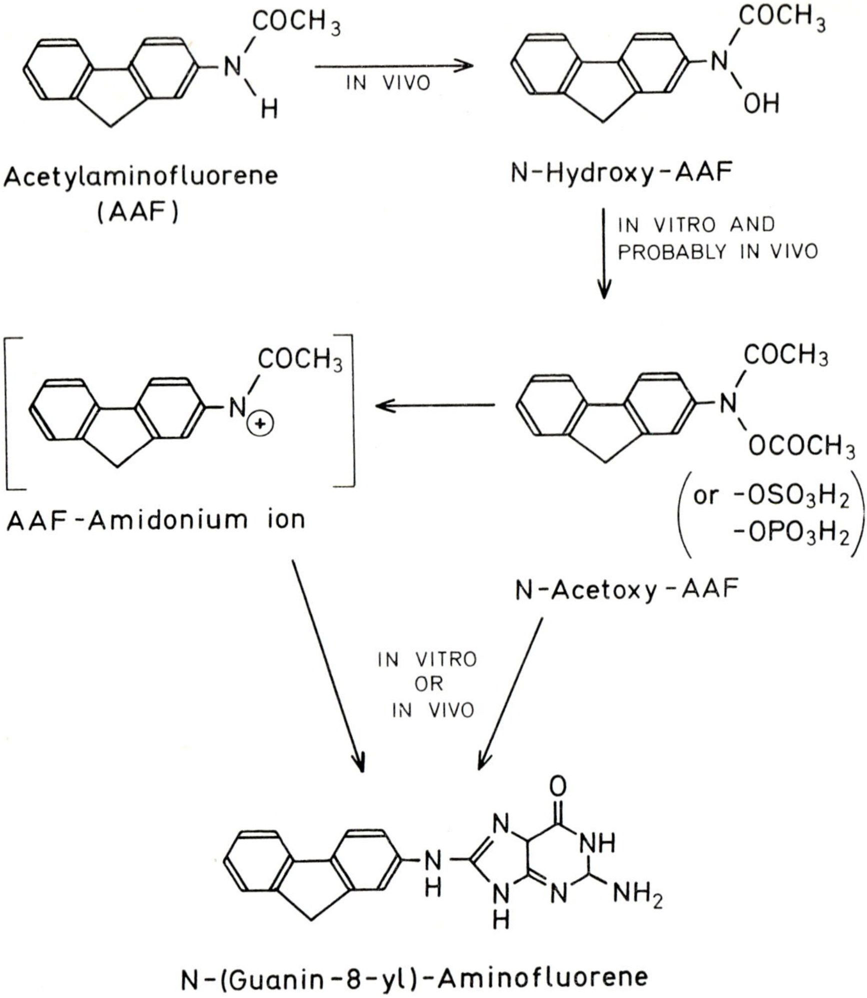

Fig. 10.5. Metabolic activation of 2-acetylaminofluorene (AAF) and product of reaction with nucleic acids *in vivo* and *in vitro*.

which, by analogy with the activation of *N*-hydroxyacetylaminofluorene, is also thought to be further esterified *in vivo* though the sites of reaction of 4NQO with DNA still remains to be elucidated.

Polycyclic hydrocarbons.

The chemically inert but potent carcinogenic polycyclic hydrocarbons undergo extensive metabolism in experimental animals where they are excreted as phenols and dihydrodiols and their corresponding conjugates with glucuronic and sulphuric acid (for review see Boyland, 1969[76]). Boyland (1950)[77] suggested many years ago that an epoxide may be an intermediate in the formation of these products. Direct evidence for this view has recently been obtained since Grover *et al.* (1971)[78] described the formation of epoxides as NADPH-dependent microsomal mixed oxidase metabolites from phenanthrene, benz(*a*)anthracene and dibenz(*a,h*)anthracene. These metabolites can be converted under appropriate conditions into the corresponding dihydrodiol, phenol or glutathione derivatives. The K-region epoxides derived from phenanthrene and dibenz(*a,h*)anthracene were found to be active alkylating agents that reacted chemically with nucleic acids (Grover and Sims (1970)[79]). They also bound more extensively to DNA, RNA and protein of cells in culture than the parent hydrocarbons (Grover, Forrester and Sims, 1971[80]). Although the various K-region epoxides which have been tested were less potent carcinogens in experimental animals than the parent hydrocarbons (Miller and Miller, 1967[81]; Boyland and Sims, 1967[82]; Van Duuren *et al.*, 1967[83]), they have been reported to produce malignant transformation of both hamster embryo cells and a clone of mouse ventral prostate cells in culture more effectively than parent hydrocarbons (Grover *et al.,* 1971[84]). The corresponding K-region cis-dihydrodiols of benz(*a*)anthracene or dibenz(*a,h*) anthracene which are not themselves chemically reactive were also effective in producing transformation *in vitro*, possibly due to further metabolism to reactive intermediates on double bonds other than that of the K-region. The K-region phenols did not, however, produce a significant number of transformed colonies but were the most toxic derivatives tested. It is arguable that these *in vitro* systems are more suitable for testing proximate reactive carcinogens than whole animals since there would be a greater probability that under these conditions they could react with cellular constituents. In this connection it is possible that the ultimate carcinogen may not prove to be carcinogenic in any system if it fails, possibly due to an unfavourable charge, to penetrate cell membranes. Such an explanation may account for the failure of the N-sulphate of AAF to induce tumours at the site of injection in the rat (DeBaun, 1968[85]).

Production of a carbonium ion has been proposed as an alternative mechanism of metabolic activation of hydrocarbons (Dipple *et al.,* 1968[86]). 7-Bromomethylbenz(*a*)anthracene and 7-bromomethyl-12-methylbenz(*a*)-anthracene were synthesized as model compounds capable of generating such species and their carcinogenicites and reactions with nucleic acids examined (Dipple and Slade, 1970, 1971[87, 88]; Dipple *et al.*, 1971[89]). It appears that, in dimethylacetamide solution, 7-bromomethylbenz(*a*)anthracene reacts with nucleosides at the same positions as do methylating agents to give N-7 guanine, N-1 adenine and N-2 cytosine derivatives; but in aqueous solution, reaction with nucleosides or nucleic acids leads to substitution on the amino groups of guanine, adenine and possibly cytosine. More than 90 per cent of the total reaction products can be accounted for as these derivatives. Unambiguous syntheses of the guanine and adenine products were achieved by alternative routes and the products shown to be chromatographically indistinguishable from those formed from the bromo compound (Dipple *et al.*, 1971[89]). Pochon and Michelson, 1971[90] and Pochon *et al.* (1971)[91] studied the physical properties of polynucleotides and DNA following reaction with the same compound. These authors found that the benzanthracene residue, covalently linked *via* a CH_2 group to a purine nucleoside in DNA, is not exterior to the double helix; unlike bromine or AAF residues, it does not cause distortion or denaturation of the secondary structure requiring a change in the nucleoside conformation from the *anti* form. They therefore proposed that the carcinogen lies in the large groove of DNA with an axis parallel to the helix axis, and that reaction at C-8 of guanine residues permits such a model. Pochon *et al.* (1971)[91] also commented on the rather unexpected ability of the bromo compound to cross-link opposite strands of DNA. It is thus possible that different products were obtained under the conditions used by these two groups to account for their separate postulates.

Many groups have investigated yet another form of activation of polycyclic hydrocarbons, resulting in the formation of radical cations capable of reacting covalently with nucleic acids. Various conditions have been used to bring about the loss of an electron, including anodic oxidation, photoirradiation with a mercury arc lamp, X-irradiation, oxidation with iodine, oxygen or ferric chloride (Bergmann, 1954[92]; Ts'o and Lu, 1964[93]; Wilk and Girke, 1969[94]; Ts'o *et al.*, 1969[95]; and Kodama and Nagata, 1969–70[96]). Products consistent with reaction at the 6-position of benzo(*a*)pyrene with adenine moieties of DNA were obtained by Wilk and Girke (1969)[94]. Ts'o *et al.* (1969)[95] argue that through hydrophobic stacking, a polycyclic hydrocarbon molecule is bound tightly to the bases of DNA *via* a face-to-face mode. When the system is suitably activated, long-lived free radicals may be formed and covalent binding between hydrocarbons and bases established which will tend to enhance the hydrophobic stacking forces and weaken the selectivity of hydrogen bonding; mispairing of bases in the recognition process will result. Significantly, radical cations are formed from carcinogenic aromatic hydrocarbons more readily than from non-carcinogenic compounds. They are also formed from aromatic amines and azo dyes which suggested to Wilk and Girke (1969)[94] a common mechanism of action for these agents, namely arylation *via* the electrophilic radical cation.

Repair of damaged DNA

MECHANISMS OF DNA REPAIR

There is increasing awareness of the existence of cellular mechanisms that can modify initial damage to DNA. Our understanding of some of the processes involved has come from studies on the sensitivity of bacterial mutants to UV radiation and has been reviewed by Howard-Flanders (1968)[96] and Setlow (1968)[97]. Similar mechanisms undoubtedly exist for the repair of chemically-modified DNA in both bacterial (Papermeister and Davidson, 1964[98]; Hanawalt and Haynes, 1965[99]; Reiter and Strauss, 1965[100]; Lawley and Brookes, 1965[101]; and Kohn *et al.* 1965[56]) and mammalian cells (Roberts *et al.* 1968[102]; Ball and Roberts, 1970[103]; Roberts *et al.* 1971*a*, *b*[104, 105]; and Lieberman *et al.*, 1971*a*, *b*[106, 107]). Particularly relevant to the induction of cancer by chemicals is the realization that while such processes may permit a cell to survive otherwise lethal damage by a particular chemical, 'repair' mechanisms can themselves introduce mutations into DNA, possibly by errors of base-pairing during the repair process itself (Witkin, 1969[108]; Witkin and Farquharson, 1969)[109]. This potentially important aspect of DNA repair is still at an early stage of development.

Two different pathways have been proposed for the dark repair of UV damage in bacteria: 'excision' or 'cut and patch' repair, and 'recombination repair' (Howard–Flanders (1968)[96]). In excision repair the initial lesion of the pyrimidine dimer, is recognized, presumably through distortion of the DNA helical structure, by an enzyme (endonuclease) which introduces a single-strand break near the lesion. An exonuclease, perhaps associated with a DNA polymerase molecule, excises the dimers with degradation of the DNA and loss of deoxyribonucleoside-5'-phosphates. A gap is produced in the DAN strand into which DNA polymerase inserts new nucleotides. This latter process, called 'repair replication' or non-semi-conservative DNA synthesis, can be distinguished by suitable radioactive and density labels in DNA from normal DNA synthesis. Finally, the end of this newly-synthesized piece of DNA is joined to the pre-existing strand possibly by means of a DNA ligase. Manifestations of this form of repair have been observed in mammalian cells after UV-irradiation (Rasmussen and Painter, 1964, 1966[110, 111]), X-irradiation (Painter and Cleaver, 1967[112]) and following treatment with a variety of alkylating agents (Roberts *et al.,* 1968 and 1971[102, 105]; Fox and Fox 1969[113]; and Cleaver, 1971[114]).

Mammalian cells have also been shown to elicit what is known as unscheduled DNA synthesis after X-irradiation (Rasmussen and Painter, 1966[111]) or UV-irradiation (Painter and Cleaver, 1969[115]) or treatment with various chemical agents such as methyl methanesulphonate (Hahn *et al.*, 1968[116] and 1971[117]; and Lieberman *et al.* 1971[106, 107]) or 4-nitroquinoline-1-oxide derivatives (Stich and San, 1970[118]; Stich *et al.,* 1971[119]). This is demonstrated autoradiographically by the incorporation of labelled thymidine into the DNA of mammalian cells which are not in the DNA synthetic phase (S) of the cell cycle at the time of treatment. Unscheduled DNA synthesis and repair replication are probably manifestations of the same process.

Recombinational or post-replication repair has been shown to occur in certain excision-defective mutants of *E.coli* which enabled them to survive and form colonies after UV-irradiation even though many pyrimidine dimers remained in their DNA (Clark and Margulies, 1965[120]; Howard-Flanders and Boyce 1966[121]). It was subsequently reported by Rupp and Howard-Flanders (1968)[122] that after UV-irradiation, these excision-defective mutants synthesize DNA slowly; the newly synthesized strands had a molecular weight inversely proportional to the UV dose. Replication appeared to take place between pyrimidine dimers, each new strand terminating at a dimer in the template strand; the newly-synthesized pieces of DNA eventually became incorporated into polynucleotide chains of comparable length to those in the control. These findings were interpreted as indicating that recombination had occurred between sister duplexes formed by replication of DNA containing damaged bases such as pyrimidine dimers. The mechanism could provide the transfer of information between duplexes necessary to construct strands containing the entire base sequence of a functional chromosome, even though many dimers remain in the template strands (Howard-Flanders, Rupp and

Wilkins, 1968[123]; Smith and Meun 1970[124]). Verification of this scheme was obtained by growing cells in medium containing ^{13}C and ^{15}N, exposing them to UV-irradiation, and then growing them in [^3H]thymidine-containing medium so that part of their DNA was of hybrid density and the ^3H-label was in the light strand, (Rupp *et al.*, 1971[125]). The DNA from unirradiated cells could be denatured and separated in a caesium chloride gradient into light and heavy bands. Denatured DNA from irradiated cells did not separate into light and heavy strands but contained strands of intermediate density which separated into light and heavy components only after shearing to 5×10^5 molecular weight, thus indicating that segments of molecular weight greater than 5×10^5 had been exchanged.

Evidence for recombination-type repair has been obtained in other systems and in response to damage by various agents. Yamamoto (1967)[126] found that when phage P22 was treated with nitrogen mustard (HN_2) and assayed on a strain of *Salmonella typhimurium* lysogenic for P22l*b*, a high frequency of recombination between damaged P22 and the prophage P221*b* was found. These findings suggest that inactivation by intrastrand cross-linkage of DNA molecules initiates recombination. Other studies (Fukuda and Yamamoto, 1970[127]) indicated that bacteriophage damaged by the potent carcinogen β-propiolactone could be repaired, presumably through the combined action of bacterial excision, bacterial recombination and phage recombination enzymes. In contrast, phage inactivated by the highly carcinogenic 4-hydroxylaminoquinoline-1-oxide (4HAQO) were not repaired by the host cell though the carcinogen again enhanced the frequency of recombination between the damaged superinfecting phage P22 and the prophage 221*b* (Yamamoto *et al.*, 1970[128]). Studies of this type are invaluable in indicating not only when carcinogenic agents or their activated derivatives are able to react with DNA, but also whether the resulting lesion is recognized by a cellular repair mechanism. Mechanisms analogous to bacterial recombinational repair almost certainly exist in higher organisms and in mammalian cells. Watson (1972)[129] has recently provided evidence for recombination repair from studies of the effects of X-rays and alkylating agents on the induction of mutations in a recombination-deficient mutant of *Drosophila melanogaster*. Cleaver and Thomas (1969)[130] found that the newly-synthesized DNA in irradiated Chinese hamster cells also decreases as a function of dose. Furthermore, in both control and irradiated cells the molecular weight increased with time but in the latter case this process could be inhibited by caffeine. Rauth (1967)[171] has suggested that caffeine inhibits a DNA repair system in UV-irradiated mouse L cells but Cleaver (1969)[132] found that caffeine had no effect on non-semi-conservative DNA synthesis. It is therefore, possible that caffeine interferes with semi-conservative DNA synthesis associated with a repair process similar to that controlled by rec mutations in bacteria. Further work is clearly required in order to establish and elucidate the mechanism of recombinational repair in mammalian cells. The existence of such a repair mechanism has been inferred from a quantitative study of alkylation in sensitive and resistant Yoshida cells (Ball and Roberts, 1970[103]). These workers found no difference in two manifestations of excision repair—the loss of alkylated moieties from DNA and repair synthesis in the two cell lines. Similar investigations showed that HeLa cells showed no diminished repair synthesis which would account for their exceptional sensitivity to *N*-nitroso-*N*-methylurea, as compared with Chinese hamster cells (Roberts *et al.*, 1971*a*, *b*[104, 105]; Plant and Roberts 1971*a*, *b*[61, 62]). But other steps in excision repair may differ in these respective cell lines, or, alternatively, the specific repair of a lethal lesion in the resistant cells may be obscured by repair phenomena associated with non-lethal events (see later). It is this last consideration that makes it difficult to assign a biological role to the various mechanisms of DNA repair that have been discussed. One requires a knowledge of the precise lesion(s) in DNA responsible for a particular biological effect—whether toxicity, mutagenicity or carcinogenicity—and the extent to which it can be repaired.

INHIBITORS OF DNA REPAIR

The enhanced lethality produced by the so-called repair inhibitors referred to earlier (Rauth, 1967[131]) has been exploited by Gaudin and Yielding (1969, 1971)[133, 134] to produce a substantial decrease in the growth rate of a resistant plasmacytoma in hamsters by administering cytoxan in conjunction with caffeine or chloroquine. These investigators have extended their studies to the field of chemical carcinogenesis; they argue that co-carcinogens are analogous to repair inhibitors in that each of these groups of compounds increases the effect of other agents that can interact covalently with DNA. Certainly the evidence that all carcinogens interact covalently with cellular macromolecules is now overwhelming (Miller, 1970[27]). Furthermore, carcinogens evoke changes suggesting that repair mechanisms are activated—as found by Lieberman *et al.* (1971*a*)[106] for acetylaminofluorene derivatives, and Stich and San (1970)[118] for 4-nitroquinoline-1-oxide derivatives.

In support of this view, Gaudin, Gregg and Yielding (1971)[135] found that the repair replication occurring in irradiated normal human lymphocytes was inhibited by every co-carcinogen tested to date. Apart from the well recognized co-carcinogens like croton oil, diethylstilboestrol which increases the tumorigenic effect of X-rays (Segaloff and Maxfield, 1971[136]) also inhibited repair synthesis. The dual role of repair inhibitors is illustrated by Vitamin A which can enhance the antileukaemic effect of bis-chloroethylnitrosourea (Cohen, 1971[137]) and act as a co-carcinogen (Levij and Polliack, 1968[138]).

GENETIC FACTORS AND DNA REPAIR

The possible relevance of DNA repair processes in the aetiology of cancer was indicated by the discovery that cells cultured from patients suffering from the hereditary skin disease Xeroderma pigmentosa (XP) which results in actinic skin cancer are defective in excison repair of UV damage due to an autosomal recessive mutation (Cleaver, 1968[139]; Setlow *et al.*, 1969[140]; Bootsma *et al.*, 1970[141]). Conceivably, the failure to repair UV-induced DNA lesions in XP cells could cause a high UV-induced mutation rate and result in cancer. Since these cells are sensitive to UV light and are impaired in their ability to support the growth of UV-irradiated viruses, (Rabson *et al.*, 1969[112]; Aaronson and Lytle (1970)[143]. they can be regarded as human diploid analogues of bacterial Uvr⁻, Hcr⁻ mutants. The biochemical defect has been identified as a deficiency of a UV-specific endonuclease which initiates the excision of the UV photoproducts. Since most XP cells can perform a low level of repair replication (Bootsma *et al.*, 1970[141]; Cleaver, 1970[144]), they have been regarded as leaky mutants in which the endonuclease is present at reduced activity. These so-called mutant cells can be used to elucidate the molecular action of other agents which interact with DNA. Bacterial mutants sensitive to UV-irradiation lack the capacity to produce DNA strand scission but can perform the remaining steps in repair. Hence chemical or physical agents which induce DNA strand scission without the involvement of an endonuclease should elicit repair processes in these repair-deficient cells; by contrast, agents which react with DNA without resulting in actual breakage of DNA should not produce indications of repair. These predictions have been borne out by studies with X-rays, alkylating agents and derivatives of 4-nitroquinoline-1-oxide. Thus XP cells are not deficient in the repair of damage to DNA caused by X-rays which are known to introduce breaks directly into DNA (Cleaver, 1969[145]; Kleijer *et al.*, 1970[146]). Alkylating agents such as methyl methanesulphonate (MMS) and *N*-methyl-*N'*-nitro-*N*-nitrosoguanidine (MNNG) also induced the same level of repair replication in normal and XP cells. This is consistent with the view that these agents produce breaks in DNA non-enzymically (Lawley, 1966[36]) and agrees with experiments on the sensitivity of Uvr⁻, Hcr⁻ bacteria to MMS. Such mutants in *E.coli* (Howard–Flanders and Boyce, 1966[147]) and *B. subtilis* (Searashi and Strauss, 1968[148]) have increased sensitivity to UV light but normal sensitivity to MMS. It must be presumed therefore that repair of these non-enzymically-induced breaks as a result of MMS and MNNG treatment does not require the initial excision step that is defective in XP cells. Alternatively, different endonucleases are required to initiate excision of alkylated bases and UV photo-products; but this possibility has been discounted in bacteria (Strauss *et al.*, 1970[149]).

In contrast to these findings with methylating agents, Stich and San (1971)[150] reported that unscheduled DNA synthesis was reduced in XP cells as compared with normal cells treated with 4-nitroquinoline-l-oxide (4NQO) or 4-hydroxylaminoquinoline-l-oxide (4HAQO); this finding indicates that single strand breaks are introduced into DNA as a result of endonuclease action.

Mutation and cancer

Confirmation of the somatic mutation theory of cancer is still being actively sought despite the years that have elapsed since it was first propounded by Boveri in 1929. The general inability to demonstrate a positive correlation between carcinogenesis and mutation can now be understood in view of the need for some carcinogens to be metabolized to an ultimate carcinogen, a step that may not occur in the genetic test system. Host-mediated assays in which animals can be used to potentiate compounds in relation to their mutagenic activity have been devised to overcome these problems (Gabridge and Legator, 1969[152]; Legator and Malling, 1971[153]). Malling (1971)[154] has described a simplified system in which dimethylnitrosamine was incubated with a suspension of liver microsomes in the presence of *S.typhimurium*, the indicator organism for mutagenicity. Other studies have revealed the mutagenic effects of what are thought to be active forms of various carcinogens in various systems. Reactive synthetic esters of acetylaminofluorene and *N*-methyl-4-aminoazobenzene caused up to 100-fold increases in the frequencies of mutations in transforming DNA (Maher *et al.*, 1968[155]), while acetoxy-acetylaminofluorene caused A/T to G/C base pair transitions in T4 phage (suggesting a role for the minor adenine reaction) (Corbett *et al.*, 1970[156]), and, following injection into adult *Drosophila*, chromosome deletions and mutations leading to the production of the *Minute* phenotype (Fahmy and Fahmy, 1971[157]). Analysis of the mutagenic activity and the nature of mutational events (base pair transitions, frameshift or deletion mutations) produced by a large number of carcinogenic compounds in bacteriophage T4 has led to the general conclusion that there is no quantitative correlation between the effectiveness of a mutagen in this system and its potency as a carcinogen; nor is any single characteristic type of mutation induced by carcinogenic compounds (Corbett *et al.*, 1970[156]). On the other hand, specific deletion mutations in *Drosophila* at the X-chromosome *bobbed* (*bb*) gene, characterized by short thin bristles in the double heterozygote, was found in the case of carcinogenic polycyclic hydrocarbons, aromatic amines, alkylating agents and nitroso compounds (Fahmy and Fahmy, 1969, 1970*a*, *b*, *c*, 1971)[158 159 161, 157]). It had earlier been shown that the partial deletio of DNA within the nucleolar organizer heterochromatin X-chromosome segment associated with these mutations was at the principal site for transcription of ribosomal RNA (Ritossa *et al.* (1966*a*)[162].

Hydrocarbon K-region epoxides (the putative ultimate carcinogens) derived from potent carcinogens but not from non-carcinogenic hydrocarbons cause host range mutations of T_2h^+ bacteriophage (Cookson *et al.* (1971)[163]), possibly of the frameshift type as indicated in other suitable test systems (Ames *et al.*, 1972[164]). Models for measuring chemical mutagenesis in mammalial cell cultures have recently been developed and exploited in studies of chemical carcinogenesis (for review see Chu, 1971[165]). Chu and Malling (1968)[166] and Kao and Puck (1968)[167] initially showed that gene mutations are increased significantly over spontaneous frequencies after treating Chinese hamster cells with alkylating agents such as EMS, MMS and MNNG (*Fig.* 10.1). The former workers followed the development of resistance to 8-azaguanine which was accompanied by the loss of the enzyme hypoxanthine-guanine phosphoribosyl transferase (HG-PRT), the enzyme required to convert the purine analogue to the nucleotide and permit its incorporation into DNA with toxic consequences. Reverse mutation frequencies at the same locus could also be determined by growing cells in appropriate selective medium. The mutagenic activities of K-region epoxides of hydrocarbons have again been amply demonstrated using this system. Benz(*a*)anthracene and methylcholanthrene epoxides were appreciably more mutagenic than the corresponding phenols, while the parent hydrocarbons and corresponding *cis*- and *trans*-dihydrodiols were inactive (Huberman *et al.*, 1971[168]). Even more convincing evidence for somatic mutation in carcinogenesis would, however, come from studies of transformation and mutagenesis in the same cells.

Enzymic modification of tRNA

ISOACCEPTING tRNAS

Synthesis of protein is now known to involve the following steps (see Davidson 1969[169] for review). An amino acid (aa_1) is activated by an enzyme (E_1) in the presence of ATP to produce the appropriate activated amino acid according to th equation:

$$ATP + aa_1 + E_1 = (aa_1 - AMP)E_1 + PPi$$

Separate enzymes, aminoacyl-tRNA synthetases, are required for each amino acid. tRNA molecules are then able to recognize a particular aminoacyl-tRNA synthetase so that they can accept the appropriate amino acid according to:

$$(aa_1 - AMP)E_1 + tRNA_1 = tRNA\ aa_1 + AMP + E_1$$

It is clear, therefore, that each aminoacyl-tRNA synthetase (also called aminoacyl-tRNA ligases) must possess two binding sites. One recognizes a specific amino acid and the other recognizes and selects a specific tRNA molecule to which that amino acid becomes covalently bound. Subsequently it was found that there is more than one form of tRNA specific for a particular amino acid (Doctor *et al.*, 1961[170]); these heterogeneous tRNAs have been called isoaccepting tRNAs (Yang and Novelli, 1968a[171]). tRNA consists of about 75 nucleotides ending in the sequence pCpCpA and it is the terminal adenosine moiety to which the activated amino acid becomes attached. The tRNA molecule then carries the amino acid to the ribosomes where the coding site (the anticodon), situated in the loop or bend near the centre of the tRNA chain in an area rich in methylated bases and pseudouridine, can link to the corresponding area (the codon) on the messenger RNA; the required amino acid sequence is then finally established. In this way the genetic information contained in the DNA can code for a particular sequence of amino acids and thus for a particular protein. The mechanism for regulating this process is, however, obscure. tRNA has long been known to be rich in minor base modifications, the most common is methylation (see later) and this occurs by the action of enzymes on intact RNA. Other enzymic methods of modifying RNA have been described apart from methylation, e.g. thiolation, formation of pseudouridine, addition of isopentenyl and other alkyl moieties, and deamination. These base modifications can change the tertiary structure of tRNAs and possibly modulate their several functions. Such changes could account for the existence of the various isoaccepting tRNA species referred to above, and the possibility that they may have some functional significance in regulation and differentiation has prompted numerous investigations. Although there is little direct evidence for such controls in animal cells, various studies have revealed that the tRNAs of different kinds of cells and cells in different metabolic states are chromatographically distinguishable (Taylor *et al.*, 1967, 1971[172, 173]). The technique employed to demonstrate these differences involved charging tRNA molecules with a particular labelled amino acid by means of tRNA synthetases and other cofactors. The aminoacyl-tRNA molecules are then separated—either on methylated albumin keiselguhr (MAK) or benzoylated diethylaminocellulose (BD) columns, or by means of reverse phase chromatography (RPC) columns—to yield tRNA profiles characteristic of a particular amino acid. These studies have shown that cultured tumour cells have transfer RNA populations that differ chromatographically from those generally found in the tissue of origin as in the case of hamster cells transformed by adenovirus, Simian virus 40, or Rous sarcoma virus (Holland *et al.*, 1967[174]). Baliga *et al.* (1969)[8] reported differences in tyrosine-, histidine-, and asparagine-tRNA between Novikoff hepatoma and normal liver; Volkers and Taylor (1971)[175] and Gonano and Chiarugi (1969)[176] have found chromatographic differences between Morris hepatomas and normal liver. Mouse plasmacytoma cells which synthesize different myeloma proteins were found by Yang and Novelli (1968b)[177] to contain different seryl-tRNA populations. Gallo and Pestka (1970)[178] compared normal lymphocytes and leukaemic lymphoblasts in man and reported small but reproducible differences in leucyl-, seryl-, threonyl- and prolyl-tRNA and pronounced differences in tyrosyl- and glutaminyl-tRNA between the two cell types. A difference in tyrosyl-tRNA was again found in a comparison of human myeloma cells and normal IgM-producing blood cells which could possibly be associated with the production of λ (lambda)-type light chains (Bence–Jones proteins) by the myeloma cells. (Fujioka and Gallo, 1971[179]). Penhoet and Holland (1971)[108] examined tRNA populations with particular reference to tyrosyl-tRNAs from more than twelve tumour biopsy specimens. (It is the tyrosyl-tRNAs that have most frequently been shown to differ in tumour tissue as compared with normal tissue). Of these biopsies, one breast carcinoma contained tyrosyl-tRNA which could be distinguished from that found in normal tissues, and this was in the most rapidly growing tumour examined. The patterns of isoaccepting phenylalanine-tRNAs isolated from spleens of patients with malignant lymphoma and leukaemia were found by Mittelman (1971)[181] to differ from those in normal tissue, while another study by Yang (1971)[182] also suggests a relationship between the characteristic isoaccepting-tRNAs and the state of cellular differentiation in the tumour tissue. Thus a more malignant form of a plasma cell tumour showed a greater relative increase in aspartyl- and tyrosyl-tRNAs; while the characteristic tyrosyl-tRNAs, found in Reuber hepatoma cells but not in the normal or regenerating liver, were also detected in the liver of 20-day-old rat embryos albeit in lower quantity. The multiple isoaccepting species of tRNA may not necessarily play a role in differentiation or regulation (Taylor 1970[183]): they may reflect mutational changes occurring in non-essential regions of the tRNA molecule, or they may reflect extensive redundancy of tRNA genes as postulated by Ritossa *et al.* (1966*b*)[184] for *Drosophila melanogaster*. The difference in the isoaccepting-tRNA species, especially in seryl- and tyrosyl-tRNA in normal and leukaemic human lymphoblasts (Gallo and Pestka (1970)[178]), could be due to modifications in the minor base components of tRNA. This possibility led Gallo and Whang-Peng (1971)[185] to investigate the regulatory effect on human lymphocytes of the tRNA minor base N^6-Δ^2-(isopentenyl) adenosine (IPA) which, in yeast, is known to be situated adjacent to the anticodon. Interestingly enough analysis of the tRNA revealed that the IPA concentration of lymphosarcoma cells was 4-fold greater than in either normal or Burkitt's lymphoma cells.

tRNA METHYLASES

The original suggestion by Borek (1963[186]; Srinivasen and Borek, 1963, 1964)[187, 188]; (see reviews by Borek, 1968[189] and Sueoka and Kano Sueoka, 1970)[190] that modification of preformed tRNA by methylating enzymes may serve a regulatory function in protein synthesis has led to many studies on the role of methylation in differentiation and carcinogenesis. This hypothesis was based (i) on the observation by Berquist and Matthews (1962)[191] that tRNA from murine mammary adenocarcinoma and the S-180 ascites tumours contains more methylated purines than does tRNA from normal mouse tissue, and (ii) on reports by Farber and Magee (1960, 1962)[192, 193] that the potent hepatic carcinogens ethionine and dimethylnitrosamine methylated the RNA of the liver after administration to rats. More recently, Craddock (1969)[194] found increased levels of methylated bases in tRNA from precancerous livers of rats fed the carcinogenic agents aflatoxin and dimethylnitrosamine. These studies have been carried out on total mixed RNAs which might have obscured any changes in specific tRNAs. Related experiments by Waalkes *et al.* (1971)[195] showed that changes in tRNA methylase activity occured prior to or as an early manifestation of the malignant conversion induced in monkeys by administering *N*-nitrosodiethylamine. A rapid turnover and excretion of methylated purines, thought to be derived from tRNA, has been found in animals with thymic lymphoma and in mouse mammary carcinoma (Mandel, Srinivasan and Borek, 1966[196]) and a hamster bearing a tumour caused by adenovirus 12 (McFarlane and Shaw 1968*a*, *b*[197, 198]).

The parameters used to characterize tRNA methylases are the rate and extent of methylation, and the specific bases methylated. The position of the methylated bases in the nucleotide chain awaits further investigation. Essentially the same methods have been used to study tRNA methylases in various tissues. The soluble enzymes from the 100,000g supernatant of cellular extracts react in the presence of ^{14}C-S-adenosyl-L-methionine with a heterologous tRNA which may be methyl-deficient tRNA, normal tRNA from *E. coli B*, or yeast tRNA.

These methylating enzymes probably located in the nucleus of the cell have been shown to be species-, organ-, and base-specific. Their role in differentiation was indicated by changes during insect metamorphosis (Baliga *et al.*, 1965[199]) and during morphogenesis of the slime mould (Pillinger and Borek, 1969[200]). Craddock (1970)[201] has discussed the evidence which suggests that tRNA methylases in tumours differ from those in normal tissue. Increased levels of tRNA methylases have been reported in human mammary tumour and in rat hepatoma (Tsutsui *et al.*, 1966[7]), in mouse hepatoma (Hancock, 1967[202]), in hamster tumours induced by SV 40 virus (McFarlane and Shaw, 1968[198]; Mittelman *et al.*, 1967)[203], in C_3H mouse mammary carcinomas (Turkington and Riddle, 1970[204]), in liver and kidney homogenates from chicks infected with Marek's disease virus (Hacker and Mandel, 1969[205]; Mandel *et al.,* 1971[206]) in a neoplastic cell line in culture compared with the non-neoplastic parental line (Gantt and Evans, 1969[207]; Gantt 1971[208]), and in cultures of polyoma-transformed rat embryo cells (Gallagher *et al.,* 1971[209]). Some doubt was cast on these observations when Kaye and Leboy (1968)[210] found that the elevated methylase levels in tumour tissue could be ascribed to the stimulating effects of ammonium ions in the assay system. But Stewart and Corrance (1969)[211] subsequently used the same assay conditions as Kaye and Leboy and confirmed the elevated methylase levels in malignant tissue. Changes in the capacity and specificity of the methylases from tumours could be interpreted as primarily related to differences in growth rates and the degree of differentiation rather than to any causative factor in carcinogenesis. Thus there is a high concentration of methylase in embryonic liver (Hancock *et al.,* 1967[202]) and in mouse mammary gland after stimulation by hormones (Turkington, 1969[212]). Viale (1971)[213] excluded these possibilities by showing that unfractionated tRNAs of human brain tumours were overmethylated as compared with human normal brain. Similarly Riddick and Gallo (1970)[214] and Gallo (1971)[215] found identical methylase activity in two spontaneous murine mammary tumours which, although histologically similar, differed in growth rate. These authors also found that increased tRNA methylase activity was characteristic of immature normal cells as well as neoplastic cells. The induction of tRNA methylase in lymphocytes following mitogen stimulation to undergo transition to an undifferentiated cell 'in cycle' was thought to be consistent with this concept (Riddick and Gallo, 1971[216]). Recent work in this field has sought to determine the mechanism controlling methylase activity focusing attention on the presence of methylase inhibitors in normal adult rat tissue, (Kerr, 1970, 1971[217,218]; Kerr *et al.,* 1971[219]). Leboy (1970)[220] has reported that naturally occurring polyamines including spermine or putrescine increased several-fold the specific activity and extent of methylation of tRNA by extracts of rat organs. These findings introduce yet another complicating factor into the significance of differences in methylase activity in normal and malignant tissue. Finally, despite these intensive investigations it remains to be resolved whether such changes are a causative factor in carcinogenesis or merely epiphenomena. Nevertheless, the original postulate that methylated bases constitute a regularing mechanism of protein synthesis remains an attractive one. The alterations in methylating enzymes in embryonic and differentiating tissue are consistent with this postulate, and the aberrant methylation in tumour tissue may represent a loss of such regulating mechanisms.

Chemical modifications of RNA

The qualitative differences previously described between tRNA species from certain tumour cells and normal cells, and the extensive work indicating that tRNA may be a critical target for chemical carcinogens, has led to studies of the biochemical consequences of reactions of carcinogens with transfer RNA. Fink, Nishimura and Weinstein (1970)[221], employing a reactive derivative of AAF, *N*-acetoxy AAF, established that binding of AAF to *E.coli* tRNA produces modifications in amino acid acceptance, codon recognition and in ribosomal binding and chromatographic behaviour of specific types of tRNA. Analysis of ribonucleic acids following administration of labelled AAF indicated a higher extent of binding to tRNA than to 5S, 18S or 28S RNAs (Agarwal and Weinstein, 1970[222]) and that reaction had occurred with more than one type of tRNA. Subsequently Grunberger and Weinstein (1971)[223] determined the effect of modifying guanosine residues in several oligonucleotides or poly (U_3G) on their ability to direct the binding of specific aminoacyl-tRNAs to ribosomes. Studies with trinucleotides in which 100 per cent of the guanosine residues were substituted with AAF indicated that the modification of guanosine at either the 5′ or 3′ end of the codon completely inactivated the function of that codon in the ribosomal binding assay. AAF modification of poly (U_3G) also inhibited its template function during protein synthesis. These effects were thought to result from an inability of codons in which guanine residues were modified by AAF to interact properly with the anticodon regions of related tRNAs. An extension of these results might indicate that AAF modification would prevent normal base pairing not only during translation but also during DNA replication and transcription. If reaction occurred with mRNAs *in vivo* then their function in translation might be impaired. An effect on transcription rather than on replication of DNA was indicated from experiments of Troll *et al.*, (1968)[224] who found that DNA isolated from the livers of male rats fed AAF resulted in reduced priming activity with RNA polymerase but not with DNA polymerase. It should be stressed in attempting to understand the biological significance of these results that at the level of reaction of AAF occurring *in vivo*, relatively few mRNA or tRNA molecules would have reacted with AAF with a low probability that modification of either codon or anticodon sites would have occurred.

Gene expression and cancer

A progressive alteration in the regulation of DNA transcription appears to be a prerequisite to the development of neoplasia. Kidson and Kirby (1964)[225] were the first to produce evidence of such a change by comparing the pattern of rapidly-labelled nuclear RNA molecules (mRNA) when separated by counter current distribution; the sources of mRNA were normal mouse liver and a transplantable mouse hepatoma. Subsequently, Kidson and Kirby (1965)[226] followed the changes in pattern of liver mRNAs in rats fed on 4′-fluoro-4-dimethylaminoazobenzene. The changes were different in type and extent from those following administration of the non-carcinogenic analogue, aminoazobenzene. Early changes in mRNA were reversible, later changes were irreversible, consistent with the time of reversibility of the pathological changes induced in the liver during azo-dye feeding. Some doubts on the validity of these and other related changes induced by hormone administration, were subsequently expressed by Leader and Barry (1967)[227] and by Jackson and Sells (1968)[228], both groups questioning the ability of the countercurrent distribution technique to follow changes in gene expression. The technique of DNA-RNA hybridization and hybridization competition has therefore been favoured for the detection of differences in the products of gene transcription in normal and neoplastic cells. The presence of additional species of hybridizible nuclear RNA (nRNA) has been demonstrated in human chronic lymphocytic leukaemia cells (Nieman and Henry, 1969[229]) and in two types of transplantable breast cancer cells from mice and rats (Turkington and Self, 1970[230]). In this latter study it was shown that, in the hybridizing experiments, mouse liver RNA competed with carcinoma RNA to a somewhat greater extent than did mammary RNA. This suggested either that some of the additional species of RNA present in carcinoma RNA may also be present in liver cells, or that some RNA species which are too low in concentration in mammary cells to be detected by the method used can be detected in RNA derived from normal liver or carcinoma cells. Since unlabelled carcinoma RNA exhibited complete competition in the reaction between labelled normal RNA and DNA it was also evident that this assay procedure failed to detect any species of rapidly labelled nuclear RNA in the carcinoma cells which were not also synthesized by normal mammary cells. Turkington (1971)[231] used the same technique to demonstrate that the progression of neoplastic development—normal cells→hyperplastic alveolar nodules→ spontaneous carcinoma→serially transplantable carcinoma—is accompanied by discrete increments at each stage in the diversity of the nuclear RNA species formed. Altered regulation of transcription thus seems to be a feature of cells that have undergone a preneoplastic change, neoplastic transformation, or neoplastic progression. Krueger and McCarthy (1970)[232] followed the annealing characteristics of pulse-labelled RNA species to DNA from four different myeloma tumours, each of which produced a single homogeneous species of immunoglobulin. Rates of reaction, thermal stability and competition experiments all suggested differences among the four different tumour DNAs, a result that may indicate specific gene amplification of immunoglobulin genes. While Gottlieb and Liu (1970)[233] confirmed these findings in the same system these authors cautioned that the technique of RNA-DNA hybridization may be subject to considerable base mispairing. Therefore only those hybrid structures in which the melting temperatures (Tm) are consistent with genuine hybrid formation can be adequately interpreted. However, Shearer (1971)[234] also Shearer and Smuckler (1971)[235] failed to find any evidence for differences between DNAs of primary and transplantable rat hepatomas and normal rat liver kidney and lung, suggesting no additional gene families were derepressed during malignant transformation.

Other evidence for the role of modification of gene expression based on the induction of liver enzymes by various carcinogenic chemicals has been discussed by Gelboin (1968)[236].

Mitochondrial DNA

Mitochondrial DNA (M DNA) was initially found to exist in a simple circular form of contour length of about 5μ. Subsequently Clayton and Vinograd (1967)[237] described two more complex forms: a circular dimer form, which was a double length circular molecule, and a catenary form, in which the single length circular molecules were connected to each other like links in a chain. Clayton and Vinograd (1969)[238] then showed that the circular dimer form was present in the mitochondrial DNAs from the peripheral blood of fourteen patients with chronic granulocytic leukaemia. The frequency of circular chains correlated with the immaturity of the leukocyte distribution and it was inferred that the frequency was strikingly reduced when patients were given chemotherapy. It is possible that membrane structural proteins are among the gene products of M DNA in animal cells, and defects in the regulation in structure of such proteins in cells containing the circular dimer could contribute to the properties of the cancer cells (Clayton and Vinograd, 1969[238]). Since the formation of circular dimers or catenanes necessarily involves the cells' apparatus for opening and closing strands of DNA it is further suggested that any disproportion of these forms could result from the malfunction of enzymes involved in DNA synthesis, recombination or repair. In this connection it is interesting that Wunderlich *et al.* (1971–2)[239] found 4.5 times as much alkylation of M DNA than nuclear DNA following a single intraperitoneal injection of *N*-nitroso [^{14}C]dimethylamine to rats or hamsters. Schwaier *et al.* (1968)[240] showed that carcinogenic nitroso compounds induced cytoplasmic mutations more frequently than chromosomal mutations in yeast cells.

References

1. Furth, J. and Kahn, M. C., *Am. J. Cancer*, **31,** 276 (1937).
2. Ishibashi, K., *Gann*, **41,** 1 (1950).
3. Furth, J., *Cancer Res.*, **23,** 21 (1963).
4. Atkin, N. B., In 'Genetic Concepts of Neoplasia', 36, 23rd Annual Symp. on Fundamental Cancer Res. Houston (1969).
5. Fialkow, P. J., Klein, G., Gartler, S. M. and Clifford, P., *Lancet*, 384 (1970).
6. Fialkow, P. J., Martin, G. M., Klein, G., Clifford, P. and Singh, S., *Int. J. Cancer*, **9,** 133 (1972).
7. Tsutsui, E., Srinivasan, P. R. and Borek, E., *Proc. Nat. Acad. Sci. U.S.A.*, **56,** 1003 (1966).
8. Baliga, B. S., Borek, E., Weinstein, I. B. and Srinivasan, P. R., *Proc. Nat. Acad. Sci. U.S.A.,* **62,** 899 (1969).
9. Jacob, F. and Monod, J., *J. Mol. Biol.*, **3,** 318 (1961).
10. Pitot, H. C. and Heidelberger, C., *Cancer Res.*, **23,** 1694 (1963).
11. Farber, E., *Cancer Res.*, **28,** 1859 (1968).
12. Foulds, L., *Neoplastic Development*, Vol. **I**. Academic Press, London 1969.
13. Earle, W. R. and Nettleship, A., *J. Natl. Cancer Inst.*, **4,** 213 (1943).
14. Gey, G. O., Gey, M. K., Firor, W. M. and Self, W. O., Acta. *Un. Int. Cancer*, **6,** 706 (1949).
15. Berwald, Y. and Sachs, L., *Nature*, **200,** 1182 (1963).
16. Huberman, E. and Sachs, L., *Proc. Nat. Acad. Sci.* (*U.S.A.*), **56,** 1123 (1966).
17. Chen, T. T. and Heidelberger, C., *J. Nat. Cancer Inst.*, **42,** 903 (1969 *a*).
18. Chen, T. T. and Heidelberger, C., *J. Nat. Cancer Inst.,* **42,** 915 (1969 *b*).
19. Chen, T. T. and Heidelberger, C., *Int. J. Cancer*, **4,** 166 (1969 *c*).
20. Mondal, S. and Heidelberger, C., *Proc. Nat. Acad. Sci.* (*U.S.A.*), **65,** 219 (1970).
21. Grover, P. L., Sims, P., Huberman, E., Marquardt, H., Kuroki, T. and Heidelberger, C., *Proc. Nat. Acad. Sci. U.S.A.*, **68,** 1098 (1971).

22. DiPaolo, J. A., Donovan, P. and Nelson, R., *J. Nat. Cancer Inst.*, **42,** 867 (1969).
23. DiPaolo, J. A., Nelson, R. L. and Donovan, P. J., *Nature*, **235,** 278 (1972).
24. Macpherson, I., *Advances in Cancer Research*, Vol. **13,** 169 (1970).
25. Miller, J. A. and Miller, E. C., *Lab. Invest.*, **15,** 217 (1966).
26. Miller, J. A. and Miller, E. C., *J. Nat. Cancer Inst.*, **47,** V (1971).
27. Miller, J. A., *Cancer Research*, **30,** 554 (1970).
28. Brookes, P. and Lawley, P. D., *Nature*, **202,** 781 (1964).
29. Boutwell, R. K., Colburn, N. H. and Muckerman, C. C., *Ann. N.Y. Acad. Sci.*, **163,** 751 (1969).
30. Dingman, C. W. and Sporn, M. B., *Cancer Res.*, **27,** 938 (1967).
31. Roberts, J. J. and Warwick, G. P., *Int. J. Cancer*, **1,** 179 (1966).
32. Roberts, J. J., *The Jerusalem Symposia on Quantum Chemistry and Biochemistry* (ed. E. D. Bergmann and B. Pullman)' Jerusalem Israel **1,** 224 (1969).
33. Swann, P. F. and Magee, P. N., *Biochem. J.*, **110,** 39 (1968).
34. Den Engelse, L., Bentvelzen, A. J. and Emmelot, P., *Chem.-Biol. Interactions*, **1,** 395 (1969–70).
35. Matsushima, T. and Weisburger, J. H., *Chem.-Biol. Interactions*, **1,** 211 (1969–70).
36. Lawley, P. D., *Progr. Nucl. Acid Res. and Mol. Biol.*, **5,** 89 (1966).
37. Ross, W. C. J., *Biological alkylating agents*, Butterworth and Co., London (1962).
38. Loveless, A., *Nature*, **223,** 206 (1969).
39. Lawley, P. D., Shah, S. A. and Orr, D. J., *Chem.-Biol. Interactions*, **5,** 431 (1972).
40. Lawley, P. D. and Shah, S. A. *Biochem J.*, **128** 117 (1972).
41. Ludlum, D. B., *Biochim. Biophys. Acta*, **142,** 282 (1967).
42. Rhaese, H. J. and Freese, E., *Biochim. Biophys. Acta*, **190,** 418 (1969).
43. Loveless, A. and Hampton, C. L., *Mutation Res.*, **7,** 1 (1969).
44. Singer, B. and Fraenkel-Conrat, H., *Biochemistry*, **8,** 3266 (1969).
45. Lawley, P. D., Lethbridge, J. H., Edwards, P. A. and Shooter, K. V., *J. Mol. Biol.*, **39,** 181 (1969).
46. Loveless, A., *Genetic and Allied Effects of Alkylating Agents*, Butterworth and Co., London (1966).
47. Malling, H. V. and de Serres, F. J., *Ann. N.Y. Acad. Sci.*, **163,** 788 (1969).
48. Wilhelm, R. C., Ludlum, D. B., *Science*, **153,** 1403 (1966).
49. Ludlum, D. B., *J. Biol. Chem.*, **245,** 477 (1970 *a*).
50. Ludlum, D. B. and Wilhelm, R. C., *J. Biol. Chem.*, **243,** 2750 (1968).
51. Ludlum, D. B., *Biochim. Biophys. Acta*, **213,** 142 (1970*b*).
52. Singer, B. and Fraenkel-Conrat, H., *Biochemistry*, **9,** 3694 (1970).
53. Ludlum, D. B., *Biochim. Biophys. Acta*, **247,** 412 (1971).
54. Troll, W., Rinde, E. and Day, P., *Biochim. Biophys. Acta*, **174,** 211 (1969).
55. Geiduschek, E. P., *Proc. Nat. Acad. Sci.* (*U.S.A.*), **47,** 950 (1961).
56. Kohn, K. W., Steigbigel, N. H. and Spears, C. L., *Proc. Nat. Acad. Sci. U.S.A.*, **53,** 1154 (1965).
57. Venitt, S., *Biochem. Biophys. Res. Commun.*, **31,** 355 (1968).
58. Ball, C. and Roberts, J. J., *Chem.-Biol. Interactions*, **4,** 297 (1971–72).
59. Yamamoto, N., Naito, T. and Shimkin, M. B., *Cancer Research*, **26,** 2301 (1966).
60. Roberts, J. J., Brent, T. P. and Crathorn, A. R., *Europ. J. Cancer*, **7,** 515 (1971).
61. Plant, J. E. and Roberts, J. J., *Chem.-Biol. Interactions*, **3,** 337 (1971 *a*).

62. Plant, J. E. and Roberts, J. J., *Chem.-Biol. Interactions*, **3,** 343 (1971 *b*).
63. Magee, P. N. and Barnes, J. M., *Advances Cancer Res.*, **10,** 164. ed. G. Klein and S. Weinhouse, Academic Press, New York and London.
64. Matsumoto, H. and Higa, H. H., *Biochem. J.*, **98,** 20C (1966).
65. Nagata, U. and Marsumoto, H., *Proc. Soc. Expl. Biol. Med.*, **132,** 383 (1969).
66. Mattocks, A. R., *Nature*, **217,** 723 (1968).
67. Culvenor, C. C. J., Downing, D. T., Edgar, J. A. and Jago, M. V., *Ann. N.Y. Acad. Sci.*, **163,** 837 (1969).
68. Ortwerth, B. J. and Novelli, G. D., *Cancer Res.*, **29,** 380 (1969).
69. Kriek, E., Miller, J. A., Juhl, U. and Miller, E. C., *Biochemistry*, **6,** 177 (1967).
70. Kriek, E., *The Jerusalem Symposia on Quantum Chemistry and Biochemistry* (ed. E. D. Bergmann and B. Pullman). Jerusalem Israel, **1,** 136 (1969 *a*).
71. Kriek, E., *Chem-Biol Interactions*, **1,** 1 (1969 *b*).
72. DeBaun, J. R., Miller, E. C. and Miller, J. A., *Cancer Res.*, **30,** 577 (1970).
73. Kapuler, A. M. and Michelson, A. M., *Biochim. Biophys. Acta*, **232,** 436 (1971).
74. Weinstein, I. B. In 'Genetic concepts and neoplasia' 23rd Annual Symposium on Fundamental Cancer Res., Houston 1969 p. 380.
75. Matsushima, T., Kobuna, I., Fukuoka, F. and Sugimura, T., *Gann*, **59,** 247 (1968).
76. Boyland, E., *The Jerusalem Symposia on Quantum Chemistry and Biochemistry* (ed. E. D. Bergmann and B. Pullman). Jerusalem, Israel, **1,** 25 (1969).
77. Boyland, E., 'The Biological Significance of Metabolism of Polycyclic Compounds.' *Symp. Biochem. Soc.*, **5,** 40 (1950).
78. Grover, P. L., Hewer, A. and Sims, P., *FEBS letters*, **18,** 76 (1971).
79. Grover, P. L. and Sims, P., *Biochem. Pharmacol.*, **19,** 2251 (1970).
80. Grover, P. L., Forrester, J. A. and Sims, P., *Biochem. Pharmacol.*, **20,** 1297 (1971).
81. Miller, E. C. and Miller, J. A., *Proc. Soc expl. Biol. Med.*, **124,** 915 (1967).
82. Boyland, E. and Sims, P., *Int. J. Cancer*, **2,** 500 (1967).
83. Van Duuren, B. L., Langseth, L., Goldschmidt, B. M. and Orris, L., *J. Nat. Cancer Inst.*, **39,** 1217 (1967).
84. Grover, P. L., Sims, P., Huberman, E., Marquardt, H., Kuroki, T. and Heidelberger, C., *Proc. Nat. Acad. Sci. (U.S.A.)*, **68,** 1098 (1971).
85. DeBaun, J. R., Rowley, J. Y., Miller, E. C. and Miller, J. A., *Proc. Soc. Expl. Biol. Med.*, **129,** 268 (1968).
86. Dipple, A., Lawley, P. D. and Brookes, P., *Europ. J. Cancer*, **4,** 493 (1968).
87. Dipple, A. and Slade, T., *Europ. J. Cancer*, **6,** 417 (1970).
88. Dipple, A. and Slade, T., *Europ. J. Cancer*, **7,** 473 (1971).
89. Dipple, A., Brookes, P., Mackintosh, D. S. and Rayman, M. P., *Biochemistry*, **10,** 4323 (1971).
90. Pochon, F. and Michelson, A. M., *Europ. J. Biochem.*, **21,** 144 (1971).
91. Pochon, F., Brookes, P. and Michelson, A. M., *Europ. J. Biochem.*, **21,** 154 (1971).
92. Bergmann, I., *Trans. Faraday Soc.*, **50,** 829 (1954).
93. Ts'o, P. O. P. and Lu, P., *Proc. Nat. Acad. Sci.* (*U.S.A.*), **51,** 272 (1964).
94. Wilk, M. and Girke, W., *The Jerusalem Symposia on Quantum Chemistry and Biochemistry* (ed. E. D. Bergmann and B. Pullman). Jerusalem Israel, **1,** 91 (1969).

95. Ts'o, P. O. P., Lesko, S. A. and Umans, R. S., *The Jerusalem Symposia on Quantum Chemistry and Biochemistry* (ed. E. D. Bergmann and B. Pullman). Jerusalem Israel, **1**, 106 (1969).
96. Howard-Flanders, P., *Ann. Rev. Biochemistry*, **37**, 175 (1968).
97. Setlow, R. B., *Progr. Nucl. Acid Res. Mol. Biol.*, **8**, 257 (1968).
98. Papermeister, B. and Davidson, C. L., *Biochem. Biophys. Res. Commun.*, **17**, 608 (1964).
99. Hanawalt, P. and Haynes, R. H., *Biochem. Biophys. Res. Commun.*, **19**, 462 (1965).
100. Reiter, H. and Strauss, B., *J. Mol. Biol.*, **14**, 179 (1965).
101. Lawley, P. D. and Brookes, P., *J. Mol. Biol.*, **25**, 143 (1967).
102. Roberts, J. J., Crathorn, A. R. and Brent, T. P., Nature ,**218**, 970 (1968).
103. Ball, C. R. and Roberts, J. J., *Chem.-Biol. Interactions*, **2**, 321 (1970).
104. Roberts, J. J., Pascoe, J. M., Plant, J. E., Sturrock, J. E. and Crathorn, A. R., *Chem.-Biol. Interactions*, **3**, 29 (1971).
105. Roberts, J. J., Pascoe, J., Smith, B. A. and Crathorn, A. R., *Chem.-Biol. Interactions*, **3**, 49 (1971).
106. Lieberman, M. W., Baney, R. N., Lee, R. E., Sell, S. and Farber, E., *Cancer Res.*, **31**, 1297 (1971).
107. Lieberman, M. W., Sell, S., Farber, E., *Cancer Res.*, **31**, 1307 (1971).
108. Witkin, E. M., *Proc. 12th Intern. Congr. Genet.*, **3**, 225 (1969).
109. Witkin, E. M. and Farquharsen, E. L., *Ciba Foundation Symposium on Mutations as a Cellular Process*, Churchill, London, 36, (1969).
110. Rasmussen, R. E. and Painter, R. B., *Nature*, **203**, 1360 (1964).
111. Rasmussen, R. E. and Painter, R. B., *J. Cell Biol.*, **29**, 11 (1966).
112. Painter, R. B. and Cleaver, J. E., *Nature*, **216**, 369 (1967).
113. Fox, B. W. and Fox, M., *Mutation Res.*, **8**, 629 (1969).
114. Cleaver, J. E., *Mutation Res.*, **12**, 453 (1971).
115. Painter, R. B. and Cleaver, J. E., *Radiation Res.* **37**, 451 (1969).
116. Hahn, G. M., Yang, S. J. and Parker, V., *Nature*, **220**, 1142 (1968).
117. Hahn, G. M., King, D., Yang, S. J., *Nature, New Biol.*, **230**, 242 (1971).
118. Stich, H. F. and San, R. H. C., *Mutation Res.*, **10**, 389 (1970).
119. Stich, H. F., San, R. H. C. and Kawazoe, Y., *Nature*, **229**, 416 (1971).
120. Clark, A. J. and Margulies, A. D., *Proc. Nat. Acad. Sci. Wash.*, **53**, 451 (1965).
121. Howard-Flanders, P. and Boyce, R. P., *Radiation Res. Suppl.* 6 156 (1969).
122. Rupp, W. D. and Howard-Flanders, P., *J. Mol. Biol.*, **31**, 291 (1968).
123. Howard-Flanders, P., Rupp, W. D. and Wilkins, B. M., Replication and Recombination of genetic material. ed. by W. J. Peacock and R. D. Brock, p. 142, Canberra: Australian Academy of Sciences.
124. Smith, K. C. and Meun, D. H. C., *J. Mol. Biol.*, **51**, 459 (1970).
125. Rupp, W. D., Wild III, C. E., Reno, D. L. and Howard-Flanders, P., *J. Mol. Biol.*, **61**, 25 (1971).
126. Yamamoto, N., *Biochem. Biophys. Res. Commun.*, **27**, 263
127. Fukuda, S. and Yamamoto, N., *Cancer Research*, **30**, 830 (1970).
128. Yamamoto, N., Fukuda, S., Takebe, H., *Cancer Res.*, **30**, 2532 (1970).
129. Watson, W. A. F., *Mutations Res.*, **14**, 299 (1972).
130. Cleaver, J. E. and Thomas, G. H., *Biochem. Biophys. Res. Commun.*, **36**, 203 (1969).
131. Rauth, A. M., *Radiation Res.*, **31**, 121 (1967).
132. Cleaver, J. E., *Radiation Res.*, **37**, 334 (1969).
133. Gaudin, D. and Yielding, K. L., *Proc. Soc. Exptl. Biol. Med.*, **131**, 1413 (1969).

134. Gaudin, D., Yielding, K. L., Stabler, A. and Brown, J., *Proc. Soc. Exptl. Biol. Med.*, **137,** 202 (1971).
135. Gaudin, D., Gregg, R. S. and Yielding, K. L., *Biochem. Biophys. Res. Commun,.* **45,** 630 (1971).
136. Segaloff, A. and Maxfield, W. S., *Cancer Res.*, **31,** 166 (1971).
137. Cohen, M. H., *Proc. Am. Assoc. Cancer Res.*, **12,** 69 (1971).
138. Levij, I. S. and Polliack, A., *Cancer*, **22,** 300 (1968).
139. Cleaver, J. E., *Nature*, **218,** 652 (1968).
140. Setlow, R. B., Regan, J. D., German, J. and Carrier, W. L., *Proc. Nat. Acad, Sci. U.S.A.*, **64,** 1035 (1969).
141. Bootsma, D., Mulder, M. P., Pot, F. and Cohen, J. A., *Mutation Res.*, **9,** 507 (1970).
142. Rabson, A. S., Tyrrell, S. A. and Legallais, F. Y., *Proc. Soc. expl. Biol. Med.*, **132,** 802 (1969).
143. Aaronson, S. A. and Lytle, C. D., *Nature*, **228,** 359 (1970).
144. Cleaver, J. E., *Intern. J. Radiat. Biol.*, **18,** 557 (1970).
145. Cleaver, J. E., *Proc. Nat. Acad. Sci.* (*U.S.A.*), **63,** 428 (1969).
146. Kleijer, W. J., Lohman, P. H. M., Mulder, M. P. and Bootsma, D., *Mutation Res.*, **9,** 517 (1970).
147. Howard-Flanders, P. and Boyce, R., *Radiation Res.*, suppl. 6, 156 (1966).
148. Searashi, T. and Strauss, B., *Biochem. Biophys. Res. Commun.*, **20,** 680 (1965).
149. Strauss, B., Coyle, M., Hill, T., Myers, T. and Prokash, L., Symposium on the Genetics of Industrial Microorganisms Academic, Prague (1970).
150. Stich, H. F. and San, R. H. C., *Mutation Res.*, **13,** 279 (1971).
151. Boveri, T., *The Origin of Malignant Tumours* (translated by M. Boveri) Williams and Williams, Baltimore (1929).
152. Gabridge, M. G. and Legator, M. S., *Proc. Soc. expl. Biol. Med.,* **130,** 831 (1969).
153. Legator, M. S. and Malling, H. V., In 'Chemical Mutagens' Vol. II p. 569 ed. A. Hollaender Plenum Press New York—London 1971.
154. Malling, H. V., *Mutation Res.* **13,** 425 (1971).
155. Maher, V. M., Miller, E. C., Miller, J. A. and Szybalski, W., *Mol. Pharmacol.*, **4,** 411 (1968).
156. Corbett, J. H., Heidelberger, C. and Dove, W. F., *Mol. Pharmacol.*, **6,** 667 (1970).
157. Fahmy, O. G. and Fahmy, M. J., *Mutation Res.*, **13,** 19 (1971).
158. Fahmy, O. G. and Fahmy, M. J., *Nature*, **224,** 1328 (1969).
159. Fahmy, O. G. and Fahmy, M. J., *Int. J. Cancer*, **6,** 250 (1970 *a*).
160. Fahmy, O. G. and Fahmy, M. J., *Mutation Res.*, **9,** 239 (1970 *b*).
161. Fahmy, O. G. and Fahmy, M. J , *Cancer Res.*, **30,** 195 (1970 *c*).
162. Ritossa, F. M., Atwood, K. C., Spiegelman, S., Genetics, **54,** 819 (1966 *a*).
163. Cookson, M. J., Sims, P., Grover, P. L., *Nature, New Biol.*, **234,** 186 (1971).
164. Ames, B. N., Sims, P. and Grover, P. L., *Science*, **176,** 47 (1972).
165. Chu, E. H. Y., In 'Chemical Mutagens' Vol. **II,** p. 411 ed. A. Hollaender Plenum Press New York—London 1971.
166. Chu, E. H. Y. and Malling, H. V., *Proc. Nat. Acad. Sci.* (*U.S.A.*), **61,** 1306 (1968).
167. Kao, F. T. and Puck, T. T., *Proc. Nat. Acad. Sci.* (*U.S.A.*), **60,** 1275 (1968).
168. Huberman, E., Aspiras, L., Heidelberger, C., Grover, P. L. and Sims, P., *Proc. Nat. Acad. Sci.* (*U.S.A.*), **68,** 3195 (1971).
169. Davidson, J. N., *The Biochemistry of the Nucleic Acids,* 6th Ed. 1969 London Methuen.

170. Doctor, B. P., Apgar, J. and Holley, R. W., *J. Biol. Chem.*, **236**, 1117 (1961).
171. Yang, W. K. and Novelli, G. D., *Proc. Nat. Acad. Sci.* (*U.S.A.*), **59**, 208 (1968 *a*).
172. Taylor, M. W., Granger, G. A., Buck, C. A. and Holland, J. J., *Proc. Nat. Acad. Sci.* (*U.S.A.*), **47**, 1712 (1967).
173. Taylor, M. W., Volkers, S. A. S., Choe, B. K. and Zeikus, J. G., *Cancer Res.*, **31**, 688 (1971).
174. Holland, J. J., Taylor, M. W., and Buck, C. A., *Proc. Nat. Acad. Sci* (*U.S.A.*), **58**, 2437 (1967).
175. Volkers. S. A. and Taylor, M. W., *Biochemistry*, **10**, 488 (1971).
176. Gonano, F., Chiarugi, V. P., *Exp. molec. Path.*, **10**, 99 (1969).
177. Yang, W. K. and Novelli, G. D., *Biochem. Biophys. Res. Commun.*, **31**, 534 (1968 *b*).
178. Gallo, R. C. and Pestka, S. J., *J. Mol. Biol.*, **52**, 195 (1970).
179. Fujioka, S. and Gallo, R. C., *Blood*, **38**, 246 (1971).
180. Penhoet, E. E. and Holland, J. J., *J. Nat. Cancer Inst.*, **47**, 1173 (1971).
181. Mittelman, H., *Cancer Res.*, **31**, 647 (1971).
182. Yang, W. K., *Cancer Res.*, **31**, 639 (1971).
183. Taylor, M. W., *Cancer Res.*, **30**, 2463 (1970).
184. Ritossa, F. M., Atwood, K. L., and Spiegelman, S., *Genetics*, **54**, 663 (1966*b*).
185. Gallo, R. C. and Whang-Peng, J., in Biological effects of polynucleotides ed. R. L. Beers and W. Braun, Springer-Verlag, N. Y. 303 (1971).
186. Borek, E., Cold Spring Harbor Symposia on Quantitative Biology, **28**, 139 (1963).
187. Srinivasan, P. R. and Borek, E., *Proc. Nat. Acad. Sci.* (*U.S.A.*), **49**, 529 (1963).
188. Srinivasan, P. R. and Borek, E., *Science*, **145**, 548 (1964).
189. Borek, E., Exploitable Molecular Mechanisms and Neoplasia, 22nd Annual Symposium on Fundamental Cancer Research, Houson, 163 (1968).
190. Sueoka, N. and Kano-Sueoka, T., *Progr. Nucleic Acid Res. Mol. Biol.*, **10**, 23 (1970).
191. Berquist, P. L. and Matthews, R. E. F., *Biochem. J.*, **85**, 305 (1962).
192. Farber, E. and Magee, P. N., *Biochem. J.*, **76**, 58P (1960).
193. Magee, P. N. and Farber, E., *Biochem. J.*, **83**, 114 (1962).
194. Craddock, V. M., *Biochim. Biophys. Acta*, **195**, 351 (1969).
195. Waalkes, T. P., Adamson, R. H., O'Gara, R. W. and Gallo, R. C., *Cancer Res.*, **31**, 1069 (1971).
196. Mandel, L. R., Srinivasan, P. R. and Borek, E., *Nature*, **209**, 586 (1966).
197. McFarlane, E. S. and Shaw, G. H., *Canadian J. Microbiol.*, **14**, 185 (1968 *a*).
198. McFarlane, E. S. and Shaw, G. H., *Canadian J. Microbiol.*, **14**, 499 (1968 *b*).
199. Baliga, B. S., Srinivasan, P. R. and Borek, E., *Nature*, **208**, 555 (1965).
200. Pillinger, D. and Borek, E., *Proc. Nat. Acad. Sci.* (*U.S.A.*), **62**, 1145 (1969).
201. Craddock, V. M., *Nature*, **228**, 1264 (1970).
202. Hancock, R. L., *Cancer Res.*, **27**, 646 (1967).
203. Mittelman, A., Hall, R. H., Yohn, D. S. and Grace, T., *Cancer Res.*, **27**, 1409 (1967).
204. Turkington, R. W. and Riddle, M., *Cancer Res.*, **30**, 650 (1970).
205. Hacker, B. and Mandel, L. R., *Biochim. Biophys. Acta*, **190**, 38 (1969).
206. Mandel, L. R., Hacker, B., and Maag, T. A., *Cancer Res.*, **31**, 613 (1971).
207. Gantt, R. R. and Evans, V. J., *Cancer Res.*, **29**, 536 (1969).
208. Gantt, R. R., *Cancer Res.*, **31**, 609 (1971).

209. Gallagher, R. E., Ting, R. C. Y. and Gallo, R. C., *Proc. Soc. Expl. Biol. Med.*, **136,** 819 (1971).
210. Kaye, A. M. and Leboy, P. S., *Biochim. Biophys. Acta*, **157,** 289 (1968).
211. Stewart, M. J. and Corrance, M. H., *Cancer Res.*, **29,** 1642 (1969).
212. Turkington, R. W., *J. Biol. Chem.*, **244,** 5140–5148 (1969).
213. Viale, G. L., *Cancer Res.*, **31,** 605 (1971).
214. Riddick, D. H. and Gallo, R. C., *Cancer Res.*, **30,** 2484 (1970).
215. Gallo, R. C., *Cancer Res.*, **31,** 621 (1971).
216. Riddick, D. H. and Gallo, R. C., *Blood*, **37,** 282 (1971).
217. Kerr, S. J., *Biochemistry*, **9,** 690 (1970).
218. Kerr, S. J., *Proc. Nat. Acad., Sci. U.S.A.,* **68,** 406 (1971).
219. Kerr, S. J., Sharma, O. K. and Borek, E., *Cancer Res.*, **31,** 633 (1971).
220. Leboy, P. S., *Biochemistry*, **9,** 1577 (1970).
221. Fink, L. M., Nishimura, S. and Weinstein, I. B., *Biochemistry*, **9,** 496 (1970).
222. Agarwal, M. K. and Weinstein, I. B., *Biochemistry*, **9,** 503 (1970).
223. Grunberger, D. and Weinstein, I. B., *J. Biol. Chem.,* **246,** 1123 (1971).
224. Troll, W., Belman, S., Berkowitz, E., Chmielewicz, Z. F., Ambrus, J. L. and Bardos, T. J., *Biochim. Biophys. Acta*, **157,** 16 (1968).
225. Kidson, C. and Kirby, K. S., *Cancer Res.*, **24,** 1604 (1964).
226. Kidson, C. and Kirby, K. S., *Cancer Res.*, **25,** 472 (1965).
227. Leader, D. P. and Barry, J. M., *Nature*, **215,** 1374 (1967).
228. Jackson, C. D. and Sells, B. H., *Biochim. Biophys. Acta*, **155,** 417 (1968).
229. Neimann, P. E. and Henry, P. H., *Biochemistry*, **8,** 275 (1969).
230. Turkington, R. W. and Self, D. J., *Cancer Res.*, **30,** 1833 (1970).
231. Turkington, R. W., *Cancer Res.*, **31,** 644 (1971).
232. Kreuger, R. G. and McCarthy, B. J., *Biochem. Biophys. Res. Commun.*, **41,** 944 (1970).
233. Gottlieb, A. A. and Liu, T., 10th International Cancer Congress, Houston, 376 (1970).
234. Shearer, R. W., *Biochem. Biophys. Res. Commun.*, **43,** 1324 (1971).
235. Shearer, R. W. and Smuckler, E. A., *Cancer Res.*, **31,** 2104 (1971).
236. Gelboin, H. V., Exploitable Molecular Mechanisms in Neoplasia 22nd Annual Symposium on Fundamental Cancer Research, Houston (1968).
237. Clayton, D. A. and Vinograd, J., *Nature*, **216,** 652 (1967).
238. Clayton, D. A. and Vinograd, J., *Proc. Nat. Acad. Sci.* (*U.S.A.*), **62,** 1077 (1969).
239. Wunderlich, W., Tetzlaff, I. and Graffi, A., *Chem.-Biol. Interactions*, **4,** 81 (1971–72).
240. Schwaier, R., Nashed, N. and Zimmermann, F. K., *Mol. Gen. Genet.*, **102,** 290 (1968).

APPENDIX to Chapter 10

Reaction of carcinogens with nucleic acids: role of DNA replication and DNA repair

Recent investigations on the binding of carcinogens to nucleic acids have sought a correlation between reactions at *particular sites* in DNA (rather than with overall DNA interactions) and tumour incidence. They have also considered the relative stabilities of these products and the consequences of DNA replication on such damaged templates. Thus O'Connor *et al.* (1973)[1] compared the reaction of the methylating hepatocarcinogen *N*, *N*-dimethylnitrosamine (DMN) with that of another methylating agent, methyl methanesulphonate, which is not a rat liver carcinogen. O^6-Alkylguanine moieties in DNA and unidentified acid-labile products were formed with the nitroso compound but were undetected or in low yield with the alkyl sulphonate. From a similar study, Craddock (1973)[2] also argued that O^6-methylguanine may be a necessary but not sufficient cause of carcinogenesis. The same proportion of O^6-methylguanine was found in the DNA isolated from intact and from regenerating liver. However, liver carcinogenesis only ensues if DMN is given during the period of restorative hyperplasia after partial hepatectomy (Craddock, 1973[3]) or following chronic feeding to adult rats (Magee and Barnes, 1956, 1962[4]) when increased turnover of DNA occurs. It seems likely therefore that replication of DNA containing O^6-methylguanine moieties is an important prerequisite for alkylation-induced carcinogenesis. It is therefore of interest that Borchert *et al.* (1973*a*, *b*)[5,6] have implicated reaction with the O^6-position of guanine with another carcinogen. They have shown that metabolism of the naturally occurring carcinogen, safrole, yields a conjugate of 1′-hydroxysafrole (*Fig. 6*), a compound which was subsequently shown to be a proximate carcinogen. The synthetic 1′-acetoxysafrole, also shown to be a carcinogen, was a powerful electrophile which reacted with guanosine monophosphate. Degradation to the nucleoside, followed by acetylation, yielded a product whose properties were consistent with its characterization as *O*-6-(isosafrol-3′-yl)-*N*-2-acetylguanosine-2′, 3′, 5′-triacetate (*Fig. 10.6*).

The vital role of cell division in carcinogenesis—first emphasized by Laws (1959)[7], following his observation that acetylaminofluorene (AAF)-induced liver cancer was increased following partial hepatectomy—has become apparent in numerous other studies with agents such including urethan, (Pound, 1968[8]; Chernozemski and Warwick, 1970[9]), UV irradiation, (Pound 1970[10]) and azo dyes (Hughes, 1969/70[11]; Warwick, 1969[12]).

More recently Pound *et al.* (1973)[13] administered DMN to rats during a period of liver regeneration that followed a necrotizing dose of the hepatotoxin carbon tetrachloride; the compound is not itself carcinogenic. The

Not all agree that it is synthesis of DNA that important.

results were consistent with the view that DMN was a more effective carcinogen when reacting with cells synthesizing DNA than with cells at mitosis. Numerous small foci of proliferating tumour cells were observed after treatment with DMN and these were thought to be similar in origin to the groups of cells found after administration of diethylnitrosourea (DEN) (Gössner and Friedrick-Freksa, 1964[14]; Friedrick-Freksa, Gössner and Börner, 1969[15]). These lesions were also increased in number when DEN was given after partial hepatectomy (Scherer and Hoffman, 1971[16]). The incidence of kidney tumours in rats induced by DMN can be increased by unilateral nephrectomy (Ito *et al.*, 1969[17]) presumably also as a consequence of stimulated cell division and DNA synthesis.

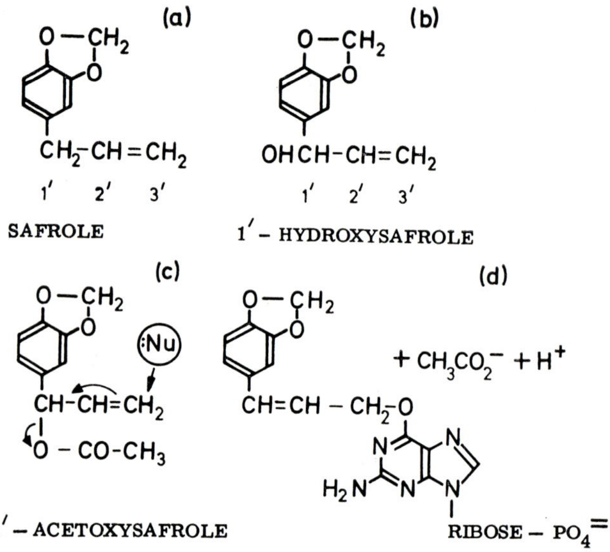

Fig. 10.6. Chemical structures of (*a*) safrole; (*b*) l′-hydroxysafrole, the presumed proximate carcinogenic metabolite of (*a*); (*c*) l′-acetoxysafrole, a synthetic electrophilic derivative of (*b*), being attacked by the nucleophile, :Nu. (*d*) The tentatively identified products of reaction of (*c*) and guanosine monophosphate (Borchert *et al.*, 1973*a*, *b*[5], [6])

The higher incidence of liver tumours induced by AAF in male hooded rats as compared to that in female rats can be correlated with the higher levels of *N*-hydroxy-AAF sulphotransferase in male rats during AAF feeding (Jackson and Irving, 1972[18]). This enzyme catalyses the formation of the reactive AAF-*N*-sulphate ester, which is thought to be responsible for the binding of AAF to liver cells (Weisberger *et al.*, 1972[19]). Jackson and Irving quantitated the amount of cell proliferation in the two series and found the mitotic index and incorporation of tritiated thymidine in livers of female rats was low and constant; thymidine incorporation and mitotic index in livers of male rats exhibited a marked increase three weeks after the rats were placed on a diet containing AAF. These pathological changes were not associated with any difference in the binding of the carcinogen to hepatic DNA in the two series (Irving and Veazey, 1971[20]), but they could be related to the difference which was noted in the proportions of the various reaction products which were present in the respective DNAs. Subsequently, Jackson and Irving (1973)[21] showed that partial hepatectomy of female rats during AAF feeding did induce hepatotoxic effects and the formation of hyperplastic nodules. Nevertheless, these nodules failed to develop into carcinomas—a finding which was thought to indicate that some factor, other than a difference in cell proliferation, might also be reponsible for the greater susceptibility of male rats to AAF carcinogenesis. Albert *et al.* (1972)[22] also studied cell loss and cell proliferation induced in rat liver by various doses of AAF in relation to tumour induction; they found that the increase in parenchymal cell replication rate correlated well with the tumour incidence.

Adamson *et al.* (1971)[23] showed that the increased susceptibility of a replicating cell to the tumorigenic action of methylcholanthrene was not associated with any augmented DNA binding. Binding of carcinogen was nearly equal in pre-existing and in newly-synthesized DNA in the preneoplastic nodule of the mouse mammary gland (Banerjee *et al.*, 1973[24]. This observation and that of Craddock[2] (see earlier) may be contrasted with that of Marquardt *et al.* (1971)[25,26] who found that liver DNA became more susceptible to the binding of DMBA when in the replicative phase, as in the regenerating liver.

It seems likely from the evidence available that replication of DNA containing modified bases could lead to amplification of this DNA damage in the daughter cell DNA; and some of this damage could result in altered gene expression and cancer. Hence the stability of substituents on DNA will be important in relation to the time following treatment with carcinogens when DNA synthesis is stimulated, possibly due to cell regeneration occurring as a consequence of induced necrosis in a particular tissue. Excision repair of DNA which has been damaged by reaction with a number of carcinogenic compounds has been clearly demonstrated (see earlier): moreover, and as discussed previously, such repair is under genetic control. Studies on cells from patients with xeroderma pigmentosa (Stich *et al.*, 1973[27]) have demonstrated their decreased DNA repair and enhanced sensitivity to damage by a number of carcinogens. However some substituents on DNA are not readily excised as evidenced by the further examples of persistent binding of carcinogens to DNA which have been noted (Marquardt, 1972[26]; Kriek, 1972[28]; Janss *et al.*, 1972[29]). The efficiency of the post-DNA replication repair process (see earlier) will therefore also be important in controlling the genetic damage which could follow DNA replication on a damaged template. The role this mechanism may play in the recovery of cells from the lethal, mutagenic and chromosome damaging effects of DNA interactions is indicated by the effect of the DNA repair inhibitor caffeine on treated cells. Caffeine is currently thought to inhibit this particular repair process (see earlier, and Roberts *et al.*, 1973[30]). Thus post-treatment incubation in caffeine enhances the lethal effects of a number of agents (see earlier), and also increases the incidence of chromosome aberrations induced by mitomycin C or alkylation (Hartley-Asp and Kihlman, 1971[31]; Kihlman *et al.*, 1973[32]; Roberts *et al.*, 1973[30]) and enhances *N*-methyl-*N*-nitrosourea-induced mutation in Chinese hamster cells (Roberts *et al.*, 1973[30]). These findings tend to support the view that inhibitors of DNA repair may act as co-carcinogens.

An alternative, but related, role for DNA repair processes in cancer initiation was suggested by the observation that viral transformation of cells is enhanced by agents which are known to disrupt the genetic integrity of a cell (Casto, 1973[33]). It is envisaged that this could result from the initiation of DNA repair processes which facilitate the incorporation of a viral genome into host cell DNA (Casto, 1973[33]).

Gene expression and cancer

Alterations in cell phenotype which are characteristic of tumour tissue and manifested by the production of tumour specific antigens and antigens characteristic of embryonic tissue (see Chapter 7) may be due either to an alteration of the genotype by the mechanisms discussed above, or by an alteration of transcription or translation. As discussed earlier, attempts to show a derepression of genes, with transcription of RNAs not made in the normal tissue, gave conflicting results. Some investigators have observed certain deletions in the spectrum of nuclear RNA (nRNA) species in rat hepatoma as compared to normal liver; others have found a deletion and a simultaneous addition of the nRNA population; while in yet other studies only the addition of new hybridizible sequences has been detected. Possible explanations for these conflicting findings in studies designed to demonstrate suppression or derepression during tumour initiation have been considered by Muramatsu *et al.* (1973)[34] and Garrett *et al.* (1973)[35]. The various discrepancies were partly attributed to differences in the tumours examined and in the limitations of the DNA-RNA hybridization techniques. The hybridization studies at present measure only RNA sequences transcribed from reiterated sequences of the genome, possibly those sequences repeated 10,000 or 50,000 times. The function of such sequences is not understood at the present time. The failure to demonstrate derepression of gene families in tumours, which are not active in normal liver, led Shearer and Smuckler (1972)[36] to concentrate on the next step in the gene to protein sequence; these workers investigated the changes in transport of RNA from the nucleus to its site of translation in the cytoplasm. Shearer and Smuckler demonstrated that RNA base sequences not found in the cytoplasm in normal cells were present in the cytoplasm of primary rat hepatomas induced by azo-dyes. The migration of RNA out of the tumour nucleus was an early consequence of feeding a carcinogenic azo-dye but not of feeding a non-carcinogenic analogue. Confirmation of this phenomenon was obtained by Garrett *et al.* (1973)[35] who found a qualitative loss of nuclear RNA species in the livers of rats treated for 10 weeks with diethylnitrosamine. These losses coincided with the first appearance of histologically identifiable hepatomas. The failure to find changes in RNA sequences detectable in the nucleus therefore led to the postulate that alteration of nuclear to cytoplasmic transport rather than alteration in transcription is the primary event in the initiation of neoplastic transformation in hepatic tissue.

Conclusions

It is only a little over ten years since binding of a carcinogen to DNA *in vivo* was unequivocally demonstrated and a product characterized. Since that time almost all known carcinogens have been shown to be capable of binding to nucleic acids in receptive animal tissues, either as a consequence of direct chemical reaction or following metabolism to reactive metabolites. These studies have generally confirmed the view that initial interaction with DNA is likely to be an essential prerequisite for tumour initiation by chemical agents. But it is equally apparent that innumerable other factors, such as the DNA replicative state. its repair potential and the hormonal status of the host are likely to be promotional factors which determine the eventual neoplastic outcome to these interactions. Other separate investigations have discussed the RNA modifications associated with the phenotypic change to the tumour cell. Future studies in the field of chemical carcinogenesis will hopefully lead to an understanding of the link between the former, possibly mutagenic, events in DNA and these latter changes.

References (Appendix)

1. O'Connor P. J., Capps, M. J. and Craig, A. W. *Br. J. Cancer*, **27,** 153 (1973).
2. Craddock, V. M. *Biochim. Biophys. Acta*, **312,** 202 (1973).
3. Craddock, V. M. *J. Nat. Cancer Inst.*, **47,** 899 (1971).
4. Magee, P. N. and Barnes, J. M. *J. Path. Bact.*, **84,** 19 (1962). *Brit. J. Cancer*, **10,** 114 (1956).
5. Borchert, P., Wislocki, P. G., Miller, J. A. and Miller, E. C. *Cancer Res.*, **33,** 575 (1973).
6. Borchert, P., Miller, J. A., Miller, E. C. and Shires, T. K. *Cancer Res.*, **33,** 590 (1973).
7. Laws, J. O. *Brit. J. Cancer*, **13,** 669 (1959).
8. Pound, A. W. *New Zealand Med. J.*, **67,** 88 (1968).
9. Chernozemski, I. N. and Warwick, G. P. *Cancer Res.*, **30,** 2685 (1970).
10. Pound, A. W. *Pathology*, **2,** 269 (1970).
11. Hughes, P. E. *Chem.-Biol. Interactions*, **1,** 301 (1969/70).
12. Warwick, G. P. The Jerusalem Symposia on Quantum Chemistry and Biochemistry (ed. E. D. Bergmann and B. Pullman) Jerusalem, Israel, **1**, 218 (1969).
    Jerusalem, Israel Academy of Sciences and Humanities.
13. Pound, A. W., Lawson, T. A. and Horn, L. *Brit. J. Cancer*, **27,** 451 (1973).
14. Gössner, W. and Friederick-Freksa, H. Z. *Nat.*, **19,** 862 (1964).
15. Friedrick-Freksa, H., Gössner, W. and Börner, P., Z. *Krebsforsch*, **72,** 226 (1969).
16. Scherer, E. and Hoffman, M. *Evr. J. Cancer*, **7,** 369 (1971).
17. Ito, N., Hiasa, Y., Tamai, A., and Yoshida, K. *Gann*, **60,** 319 (1969).
18. Jackson, C. D. and Irving, C. C. *Cancer Res.*, **32.** 1590 (1972).
19. Weisberger, J. H., Yamamoto, R. S., Williams, G. M., Grantham, P. H., Matsushima, T. and Weisberger, E. K. *Cancer Res.*, **32,** 491 (1972).
20. Irving, C. C. and Veazey, R. A. *Cancer Res.*, **31,** 19, (1971).
21. Jackson, C. D., and Irving, C. C. *Cancer Res.*, **33,** 397 (1973).

22. Albert, R. E., Burns, F. J., Bilger, L., Gardner, D., and Troll, W. *Cancer Res.*, **32,** 2172 (1972).
23. Adamson, R., Banerjee, M. R. and Medina, D. *J. Nat. Cancer Inst.*, **46,** 899 (1971).
24. Banerjee, M. R., Kinder, D. L. and Wagner, J. E. *Cancer Res.*, **33,** 862 (1973).
25. Marquardt, H., Bendich, A., Philips, F. S. and Hoffman, D. *Chem.-Biol., Interactions*, **3,** 1 (1971).
26. Marquardt, H., Philips, F. S. and Bendich, A., *Cancer Res.*, **32,** 1810 (1972).
27. Stich, H. F., San, R. H. C., and Kawazoe, Y. *Mutation Res.*, **17,** 127 (1973).
28. Kriek, E., *Cancer Res.*, **32,** 2042 (1972)...
29. Janss, D. H., Moon, R. C. and Irving, C. C. *Cancer Res.*, **32,** 254 (1972).
30. Roberts, J. J., Sturrock, J. E. and Ward, K. N. *Mutation Res.*, **26,** 129 (1974).
31. Hartley-Asp, B., and Kihlman, B. A., *Hereditas*, **69,** 326 (1971).
32. Kihlman, B. A., Sturelid, S., Hartley-Asp. B. and Nilsson, K. *Mutation Res.*, **17,** 271 (1973).
33. Casto, B. C. *Cancer Res.*, **33,** 402 (1973).
34. Muramatsu, M., Nemoto, N., Inui, N. and Takayama, S., *Cancer Res.*, **33,** 739 (1973).
35. Garrett, C. T., Katz, C., Moore, R. E. and Pitot, H. C., *Cancer Res.*, **33,** 1662 (1973).
36. Shearer, R. W. and Smuckler, E. A. *Cancer Res.*, **32,** 339 (1972).

Chapter **11**

THE ROLE OF VIRUSES IN CANCER

K. E. K. Rowson, M.D., Dip.Bact., M.R.C.Path.
Senior Lecturer in Clinical Pathology (Virology), Institute of Laryngology and Otology, London

---

It appears increasingly likely that viruses play an important role in the causation of at least some malignant tumours in man. The history of tumour viruses goes back to the observation made in the last century that human warts could be transmitted by direct or indirect contact between one man and another (see review by Rowson and Mahy, 1967[1]), but serious investigation of tumour viruses may be considered to start with the report in 1908 that the erythromyeloblastic leukaemia of chickens could be transmitted by a cell-free filtrate. The study of tumour viruses can be divided into three phases. In the first, from 1908 until the discovery of polyoma virus in 1953, research into tumour viruses consisted mainly of qualitative experiments in which tissue extracts, usually prepared from tumours, were injected into animals which were then observed for the development of neoplasms. By this simple procedure viruses were demonstrated to produce tumours in birds, mammals and amphibia but little progress was made in elucidating the underlying cellular processes. The reason was, of course, that the tumour viruses identified, prior to the discovery of polyoma virus, were unusually difficult to work with in the laboratory. It was not until the discovery of polyoma virus and the recognition that simian virus 40 (SV_{40}) and certain adenoviruses were oncogenic, that viruses were available which were suitable for the study of the interaction between cells and viruses. It is now accepted that all, or at least part of the viral nucleic acid is incorporated into the genetic information of the cell and codes for the production of a number of new antigens; these alter the behaviour of the cell and give it the properties of a tumour cell. However, we do not know what the alteration is which gives the tumour cell its neoplastic property. This remains to be discovered and, equally important, there is still much to learn about the interaction between the tumour cell and the immunological system of the animal—the neoplastic cell has new antigens which can be recognized by the immune system as foreign but do not lead to the rejection of the tumour cells. The study of the interaction between the tumour and the whole animal is the third phase of tumour virus research and it is one of the most active fields of cancer investigation at the present time.

For many years tumour viruses were regarded as curiosities, unlikely to be of much significance in the causation of tumours. Cancer did not have the epidemiological features of most typical infectious diseases with their relatively short incubation periods and the high probability that disease would follow infection. But a number of infectious diseases are now known in which the incubation period is measured in years and there is no difficulty in visualizing an infectious disease with a sporadic incidence such as that of most tumours. Although we have no definite proof that any malignant tumours in man are due to the action of a virus, the idea that some of the tumours might be virus-induced is challenging. Cancer is a complex disease and there is increasing evidence that multiple factors are implicated in the development of tumours. Viruses and other agents may equally combine to bring about the neoplastic change or modify the hosts response to the tumour cells (Roe and Rowson, 1968[2], Southam *et al.,* 1969[3]).

The tumour viruses

In 1908 Ellermann and Bang[4] reported that the erythromyeloblastic leukaemia of chickens could be transmitted by the inoculation of a cell-free filtrate. This fundamental observation was subsequently confirmed but did not attract much attention at the time: it was thought to indicate that the disease was infectious and therefore not neoplastic, rather than that it was a neoplastic disease due to a virus. In 1910 Rous[5] transmitted a fowl sarcoma by means of a cell-free filtrate. Originating spontaneously in a Plymouth Rock hen, the sarcoma had been transmitted several times by cell grafts before a cell-free passage was attempted. Previous efforts to transmit rat, mouse and dog tumours by cell-free extracts had not been successful, and the results with the fowl tumour must have been a great surprise. But Rous was able to confirm his observations (Rous, 1911[6]) and he subsequently transmitted other fowl tumours with cell-free filtrates (Rous, 1914[7]). For many years it was thought that virus-induced tumours were confined to fowls. It is true that both human and canine warts had been transmitted by tissue extracts even before the experiments with fowl tumours, but warts are benign tumours, and little interest seems to have been taken in them. Nevertheless, in 1919 Wile and Kingery[8] had shown that human warts could be serially transmitted in volunteers, by the intradermal injection of cell-free extracts from freshly removed warts.

It was not until 1932 that the number and host range of tumour viruses began to expand. In that year Shope shot a wild cottontail rabbit near Princeton, New Jersey, and found under the skin of the front and hind paws small nodules which proved to be fibromas. These tumours were transmitted to domestic and cottontail rabbits by cell-free tumour extracts (Shope, 1932[9]). Tumours developed promptly after injection of such extracts and grew rapidly for a time; but they soon stopped growing and often regressed. In the following year Shope (1933)[10] described another tumour of the cottontail rabbit: this was a papilloma which could again be transmitted by cell-free tumour extracts to domestic and cottontail rabbits—but although the tumours often regressed they also quite frequently developed into invasive carcinomas. These were the first malignant mammalian tumours apparently induced by a virus, but as no virus could be extracted from them it was suggested that the virus was only responsible for the papilloma and not for the carcinoma. It was, however, possible to demonstrate viral antigen in the carcinoma cells even though they contained no infective virus.

The next oncogenic virus to be discovered was the mouse mammary tumour virus. Pure inbred lines of mice had been developed with a very high incidence of mammary tumours: this high incidence was independent of all known external factors and appeared to be a genetic characteristic of the mouse strain. But when high and low mammary tumour strains were crossed it was found that F_1 females which had mothers from the strain with a high tumour incidence developed many mammary tumours; F_1 females with mothers from the strain with a low tumour rate developed few tumours. It was therefore clear that there was some extra-chromosomal factor being passed from mother to daughter in the lines of mice with a high mammary tumour rate. This factor could have been transmitted in the cytoplasm of the ovum, across the placenta, or after birth via the milk. Bittner[11,12,13,14] chose to investigate the last of these possibilities. He removed three litters of strain A mice (with a high incidence of mammary tumours) from their mothers when they were less than 24 hours old, and gave them to foster-mothers of the CBA strain which has a low mammary tumour rate. There were nine females in the three foster-nursed litters, and only three of them developed mammary tumours; the expected incidence in strain A mice is seven or eight. A similar reduction in the incidence of mammary tumours was observed among their descendants (Bittner, 1936[11]). These results were confirmed, and it was found that the converse was also true. Mice of a strain with a low mammary tumour incidence, foster-nursed by mothers from a strain with a high mammary tumour rate, developed more mammary tumours than expected (Bittner, 1939, 1940[12,13]). It was thus possible to alter the mammary tumour incidence in a strain of mice, not only in the mice which were foster-nursed, but also in their descendants. Mammary cancer in mice was therefore shown to be a communicable disease whose causative agent was transmitted in the milk. This agent was later found to pass through bacteria-proof filters (Bittner, 1942[14]) and could therefore reasonably be regarded as a virus. But Bittner's findings were so novel and unacceptable that the terms 'milk factor' or 'milk influence' were widely used to describe the mammary tumour virus.

At about the time that Bittner was working on the mammary tumour virus, Lucké was investigating the frog kidney carcinoma, the cells of which have striking acidophilic intranuclear inclusion bodies. Lucké was able to transmit renal carcinoma by inoculating tumour tissue which had been dessicated or stored in 50 per cent glycerine for three weeks. The tumours occurred in the kidneys, not at the injection site, and Lucké concluded that the cause was a virus (Lucké, 1938[15]) though this view was not finally confirmed until 1956 (Duryee, 1956[16]).

The next neoplastic disease shown to be transmissable by a cell-free extract was mouse leukaemia, a disease very similar to human leukaemia (Furth *et al.*, 1935[17]) and thus of great interest. Many attempts had been made to transmit mouse leukaemia, but all failed until the successful transmission reported by Gross[18] in 1951. The reason for Gross's success was that he injected his extract of leukaemic tissue into newborn mice, a technique which had recently been introduced to isolate coxsackie viruses. His observations were confirmed with some difficulty, and many other strains of mouse leukaemia virus later identified. Surprisingly, many of them have been isolated from solid tumours in non-leukaemic mice. Some of these viruses are very similar to that isolated by Gross, producing a lymphocytic leukaemia indistinguishable from the spontaneous disease in AK or C58 mice. Others produce different types of leukaemia (see reviews by Dmochowshi, 1960[19]; Gross, 1961[20]; Miller, 1961[21]; Sinkovics, 1962[22]; Stansley, 1963[23]; Moloney, 1964[24]; Gross, 1964[25, 26] and 1970[27]; Boiron *et al.*, 1967[28]; Dougherty and Di Stefano, 1969[29]; Pasternak, 1969[30]).

While working on mouse leukaemia, Gross and Stewart independently observed that suckling mice inoculated with extracts of leukaemic tissue from AK strain mice developed parotid gland tumours (Gross, 1953[31]; Stewart, 1953[32]). At first it was considered that these tumours were caused by the leukaemogenic virus, but it soon became clear that two viruses were present in the extracts of leukaemic tissue—one could be propagated rapidly in mouse embryo tissue culture with destruction of the cells, was ether-resistant, and gave rise to solid tumours when injected into suckling mice; the other caused no cytopathic effect in tissue culture, was ether-sensitive and produced only leukaemia when inoculated into baby mice. The fact that the new virus was first isolated from leukaemic tissue was purely fortuitous, and other strains have since been isolated from a mammary carcinoma (McCulloch *et al.*, 1959[33]) and from apparently normal tissues of wild mice (Huebner *et al.*, 1962[34]). Polyoma virus, as it was called, was immediately recognized to be very different from the tumour viruses previously discovered. They all appeared to be species-specific and produced only one type of tumour, whereas polyoma virus gave rise to a great variety of tumours in many species: in a group of 117 mice inoculated soon after birth, Stewart, Eddy and Borgese (1958)[35] identified twenty-three different types of neoplasms. The number of susceptible species was equally remarkable. In addition to mice, hamsters (Chinese and Syrian), rats, rabbits, guinea-pigs, ferrets and the multimammate mouse *Rattus* (*Mastomys*) *natalensis* were all susceptible to the action of polyoma. But the most important property was the ease with which the virus could be handled in tissue culture systems and studied by serological methods. Work on this virus was also facilitated by its ability to agglutinate erythrocytes of many species (Sachs *et al.*, 1959[36]); the virus attaches to red cells by adsorbing to the same mucoprotein type of receptor site as influenza virus. The receptors on the red cells can be destroyed by the receptor-destroying enzyme of *Vibrio cholerae* or by influenza virus, but polyoma virus does not itself destroy the receptors (Hartley *et al.*, 1959[37]). Treatment of tissue culture cells with receptor-destroying enzyme also reduces their susceptibility to polyoma virus infection, so presumably the mucoprotein receptors destroyed by the enzyme are involved in the entry of the virus into nucleated cells (Rowe, 1961[38]).

Unlike the earlier tumour viruses, polyoma appeared to have many characteristics in common with those viruses which either produce non-neoplastic diseases, or are orphan viruses. This must have suggested to many workers that some of the viruses already known might, under certain conditions, induce tumours. One of the problems in preparing virus vaccines in monkey kidney tissue-cultures is the large number of contaminating 'orphan' viruses. The possibility that some of these simian viruses could produce tumours was investigated by Eddy and her colleagues (Eddy *et al.*, 1961)[39]. Extracts from cultures of (pooled) rhesus monkey kidney cells were inoculated into newborn hamsters and, after one hundred and eighteen days, undifferentiated sarcomas appeared at the injection sites. Similar tumours were also found in the lungs and kidneys of a few animals. Cell-free extracts prepared from these sarcomas were injected into newborn hamsters but tumours did not develop. Tissue cultures were made from the tumour tissue, and a cell-free extract prepared from these cultures induced subcutaneous sarcomas on inoculation into hamsters. The tumour cultures showed no cytopathic effect, but when the culture medium was transferred to grivet monkey cultures, cytoplasmic vacuoles were found in the cells, similar to those observed by Sweet and Hilleman (1960)[40] with simian virus 40 (SV40). The new tumour virus indeed proved to be SV40 (Eddy *et al.*, 1962[41]; Girardi *et al.*, 1962[42]) which, although often found in tissue cultures of rhesus and cynomalgus monkey kidneys, does not produce a cytopathic effect in them.

When SV40 was injected intracerebrally into newborn hamsters, ependymomas were produced (Gerber and Kirschstein, 1962[43]), the first gliomas of viral origin to be reported. Similar tumours have been observed following the subcutaneous injection of SV40 into newborn *Rattus* (*mastomys*) *natalensis* (Rabson *et al.* 1962[44]). Mastomys and hamsters are so far the only species in which SV40 has been shown to induce tumours. Newborn rats, mice, guinea pigs and rabbits have been observed for many months after the injection of SV40, but tumours have not appeared (Eddy, 1962, 1964[45,46]). Man is susceptible to infection with SV40, and was frequently infected by contaminated virus vaccines prepared from monkey kidney tissue cultures before this danger was recognized. Formalized vaccines also contain live SV40: the virus is inactivated more slowly than poliovirus and contains a fraction which may resist inactivation under the conditions used for vaccine preparation (Gerber *et al.*, 1961[47]). SV40 has been administered to adults and children by mouth with live attenuated poliovirus vaccine, and by injection with inactivated poliovirus and adenovirus vaccines; it has also been given intranasally to volunteers (Morris *et al.*, 1961[48]). When virus is given by mouth, antibodies to SV40 have not been found in the serum but the virus may be excreted in the stools of young infants for as long as five weeks after one oral dose (Melnick and Stinebaugh, 1962[49]), and there must therefore have been infection even though antibodies were not produced. The volunteers given SV40 intranasally developed antibodies, and the virus was re-isolated from throat washings in some of them seven to eleven days after infection. Parenteral injection of formalinized vaccines containing live SV40 has been followed by the development of high antibody titres. No harmful short-term effects of infection with SV40 have been detected in man. SV40 does, however, produce cell transformation in tissue cultures of human cells (Shein and Enders, 1962[50,51]; Koprowski *et al.*, 1962[52]; Jensen *et al.*, 1963[53]; Shein *et al.*, 1964[54]; Jensen *et al.*, 1964[55]) and it is conceivable that it might produce tumours if given in large doses to infants.

The incidence of malignant disease in persons under twenty-five years of age in the U.S.A. has therefore been studied for the four years following the introduction of poliovirus vaccination, but no effect attributable to SV40 has been detected. Different States received vaccine batches containing different amounts of SV40, and the tumour incidence in these groups has not been significantly different (Fraumeni *et al.*, 1963[56]). It should be borne in mind that a carcinogenic effect would not have been detected if the latent period was long, if the dose of virus were too low, or if the children involved were beyond the age of susceptibility.

The next virus found to be oncogenic by the method of injecting previously known viruses into newborn hamsters was the human adenovirus type 12. Trentin, Yabe and Taylor (1962)[57] inoculated human adenoviruses of types 2, 3, 7, 7a, 9, 11, 12 and 14 into groups of animals; eight of the ten hamsters receiving type 12 virus developed local injection-site sarcomas after a latent period of one to three months. The tumours could be transmitted, and they grew progressively when transplanted to young adult hamsters. No neoplasms developed in hamsters injected with the other adenovirus types. Huebner, Rowe and Lane (1962)[58] tested different strains of adenovirus type 12, and demonstrated that the ability to produce tumours in hamsters was a general property of type 12 strains. They also found that type 18 would produce tumours, but tumours were not obtained with human types 1–11, 14, 15, 17–28 nor with simian, bovine or mouse adenoviruses. Subsequent work has, however, shown that many human and animal adenoviruses can induce tumours on injection into new born hamsters. The oncogenic human adenoviruses may be divided into group A comprising types 12, 18 and 31 which are highly oncogenic, and group B consisting of types 3, 7, 14, 16 and 21 which are weakly oncogenic (Trentin *et al.*, 1968[59]). Some of the human adenoviruses which are apparently not oncogenic when injected into newborn hamsters can transform rat or hamster cells in tissue culture. These transformed rat cells do not induce tumours on injection into rats unless the rats are treated with cortisone, perhaps because of strong virus-induced antigens(s) causing rejection of the transformed cells (McAllister *et al.*, 1969[60]). Human adenovirus type 12 has been shown to produce tumours in rats (Huebner *et al.*, 1963[61]), mice of certain strains (Yabe *et al.*, 1964[62]), and *mastomys* (Rabson *et al.*, 1764[67]), but these species are less susceptible than hamsters. Viral replication cannot be demonstrated in hamster tissues after virus injection and the tumours have not been found to contain any infective virus; but they do contain virus coded antigens (Huebner *et al.*, 1963, 1964[61,64]). The occurrence of virus-specific non-virion T antigens in virus induced tumours and the presence of antibodies to these antigens in tumour bearing animals provided the basis for a method for assessing the possible role of adenoviruses in human patients with tumours (Huebner 1967[65]). Although the results of serological surveys using semi-purified T antigens have not provided any evidence that adenoviruses are associated with human tumours (Gilden *et al.*, 1970[66]), human cells in culture can be transformed by adenovirus type 12 (Shaw and McFarlane 1969[67]) and by the chicken-embryo-lethal-orphan (CELO) virus which is an avian adenovirus (Anderson *et al.*, 1969[68]). It seems that adenoviruses are potentially oncogenic for man but probably do not produce tumours under natural conditions. Oncogenicity appears to be a common property of both human and animal adenoviruses. Of eighteen adenoviruses of simian origin tested by Hull and his co-workers (1965)[69] six induced tumours in hamsters. SA7 isolated from a Cercopithecus aethiops monkey was particularly potent. Other animal adenoviruses shown to be oncogenic are bovine adenovirus type 3 (Darbyshire, 1966)[70], chicken-embryo lethal-orphan virus (Sarma *et al.*, 1965[71]) and canine adenoviruses (Sarma *et al.*, 1969)[72], Dulac *et al.*, 1769[73]).

In the last few years it has been found that a number of viruses cannot replicate unless the cell they infect is also infected by a helper virus. These so-called defective viruses lack some of the information necessary for replication, a deficiency that is made good by the helper virus (Rowe, 1967[74]; Rapp, 1969[75]). The degree of defectiveness is variable. Many stocks of human and animal adenoviruses are mixed with an adeno-associated virus (Hoggan, 1970[76]) which can only multiply in cells infected by an adenovirus. The adeno-associated virus infects humans but is not known to cause disease, and antibodies to the virus are not more frequent in patients with tumours than in other groups (Sprecher-Goldberger *et al.*, 1970[77]). The human adenoviruses are themselves defective, but to a lesser degree. They can replicate in human cells without a helper virus, but in green monkey kidney cells the help of SV40 virus is required for the production of infective virus. The interaction between certain adenoviruses and SV40 is more complex than simple complementation (Rapp and Melnick, 1966[78]). A hybrid virus can be produced that is phenotypically an adenovirus but contains a part of the SV40 genome. The hybrid virus does not give rise to SV40 virus particles but the presence of SV40 viral DNA is revealed by the formation of SV40 tumour antigen in infected cells. Like the human adenovirus, the hybrid virus cannot replicate alone in monkey kidney cells; but the two particles together—hybrid virus and SV40— can replicate. The hybrid particle has been called PARA—an acronym for 'particle aiding replication of adenovirus'. Several different adenoviruses can substitute as helpers for PARA, and the progeny virus has the phenotype of the helper. The term transcapsidation has been used for the process by which the genetic information of one virus is carried within the capsid of an unrelated virus. By this process non-oncogenic viruses could acquire oncogenic potential, and an oncogenic virus may be able to produce tumours in new hosts.

Further work on the leukaemia viruses suggests that leukaemia in most if not all species is probably virus-induced though it is only in the fowl, mouse and cat that a viral aetiology has been proved. There is now growing evidence that leukaemia in cattle, pigs, dogs and guinea pigs is associated with a virus (see review by Jarrett 1970[79]). An interesting development has been the observation that both the Rous (fowl sarcoma) virus and the mouse sarcoma virus discovered by Harvey[80] in 1964 are defective and unable to produce their viral envelopes without assistance from one of the leukaemia viruses which acts as a helper providing information for the viral envelope. Thus the sarcoma virus has the antigenic and host-range characteristic of the helper virus. The sarcoma virus can enter a cell and transform it into a tumour cell (Aaronsen *et al.*, 1970[81]); but infective progeny are not formed in the absence of a helper virus (see review by Harvey and East, 1971[82]). The discovery of a sarcoma virus in cats (Snyder and Theilen, 1969[83]) raises the possibility that a similar relationship may exist in this species. The mouse sarcoma virus genome can be rescued from non-virus producing cells by the cat leukaemia virus (Sarma *et al.*, 1970[84]) and this process of rescue by a leukaemia virus from another species provides a possible method of demonstrating the presence of a human leukaemia virus in extracts of human leukaemic tissues (Steeves *et al.*, 1971[85]).

Among the herpes group of viruses there are a number that cause tumours in animals. The Lucké frog kidney carcinoma is caused by a herpes virus (Mizell *et al.*, 1969[86]) and so is Marek's disease, a lymphomatous condition of chickens (Churchill, 1968[87]; Epstein *et al.*, 1968)[88]. There is also a herpes virus (*Herpes Saimiri*) isolated from a squirrel monkey which causes tumours on injection into owl monkeys and marmosets (Meléndez *et al.*, 1969[89]; and 1971[90]). Herpes viruses have been found in association with tissue cultures of lymphoid tumour cells from guinea pigs (Nayak 1971[91]) and man (see review by Epstein 1970[92]). C-type virus particles are also present in the lymphoblasts of leukaemic guinea pigs (Feldman and Gross 1970[93]) and it remains to be shown what role these two viruses play in the development of leukaemia in the guinea pig. The herpes virus associated with human lymphoid tumours, the EB virus from Burkitt lymphomas, appears to be the causative agent of infectious, mononucleosis (see Carter and Penman 1969[94]) and may well play a role in the production of some human tumours (Epstein 1971[95]).

It has been suggested by Huebner and his colleagues (Huebner and Todaro, 1969[96]) that all vertebrates carry vertically transmitted genetic information for producing C-type RNA viruses. They postulate that the viral information pertaining to these C-type particles (the virogene) has a portion responsible for transforming a normal cell into a tumour cell (the oncogene) and that the virogene is transmitted from animal to animal and from cell to cell as a repressed viral genome, thus behaving more like a cellular gene than a virus. The complete C-type virus is rarely formed under natural conditions but it is commonly observed in certain inbred lines of mice such as AKR. Under natural conditions it may be more common for partial expression of the virogene to occur—i.e. for expression of the oncogene portion only: this could happen as a consequence of exposure to chemical carcinogens, radiation or merely increasing age. Whether infectious virus and/or tumour become expressed may well depend largely on genetic factors (Meier and Huebner, 1971[97]). Evidence for the existence of latent C-type viruses is rapidly increasing (Gardner *et al.*, 1971[98]) and their possible significance in the aetiology of 'spontaneous' tumours must be seriously considered.

Taxonomy of tumour viruses

Two questions asked early on in the study of tumour viruses were: Are the tumours produced by such viruses similar to tumours not known to be virus induced? And are tumour viruses similar to other viruses or do they constitute a separate group?

In answer to the first question, no one has yet observed any consistent differences between tumours that are and are not known to be caused by viruses—except that tumours produced by viruses all have a virus coded antigen specific for the particular virus, whereas chemically-induced and other tumours appear to have new antigens which are different for each tumour produced.

In answer to the second question, it is certain that tumour viruses do not form a separate group in the generally accepted classification of viruses. As can be seen in Table 11.1 there are tumour producing viruses in five of the fourteen

Table 11.1. A classification of animal viruses

Nucleic acid core	*Capsid symmetry*	*Virion naked or enveloped*	*Virus groups*	*Tumour viruses in group*
DNA	Cubic	Naked	1. Parvovirus (Picodnavirus)	———
			2. Papovavirus	Human, rabbit and bovine papilloma viruses. Polyomavirus, Vacuolating virus (SV40).
			3. Adenovirus	Many human and animal types.
		Enveloped	4. Herpesvirus	Lucké virus, Marek's disease virus, H. Saimiri, Epstein Barr virus.
	Complex	Complex coat	5. Poxvirus	Yaba virus, rabbit, squirrel and hare fibroma viruses.
RNA	Cubic	Naked	1. Picornavirus	———
			2. Reovirus	———
	Helical	Enveloped	3. Myxovirus	———
			4. Rhabdovirus	———
	Unknown	Enveloped	5. Oncornavirus	Avian, murine and feline leukaemia and sarcoma viruses.
			6. Arenavirus	———
			7. Togavirus	———
			8. Coronavirus	———

groups of viruses. Tumour viruses have only one property in common—that they produce tumours on injection into animals. They form a group rather like the respiratory viruses, all producing a similar disease but composed of viruses of many different types. However, one obvious essential for transformation of a normal cell into a tumour cell is that the cell must not be killed by the infecting virus. There are two types of non-cytocidal infection, and the tumour viruses can be divided into those such as leukaemia viruses in which the virus replicates and is released continuously by budding from the cell surface, and those like polyoma, SV40 and adenoviruses in which no infective virus is formed in the cell but the viral genome is maintained and replicated in step with the cell genome.

It seems likely that tumour viruses have nucleic acid with special characters since the ability to transform normal cells into tumour cells must depend not only on the presence of the necessary information but also on the nucleic acid being capable of integration into the genetic apparatus of the cell. If this requires any special properties these would obviously be characteristcs which could be used to identify possible tumour viruses.

The ecology of tumour viruses

Tumour viruses have often appeared to be purely laboratory phenomena but the fowl leukaemia and Marek's disease viruses are a striking exception. The neoplastic diseases they produce are of great economic importance to the poultry industry. The leukaemia viruses can be transmitted from generation to generation via the egg, and they are the only viruses known definitely to be passed in this way. Not all infected birds develop neoplastic disease, and most have a latent or silent infection. Most flocks have a variable proportion of demonstrably infected birds and it has not been easy to obtain flocks wholly free from infection, a drawback that has made the study of these viruses very difficult (see reviews by Beard, 1957[99]; Campbell, 1961[100]). It now appears that even birds without the group antigen, which has been used as a sign of infection with one of the leukosis viruses, may be carrying the virus in a latent form (Weiss *et al.,* 1971[101]).

Transmission from generation to generation in the ovum or milk is often called 'vertical transmission', whereas transmission by the more usual routes of cross-infection between individuals is called 'horizontal transmission'. Further examples of tumour viruses transmitted vertically are the mouse mammary tumour virus and the mouse leukaemia viruses which are passed from the mother to the young predominantly, if not entirely, via the milk.

The vertical transmission of virus-induced mouse leukaemia was first noticed by Gross who found that the offspring of mice injected with passage A virus had a high incidence of leukaemia (Gross, 1951[102]). Similar observations have been made with Graffi and Friend viruses in mice (Krischke and Graffii, 1962[103]; Mirand Grace, 1962[104]) and with Moloney virus in mice and rats (Salaman and Harvey, 1961, 1962[105,106]). The male appears to play no part in transmission of the virus, and not all virus-injected females, or the female descendants of virus-injected females, transmit the virus to their young. Nevertheless, a persistent high incidence of virus transmission to the ninth generation has been observed. The factors determining the success or failure of vertical transmission are unknown. The relationship between apparently spontaneous leukaemia and the leukaemia viruses is hard to assess, but the leukaemias induced by the viruses of Gross, Kaplan, Moloney, Graffi and Stansly cannot be differentiated on histological grounds from neoplasms of similar cell type occurring spontaneously (Dawe *et al.,* 1962)[107], and it is highly improbable that these viruses do not play some part in the development of the natural disease. However, in pure lines of mice with a high incidence of spontaneous leukaemia, the milk does not appear to be an important factor; the incidence of leukaemia is not reduced if the young are removed to a foster-mother of a low leukaemic strain as soon as they are born (Law, 1962[108]). It appears likely that all AKR mouse cells carry the leukaemia virus genome in an unexpressed form (Rowe *et al.*, 1971[109]). The difference between the natural and the experimental disease may be due to the fact that the viruses used in experiments have been passaged many times, and have thus been subjected to considerable selection and even contamination. The leukaemia viruses have often become more potent on passage, and other properties may also have been altered.

Horizontal transmission of the mouse leukaemia viruses, if it occurs, does not seem to be a common cause of leukaemia; but this by no means excludes its occurrence. The end result of an infection with a tumour virus depends closely on factors such as the dose of virus, the age of the animal at the time of infection, and the presence of circulating antibodies. The relationship between infection and tumour formation has been extensively studied in the case of polyoma virus. Mice only develop tumours if polyoma virus is injected during the first few days of life. As they grow older the mice rapidly become more resistant to its oncogenic effect. For a short time this resistance can be overcome by increasing the dose of virus, but soon they are completely resistant.* Such mice are, however, still susceptible to infection with polyoma virus. Infected mice excrete the virus in their saliva and urine, and the infection spreads silently in a mouse colony. The spread of infection can be readily observed by the appearance of antibodies in the plasma of infected mice. Although infection with polyoma virus is widespread among laboratory and wild mice, spontaneous polyoma-induced tumours are rare. This is probably due to the fact that mice born to uninfected mothers are unlikely to be exposed to infection until they are weaned, by which time they are too old for a small dose of virus to produce tumours. The young from polyoma-infected mothers are exposed to infection from their mothers, but are protected for the first six to eight weeks of life by maternal neutralizing anti-bodies which pass across the placenta to the foetus, and via the milk to the young (Law *et al.*, 1962[110]). Spontaneous polyoma tumours can only occur in any number for a short time while the virus is spreading rapidly after its introduction into a polyoma-free animal house (Rowe, 1961[38]). A similar situation would arise if a polyoma-free colony was introduced into an infected animal house.

Polyoma virus rarely produces tumours under natural conditions, and this may well be the usual state of affairs with tumour viruses. The human adenoviruses and SV40 have not been shown to produce tumours in man or monkeys, though they frequently infect their natural hose. On the other hand some tumour viruses, such as the Shope papilloma virus, seem to produce tumours quite commonly in their natural host. The cottontail rabbits, in which the papilloma virus occurs naturally, live in burrows and it is probable that the virus is spread by transference of infected material from the papilloma of one rabbit to the wall of the burrow and thence to the flank of another rabbit; the virus probably penetrates the skin through minor abrasions. The Shope fibroma virus and the other fibroma viruses of the pox group closely resemble myxoma virus, and may be spread by blood-sucking insects.

The virus of Marek's disease proved difficult to separate from tissues and the infective nature of the disease was questioned (see review by Biggs *et al.*, 1968[111]). But it has now been shown that infective virus is spread from the

*This resistance may later break down under special circumstances—e.g. in mice immuno-suppressed by adult thymectomy and repeated injections of antilymphocyte globulin. Gaugas *et al.* (1969)[109]a.

feather follicles and that infection is readily transmitted from one bird to another by dust (Calnek *et al.*, 1970[112]; Nazerian and Witter, 1970[113]).

In the laboratory, tumour viruses are often handled as though they could not give rise to cross-infection like other viruses. This is probably a grave mistake, for cross-infection can undoubtedly occur. Rous sarcoma virus is often considered non-contagious, but Burmester and Fontes (1960)[114] found that chicks inoculated with Rous sarcoma virus when nine days old passed the virus on to a high proportion of their uninjected cage mates. These naturally-infected chicks developed tumours after a much longer latent period than the inoculated birds. Since the factors on which the transmission of most tumour viruses depend are not known, experimental animals should always be kept strictly isolated. In this connection it is difficult to over-emphasize the importance of having experimental animals available that are free of all known viruses. The fact that there may well be unrecognized viruses present in a pathogen-free stock cannot be a reason for studying one virus in an unnecessary mixture of other viruses. Unfortunately, few viruses are as easy as polyoma virus to detect and eliminate from a mouse colony—polyoma-virus-free stock can be obtained merely by selecting breeding animals with no circulating polyoma antibodies (Salaman and Rowson (1960[115]). If Huebner's theory is true and all vertebrates carry latent oncogenes it may prove impossible to obtain animals free of these genes.

Tumour induction

The detailed sequence of events in the induction of tumours by viruses is not yet fully understood. *In vitro*, it has been shown that infected cells undergo a morphological transformation, acquire certain new properties, and can be shown to be neoplastic on inoculation into a suitable recipient animal. In *vivo*, however, it is more difficult to be sure what happens. It is clear that the fate of an individual transformed cell *in vivo* is likely to depend on host factors such as the nature of the immune response and the level of circulating hormones, but some experimental evidence has been obtained which supports the view that tumour viruses act directly on the cells whose descendants form a tumour, and that such interaction takes place within a few hours of the virus being injected (even though the tumour may not appear for several weeks or even months).

In newborn hamsters, tumour induction by polyoma virus is very rapid. Four days after inoculation, clusters of transformed cells can be seen in the kidneys in the region of the collecting tubules near the cortico-medullary junction. The focal distribution of these transformed cells suggests the possibility that they might be clones of cells, originating from single cells transformed by the virus soon after injection. In support of this theory Stoker, (1960)[116] found that the number of foci was roughly proportional to the dose of virus injected, and that the observed frequency distribution of foci in the kidneys from a group of hamsters receiving a small dose of virus approximated to a Poisson distribution. This would not have been so if the foci had been initiated by virus which had replicated after injection into the animals. The average number of cells in each focus four days after the injection of virus was estimated to be sixty-five. A clone of this number would require six generation cycles for its formation so, unless the generation time was extremely short, transformation must have occurred soon after infection. If transformation does indeed occur soon after infection, the generation time of the transformed cells will be sixteen hours—a division time found for many cells growing under optimum conditions *in vitro*. Stoker [116] also showed that, after a certain dose of virus, the proportion of hamsters with foci of transformed renal cells at nine days was the same as the proportion which went on to develop gross renal tumours; this observation suggests that no new foci of transformed cells are produced after the initial period.

Another line of enquiry indicating the rapid action of polyoma virus comes from experiments on the neutralization of tumour-producing activity of the virus by antibody. Stewart, Eddy and Stanton (1959)[117] found that polyoma virus antiserum, injected into newborn mice one hour before the virus, prevented the development of tumours; it failed to do so when injected as little as one hour after the virus. Habel and Silverberg (1960)[118] reported a similar experiment in which one day old hamsters, inoculated with polyoma virus, were injected with polyoma antiserum or normal serum at different times before or after administration of virus. Antiserum injected one hour before the virus completely protected half the hamsters against the tumour-producing activity of the virus; in the remainder there was limited development of sarcomas at the site of injection. Serum given one hour after the virus did not save any of the hamsters, but the tumours were all confined to the site of injection, and the survival time was very much prolonged. Serum given twenty-four hours after the virus was without effect. The fact that local tumours could develop at the injection site when other tumours were prevented from appearing, strongly suggests that the virus has a local action. Another experiment demonstrating the local action of polyoma virus was reported by Stanton (1960)[119] who implanted cotton pledgets subcutaneously in the axillae of eight newborn hamsters. The implants on the right side had been soaked in tissue-culture fluid containing polyoma virus, those on the left in control (polyoma-free) fluid. Six of the eight hamsters developed subcutaneous sarcoma, all of them in the right axilla. If the virus did not act locally, it is hard to see why the tumours should appear in the right axilla rather than in the left. In both these experiments, where only local tumours developed at the site of virus inoculation, the virus must have been able to enter cells at the injection site, but not more distant cells.

Polyoma virus is a potent antigen but antibodies were not elicited in the hamsters which, passively protected by polyoma antiserum, developed only local tumours. This indicates that little if any new virus was formed so the cells at the site of injection were probably transformed by the virus injected. It has also been found that hamsters which develop tumours due to the injection of SV40 or adenoviruses frequently do not develop neutralizing antibodies in their plasma, and there is no evidence that these viruses replicate in hamsters.

The study of neoplastic transformation has been made much easier by the observation that tissue cultures infected with certain tumour viruses undergo a change in morphology which seems to be associated with the conversion of normal cells into neoplastic cells. Though encountered with at least five tumour viruses, this charge has been most extensively studied with polyoma virus. When a mouse embryo tissue-culture is infected with polyoma virus, most cells support the replication of the virus and are destroyed in the process. This cytopathic effect is easily seen and is similar to that produced by many non-tumour viruses. About twenty per cent of the cells survive and can be propagated without any further gross cell destruction though such cultures usually continue to release small quantities of virus into the surrounding medium. Hamster embryo cultures infected with polyoma virus behave rather differently. There is no cytopathic effect, and little if any new virus is produced. Both the infected hamster cells and the surviving mouse cells show certain new characteristics which indicate that they have undergone neoplastic transformation. Normal cells tend to lie with their long axes parallel and form a sheet one cell thick; transformed cells lie at random, crossing one another, and tending to pile up on top of each other. The transformed cells have an increased growth-rate and the culture medium becomes acid more rapidly than in untransformed cultures. They can be propagated indefinitely, unlike freshly explanted animal cells which usually die after being subcultured for a time. Transformed cells often show chromosomal abnormalities and contain new virus-specific antigens. The cell surface shows changes in electrical charge and the cells are agglutinated by certain plant glycoproteins. (See reviews by Meyer 1971[120], and Melnick 1971[121]).

A rather similar process may occur 'spontaneously' in uninoculated tissue cultures. Usually an old slowly-growing culture suddenly starts to grow more quickly. The new rapidly growing cells are all of one morphological type and they can be more readily subcultured. The similarity between spontaneous and virus-induced transformation is striking but, although the spontaneously transformed cells are often malignant or later become so on further culture, this does not seem to be a necessary consequence of spontaneous transformation; indeed the ability to produce tumours on inoculation into animals can be lost as well as acquired by these cells (see review by Paul (1962)[122] and Macpherson 1971[123]).

The term transformation is perhaps best used to describe a change in the growth potential of a culture, without the implication that the cells have become tumour cells. The conversion of a non-tumour cell into a tumour cell can then be referred to more specifically as neoplastic transformation. The difficulty with neoplastic transformation is to know when it has taken place, because there is no clear and unqualified test for the malignant character which tumour cells possess. The only reliable test is still to inoculate cells into an immunologically compatible host animal but even this procedure is not satisfactory: as the newly formed tumour cells may contain antigens which are not present in the tissues of the isologous host, and so provoke an immunological reaction.

It would be convenient if cells which have undergone malignant transformation could be identified immediately after exposure to a virus, but this is not possible at the present time. Stoker and MacPherson (1961)[124] have used an experimental system in which a suspension of hamster embryo cells is exposed to polyoma virus, and then plated out to determine the proportion of normal and malignant cells. The cells which have become tumour cells give rise to clones that are morphologically distinct from those formed by normal cells (*Fig. 11.1*). The proportion of colonies with the neoplastic growth pattern was directly related to the dose of virus per cell, but the proportion of cells transformed in this way was always low, and a large dose of virus was required. There are several possible explanations for this low yield of cells showing neoplastic transformation. It could be that only some of the virus

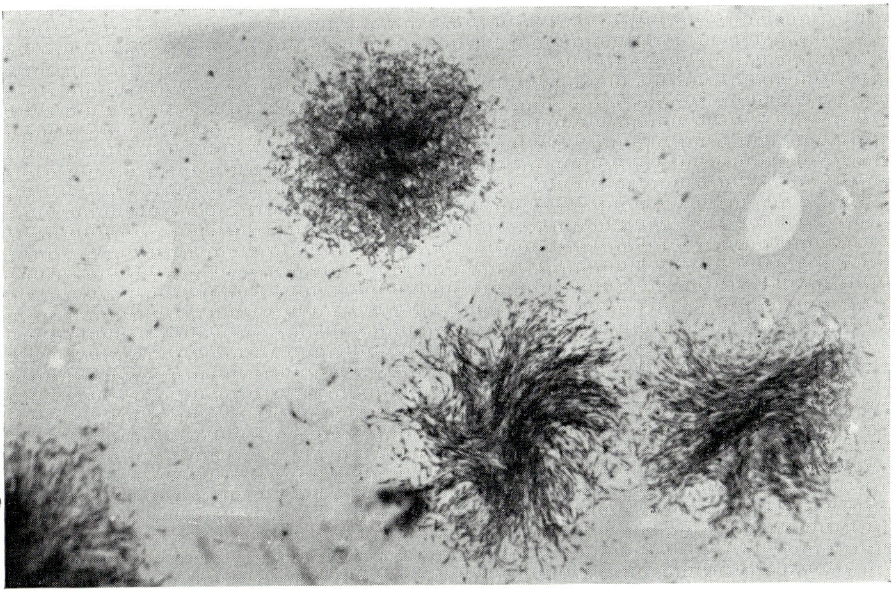

Fig. 11.1. Colonies of hamster cells developing from a suspension of cells plated out after exposure to polyoma virus. The cells in the upper colony are transformed, those in the lower ones are normal. (Photograph kindly supplied by Professor M. Stoker and previously published in Cold Spring Harbor Symposia on Quantitative Biology, Vol. XXVII, p. 377.)

particles were capable of producing neoplastic transformation or that only a few of the (mixed) population of target cells were susceptible; or that, despite an excess of competent virus and susceptible cells, there is a low probability of the virus entering a cell, or having done so, of its producing neoplastic transformation. These possibilities have been investigated by the use of the BHK21 line of hamster cells which, although transformed, have retained the orderly growth pattern of non-malignant cells and do not produce malignant tumours when injected into hamsters. Using clones of BHK21 cells, MacPherson and Stoker (1962)[125] showed that the rate of malignant transformation remained low—so the limiting factor does not appear to be a supply of genetically susceptible cells. By means of immunofluorescent staining of cells exposed to polyoma virus, Fraser and Gharpure (1962)[126] have demonstrated that all the cells take up virus though only a few are transformed. Further work using cells in agar suspension (MacPherson and Montagnier, 1964[127]) has shown that all the cells which take up virus are stimulated to divide and show some of the properties of transformed cells, but after a few divisions they lose the virus and revert to normal. In a few cells, however, the viral genome becomes integrated into the cellular genetic apparatus and the transformed state is maintained (Stoker, 1969[128]).

Apart from the placque type and dose of virus used, certain environmental factors have been found to affect the yield of transformed cells: these include the type and concentration of serum used in the culture medium (Stanners, Till and Siminovitch, 1963[129]), the concentration of magnesium ions present during the post-absorption period (Stoker and Abel, 1962[130]), the temperature of incubation of the infected cells prior to cloning (Medina and Sachs, 1963[131]), the pH of the culture medium (Kisch and Fraser, 1964[132]) and previous exposure of the cells to X-irradiation (Stoker, 1963[133]). The action of X-irradiation could be to select susceptible cells, or directly to alter cells and make them more susceptible to transformation. The latter is the more likely explanation, as the increased sensitivity to transformation lasts for only about two days after X-irradiation, and an increased rate of transformation occurs in cultures irradiated twenty-four hours after exposure to polyoma virus (Stoker, 1964[134, 135]).

How does the virus bring about neoplastic transformation? One possibility is that polyoma virus acts indirectly. If the cultures contained a very few mutant cells which were inhibited by the presence of normal cells, polyoma virus could allow these cells to grow out by infecting and altering all the others. This seems impossible as, in the line of hamster cells used by Stoker, transformed clones have never appeared when these cells have been plated out after exposure to control virus-free culture medium, whereas cells exposed to virus consistently yield transformed clones. Neoplastic transformation could still be an indirect process if the polyoma-infected cell released a new transforming substance which acted on a neighbouring cell. If this were so the transformation rate should be related to the cell density, but it is not. Even so, the indirect process could have taken place rapidly among cell clumps in the absorption tube before plating, but the transformation rate is found to be unrelated to the degree of cell clumping during exposure to the virus (Stoker and Abel, 1962[130]; Stoker 1963[133, 136]). Thus, neoplastic transformation appears to be a direct effect of the virus suspension, but the efficiency in terms of virus particles is very low, a dose of 10^4 plaque-forming units of virus being required to transform one cell (MacPherson and Montagnier, 1964[127]). That neoplastic transformation is in fact caused by the virus particles and not by some other factor in the virus preparation, rests on the following observations:

1. The transformation rate is directly related to the dose of virus used over a range of multiplicities from less than 1 up to 500 plaque-forming units per cell, above which no further increase in transformation rate is obtained (MacPherson and Montagnier, 1964[127]).
2. Receptor-destroying enzyme releases both plaque-forming virus and transforming activity from cell debris.
3. Transformation is prevented by virus antiserum, but not by DNAase.
4. In density gradients, transforming activity bands with 'full' virus particles and not with 'empty' capsids (Abel and Crawford, 1963[137]).

Rous sarcoma virus appears to be a much more efficient transforming agent than polyom virus or any of the other transforming viruses. If a sparse sheet of chick fibroblasts is exposed to a Rous sarcoma virus preparation and the cells are allowed to grow for a few days, small clumps of transformed cells can be identified and it is possible to titrate a Rous virus preparation by counting such foci (Temin and Rubin, 1958[138]).

The virus-cell relationship

It is now well established that tumour cells produced *in vivo* or *in vitro* by the small DNA viruses do not depend for their neoplastic properties on the continuing presence of complete infective virus particles. It has therefore been suggested that the viral nucleic acid is incorporated into a cell's genetic apparatus by a process in some way analogous to lysogeny in bacteria. Bacterial cells carrying a prophage are distinguished from comparable non-infected cells by (1) release of active phage, (2) resistance to superinfection with the same, or a closely related phage, and (3) production of new proteins under the influence of the prophage. The question arises: Do virus-transformed cells have comparable properties?

Tissue cultures transformed by polyoma virus or cultures of polyoma-induced tumour cells may continue to release virus in small amounts indefinitely; but this has been shown (Vogt and Dulbecco, 1962[139]) to be due to a slowly preading, cytocidal infection in a partially-resistant population of cells, and not to the spontaneous induction of a 'provirus' present in the cells. Some clones derived from single cells in these virus-producing cultures do not release virus though they retain all the properties of transformed cells. If these non-virus-producing clones are reinfected, they continue to form new virus in small amounts as before. Efforts to induce the production of polyoma virus in transformed cells by the methods which have been used for lysogenic bacteria have generally been unsuccessful (Habel and Silverberg, 1960[118]; Winocour and Sachs 1961[140]; Vogt and Dulbecco 1962[139]). Infectious polyoma virus has, however, been obtained from two lines of transformed cells—in one case from a line of rat cells by exposure to X-irradiation, mitomycin C or U.V.-irradiation (Fogel and Sachs 1969[141], 1970[142]) and in the other by an alteration in temperature from a line of mouse cells transformed by a thermosensitive mutant (Vogt, 1970)[143]. Cells transformed by SV40 resemble polyoma-transformed cells in that they neither release nor contain demonstrable infective virus (Sabin and Koch, 1963[144]), but virus can be obtained from them if the cells are grown in culture with grivet monkey-kidney cells or rabbit-kidney cells (Gerber, 1963[145]). Rabbit-kidney cells cannot be infected by intact SV40 virus but can be infected by SV40 nucleic acid. This may indicate that the transformed cells contain the viral nucleic acid, but are unable to produce whole virus particles. Growth of the tumour cells in the mixed cultures is not necessary for virus production. Virus is formed even if the tumour cells receive a lethal dose of X-irradiation before they are placed in culture with the monkey-kidney cells (Sabin and Koch, 1963[144]). Recovery of infectious virus can be enhanced by cell fusion (Harris and Watkins, 1965[145]) between SV40 transformed cells and permissive cells i.e. cells which support virus replication (Watkins and Dulbecco, 1967[146]). It has been reported that virus formation can be induced by treatment of SV40 tumour cells with proflavine, hydrogen peroxide or mytomycin C (Gerber, 1964[147]). Infective adenovirus has not been recovered from adenovirus transformed cells. The explanation for the failure to obtain infective virus from many transformed cells is not known but it may be that the cells contain only part of the genome.

In contrast to the cells transformed by the small DNA viruses, the tumour cells produced by the RNA leukaemia viruses usually seem to release virus continuously. The fowl (Rous) and mouse sarcoma viruses can, however, give rise to tumour cells which do not release virus. This is apparently because the sarcoma viruses are defective and require the aid of a second virus to produce new infective particles (Hanafusa, Hanafusa and Rubin, 1963[148], 1964[149–151]; Harvey, 1971[82]). When single foci of Rous virus-transformed cells were picked and cultured a very few were found to produce lines of cells which did not release Rous virus, or a virus of the chicken leukosis group called Rous-associated virus (RAV) (Rubin and Vogt, 1962[152]), which is always present in Rous virus preparations at a higher titre than the Rous virus itself. Though closely similar to Rous virus, this Rous-associated virus does not produce Rous tumours. It does not cause a noticeable morphological change in chick fibroblast cultures, but it induces resistance to Rous virus within a few days and this resistance is the basis for its detection and assay. If RAV is added to Rous virus-transformed cell cultures which are not releasing virus, they soon begin to produce both RAV and Rous virus. The RAV is a helper virus required by the defective Rous virus for the formation of complete virus. All non-virus producing Rous-virus transformed cells will produce complete Rous virus particles if they are superinfected with RAV or another of the fowl leukosis viruses—therefore the Rous virus genome must be maintained and replicated in the non-virus producing transformed cells. In order to produce the virus protein coat, it seems that information provided by the RAV nucleic acid is required. If this is so, the non-virus producing tumour cells should contain no Rous protein, which is the Rous antigen, and the Rous virus produced in response to superinfection with different leukosis viruses should be antigenically different. These two deductions seem to be true (Hanafusa, Hanafusa and Rubin, 1964[150]). The non-virus producing Rous tumour cells do not cause an immunological response, nor do they absorb Rous virus antibodies; and Rous viruses formed with the aid of different helper viruses are antigenically different.

The second characteristic of lysogenic bacterial cells—resistance to superinfection-cannot—readily be applied to hamster cells transformed by SV40 or adenovirus; these cells are not susceptible to the ordinary type of virus-producing infection before transformation and cannot therefore show an acquired resistance after transformation. Polyoma-transformed cells vary in their resistance to superinfection: most *in vivo* transformed cells are sensitive, while *in vitro* transformed cells are resistant. This difference in susceptibility can probably be accounted for by the fact that *in vitro* transformation takes place in the presence of large amounts of free virus, and there is therefore a considerable selection pressure in favour of cells resistant to destruction by polyoma virus; *in vivo* there is usually circulating antibody present with little free virus, and in these circumstances resistance to the virus may have no survival value. It has been shown that there is a correlation between the resistance of polyoma tumour cells to polyoma virus and to vaccinia virus (Hellström and Hellström, 1963[153]). The most likely explanation for this seems to be that the resistant cells are better interferon producers than the sensitive ones.

Though tumour cells may not always release virus or be resistant to superinfection, they do display new antigens which are specific to the virus present in the cell. Sera from animals bearing virus-induced tumours contain antibodies which react in complement fixation tests or by immunofluorescence with these new antigens ('T' antigens) which appear in the nuclei of transformed cells and productively infected cells (Habel, 1966[154]). The T antigens produced by polyoma virus, SV40 and adenoviruses do not cross-react immunologically, but the T antigens induced by the same virus in different animal species do cross-react. The T antigens are not viral structural proteins, but they are presumably viral coded products since they are virus-specific. On the surface of the virus transformed cell are further virus-specific antigens which are similar to tissue transplantation antigens and may lead to the rejection of cells inoculated into an immunized animal (see review Law, 1969[155]). Polyoma tumours are not always easy to transplant, even to another site in the same animal and, in quantitative experiments using trypsinized tumour-cell suspensions, it is possible to demonstrate a relative resistance to the growth of inoculated tumour cells in animals which have been immunized with polyoma virus (Habel 1961[156]; Sjogren, Hellström and Klein , 1961[157]). The resistance is not complete and it can be overcome if large numbers of cells are given; in resistant mice the latent period before the development of a tumour is longer than in normal mice. Resistance can be produced by the inoculation of polyoma tumour cells which are not releasing active virus, but not by virus inactivated with ultraviolet rays (Sjögren, 1961[158]; Habel, 1962[159]). The resistance appears to be of the transplantation type as it cannot be transferred with serum. The new antigen is probably present in all the tumour cells, because tumours passaged in polyoma-immune mice do not lose it, in spite of the considerable selection pressure against cells with this antigen (Hellström *et al.*, 1962[160]).

Proof of the persistence of the viral genome in transformed cells comes from the chemical identification (by nucleic acid hybridization techniques) of virus-specific nucleotide sequences in the genome of the transformed cells (see review by Dulbecco, 1969[161]; Winocour, 1971[162]). Until the recent demonstration in many tumour viruses of an RNA-dependent DNA polymerase (Temin and Mizutani 1970[163]) which can make a DNA copy from the viral RNA it was difficult to see how the viral RNA could be integrated into the cell DNA; but it now appears that both DNA and RNA tumour viruses may have a common mode of integration into the genetic apparatus of the cell.

Tumour development

If neoplastic transformation takes place after a virus is injected, what is happening during the latent period before a tumour appears? It seems likely that the tumour cells, recognized by the host as altered 'foreign' cells, excite an immunological response which prevents their rapid development and may even lead to their death. In newborn animals, antigens may elicit a degree of tolerance rather than an effective immune reaction and this may be the reason why many tumour viruses are more effective when injected into baby mice and hamsters. Polyoma virus injected into newborn mice gives rise to antibodies and some measure of resistance to the growth of tumour cells; but the response is probably slower than in adults and the balance is tipped in favour of the tumour cells which can reach the critical number required to overcome the hosts defence mechanisms. Chemical carcinogens have been shown to have some effect on the production of tumours by viruses. Newborn mice, injected with polyoma virus and later treated by the application of carcinogenic or tumour-promoting agents to the skin, develop significantly more polyoma-type tumours than mice which receive the virus alone (Rowson *et al.*, 1961[164]). The mechanism of the interaction between tumour viruses and chemical carcinogens is not clear, but it could be that the chemicals interfere with the defences of the host and allow a small number of transformed cells to develop into a tumour. A wide variety of chemical carcinogens are capable of depressing the immune response of mice to sheep erythrocytes (Malmgren *et al.*, 1952)[165], and it has been shown that 3-methylcholanthrene can interfere with homograft rejection of transplanted skin and increase the growth of transplanted tumour cells in mice (Prehn, 1963[166]). Rather surprisingly, viruses and chemical carcinogens may interact the other way round, the virus increasing the incidence of skin tumours due to a chemical carcinogen. Skin tumours produced by the application of benzo(a)pyrene appeared sooner, in larger numbers, and with a higher proportion of carcinomas, in mice which had been injected when newborn with polyoma virus than in those which had not (Rowson *et al.*, 1961)[164]. The importance of the interaction between viruses and chemical carcinogens is still difficult to assess but several examples have been reported. (See reviews by Duran-Reynals, 1963[167]; Salaman and Roe, 1964[168]; Roe and Rowson[1], 1968[2]). A number of virus infections are known to alter the immune response (See reviews by Salaman 1969[169], 1970[170]). The Friend and Rauscher leukeamia viruses depress the immune response of infected mice but the importance of this action of the virus in the development of leukaemia is uncertain. The administration of antilymphocyte serum which depresses cell-mediated immune responses, is certainly known to increase the susceptibility of young adult mice to the leukaemogenic effects of injected Moloney leukaemia virus (Law and Chang, 1971[171]).

Other factors no doubt play a part in the resistance of the host to tumour development. Cortisone, X-rays and neonatal thymectomy, for example, interfere with the immune mechanism, and there are reports which suggest that they may reduce the resistance of adult mice to the development of polyoma tumours. Wooley and Small (1957)[172] observed parotid gland tumours in mice after prolonged treatment with cortisone. It is probable that the mice were naturally infected with polyoma virus, and that treatment with cortisone permitted the growth of polyoma tumours. Law and Dawe (1960)[173] produced polyoma tumours by the injection of virus into two-month-old mice after they had received 300 r whole-body X-irradiation. Neonatal thymectomy has been shown largely to abolish the relative resistance of certain strains of mice to tumour induction by polyoma virus (Law 1965[174]).

Chang and Rasmussen (1965)[175] reported that mice infected with polyoma virus at the age of two to three weeks developed a high incidence of tumours when subjected to sound stress for three hours a day for six days, and then to avoidance-learning stress in a shuttle box for six hours a day for two weeks. The mechanism by which stress acts appears to be the suppression of interferon formation rather than by any effect on the immune defences. The importance of interferon in the ecology of the tumour viruses is difficult to assess, but both polyoma virus and Rous virus are sensitive to interferon and both stimulate the production of interferon in infected cells. Some strains of polyoma virus are more effective interferon-producers than others, and in mice the strains which produce least interferon produce the most tumours (Friedman and Rabson, 1964[176]). Interferon delays the development of Friend and Rauscher virus induced leukaemia in mice and impairs the growth of tumour cells *in vivo* and *in vitro* (Gresser *et al.*, 1969[177], 1971[178]). It seems likely that interferon acts both by suppressing viral multiplication and also directly on the cells. The interferon inducer polyinosinic polycytidylic acid (poly I poly C) may act to suppress tumour development by interferon production but it probably also acts by some other path such as the stimulation of cell mediated immunity (Weinstein *et al.,* 1971[179]). It is currently believed that one function of cell-mediated immune responses may be the prevention of neoplasia. In support of this theory treatment with immunosuppressive drugs has resulted in patients developing more malignant tumours than would have been expected but most have been of the lymphoreticular type. Why this should be is not clear but recently epithelial carcinomas of the skin have been reported in seven of fifty-one kidney allograft recipients in Australia (Walder *et al.*, 1971[180] *see also* recent paper by Hoover and Fraumeni, 1973[180a]).

Certain antibodies present in patients with tumours may block tumour cell destruction by activated lymphocytes and certain other serum factors may be capable of unblocking the cytocidal reaction (Hellström *et al.*, 1971[181]).

Normal cells cease to move and divide when they come into contact with each other, whereas tumour cells and transformed cells are not mutually inhibited. However, polyoma-transformed BHK21 cells are inhibited by normal hamster fibroblasts (Stoker, 1964[135]). If normal cells can inhibit the movement and division of transformed cells *in vivo* as well as *in vitro*, this would help to explain why some apparently malignant tumours do not invade surrounding tissues or give rise to metastases, and why some tumours appear to have a very long latent period.

Viruses and human tumours

Other than warts, there are no human tumours of proven viral origin; but it would be surprising if viruses were not responsible for some human neoplasms since tumours of proved viral origin have been found in such a wide variety of animals. Biochemically, the tissues of very different animals appear to be similar, yet the character and incidence of spontaneous tumours vary remarkably from one species to another; spontaneous tumours are common in mice and men, but rare in guinea-pigs. The mammary tumours of rats are nearly always benign, while those in man and mouse are often malignant. There must be some factor giving rise to this difference between species, and it is tempting to think that it might be susceptibility to different viruses. In mice, a high incidence of mammary tumours or leukaemia can be caused by the vertical transmission of a virus. There are many reports of human tumours observed to follow viral infections (see review by Hilleman, 1963[182]), but viral infections are common and isolated cases mean very little.

In research into human disease conditions, epidemiology often has to replace direct experimentation. The observation that certain occupations were associated with an increased incidence of certain tumours was instrumental in identifying a number of chemical carcinogens; and so with the increasing interest in tumour viruses it was natural to look for epidemiological clues to identify tumours which might be caused by infective agents. A number of studies have been made in an effort to show that the incidence of leukaemia is not random, but the results have not been convincing (Glass *et al.*, 1971[183]; Kessler and Lilienfeld, 1969[184]). Studies on the Burkitt lymphoma have been much more successful (Burkitt, 1958[185], 1963[186], 1969[187]; Burkitt and Wright, 1970[182a]). This tumour, found almost exclusively in regions of high rainfall and high temperature, occurs mainly in parts of subsaharal Africa and in New Guinea. It was originally thought to be associated with an arthropod-borne virus, but when the tumour cells were grown in culture a herpes type virus was observed in them by electron microscopy (Epstein, Henle, Achong and Barr, 1965[188]). This virus, now known as Epstein-Barr (EB) virus, is widespread and commonly infects children all over the world. In most children it causes a silent infection or perhaps mild respiratory disease with solid immunity to reinfection; but in a proportion of young adults it causes infectious mononucleosis (P.H.L.S. report, 1971[189]). The virus is not seen in Burkitt tumour cells until they have been grown in culture for some time, and even then only a small proportion of cells contain demonstrable virus particles; the virus is not released into the medium in appreciable amounts. Cells containing virus can be demonstrated, and antibodies in the serum titrated by an indirect immunofluorescence test (Henle and Henle, 1966[190]). Antibodies have been found to be common in all the populations studied in various parts of the world and they are acquired early in life by most people (Pereira *et al.*, 1969[191]; Niederman *et al.*, 1970[192]). The fact that EB virus has a world wide distribution and causes a common disease does not exclude it from being the cause of certain tumours. The main evidence linking EB virus with Burkitt's lymphoma and tumours of the post-nasal space is as follows:

(*a*) Although the virus is rarely detected in fresh tumour tissue, it appears with a high degree of regularity in cultures of tumour cells presumably when the restraining influence of the patients' antibodies is removed.

(*b*) The cell membrane of fresh and cultured Burkitt tumour cells have been shown to possess new antigens not present on the surface of bone marrow cells from the patients (Klein *et al.*, 1967[193]). These antigens are detected with live tumour cells instead of the acetone-fixed cells used in tests for EB virus antigen. The corresponding antibodies are found in the sera of patients with Burkitt's lymphoma, tumours of the post-nasal space and infectious mononucleosis. The membrane antigens are not the same as the viral antigen but appear to be induced by the virus, (see review by Klein, 1971[194]).

(*c*) Virtually all patients with confirmed Burkitt's lymphoma have EB viral antibodies, usually in high titre, whereas in normal children of similar age, sex and tribe, antibodies are usually absent or in low titre. More than 75 per cent of patients with cancer of the post-nasal space have high titres of EB virus antibodies whereas patients with other types of tumours in the nasopharynx do not. (Henle *et al.*, 1970[195]).

(*d*) EB virus appears to have a growth stimulating effect on cells in culture—which supports, but certainly does not prove, that it may be an oncogenic virus (Gerber *et al.*, 1969[196]).

If EB virus is not the cause of certain tumours but merely a passenger virus finding a favourable habitat, it is necessary to explain why Burkitt tumours provide such conditions while other lymphoreticular neoplasms do not. The factor which causes the geographical distribution of Burkitt's lymphoma and carcinoma of the post-nasal space remains to be resolved but a depression of the immune response by malaria may be a factor in precipitating the development of Burkitt's lymphoma (Burkitt 1969[187]; Burkitt and Wright 1970[187a]; Kafuko and Burkitt, 1970[197]). In support of this theory, Pike and his colleagues (1970)[198] found that thirty-six patients with Burkitt's lymphoma had a lower incidence of AS haemoglobin (Sickle cell trait) than a control group. Their results did not attain statistical significance but suggested that people with AA haemoglobin were about twice as likely to develop the lymphoma as those with AS haemoglobin. That a parasitic infection can increase susceptibility to virus-induced neoplasms is clear from an experimental study in which a concurrent infection with a murine plasmodium increased the incidence of malignant lymphoma during the six months following the injection of Moloney leukaemia virus into adult BALB/c mice (Wedderburn, 1970[199]).

Recently a number of diseases have been noted in which high levels of EB virus antibodies are more frequent than expected. In the lymphocyte-depleted phase of Hodgkin's disease, high antibody levels comparable to those found in Burkitt's lymphoma patients are common: in the more benign lymphocyte-predominant form, low antibody levels are the rules as in the control patients (Johansson *et al.*, 1970[200]; Levine *et al.*, 1971[201])*. High titres of antibody against EB virus antigens have been recorded in sarcoidosis (Hirshaut *et al.*, 1970[202]) but further studies have shown that antibody levels to herpes simplex virus and cytomegalovirus are also raised in this condition (Wahren *et al.*, 1971[203]). It thus appears likely that the raised antibody levels are due to non-specific factors and the data at present do not provide evidence of any aetiological role for EB virus in sarcoidosis. Another disease in which high levels of EB virus antibodies have been observed is systematic lupus erythematosus (Evans, Rothfield and Niederman, 1971[204]). It may be that the virus plays some non-specific role in the production of this disease or it may be that the altered immune state of the patient favours the viral infection.

Another tumour with a peculiar epidemiology is carcinoma of the uterine cervix. This tumour is almost unknown in virgins and occurs most commonly in women who have had multiple sex partners. It also has a marked

---

*Other authors have reported a normal distribution of EB virus antibodies in Hodgkin's Disease. Cf. Goldman and Aisenberg, 1970[201]a).

racial pattern being common in Christians and Hindus but rare in Jews and Moslems. These epidemiological features suggested that the cause might be a venereal disease which was to some extent prevented by circumcision. Nahmias and his colleagues found that the cervix was an important site of infection in genital herpes simplex infection, a disease which was sexually transmitted (Josey *et al.*, 1966[205]; Nahmias *et al.*, 1967[206]). They also found that the genital strain of virus was different from the oral strain (Dowdle *et al.*, 1967[207]). The finding of two serological types of Herpes simplex virus was in agreement with earlier work (Plummer, 1964[208]; Schneweis, 1962[209]) but it was now established that type 1 caused the oral lesions and type 2 the genital lesions. Serological surveys from a number of laboratories (Rawls *et al.*, 1969[210]; Sprecher-Goldberger *et al.*, 1970[211]; Nahmias *et al.*, 1970[212]; Royston and Aurelian, 1970[213]; Catalano and Johnson, 1971[214]; Rowson and Jones, 1972[215]) have shown that herpes simplex type 2 antibodies are much more common and at higher titre in women with carcinoma of the cervix than in control groups. An association between carcinoma of the cervix and type 2 virus appears to be proved but it may not be a causal relationship: two independent infections may both be transmitted in the same way or the altered cervical epithelium perhaps predisposes to herpetic infection. Recently it has been reported that a genital infection with herpes simplex type 2 can be produced in non-human primates (London *et al.*, 1971[216]) and this system may reveal if the virus has a neoplastic potential. A few tumours have been observed in hamsters following the injection of a very large number of new-born animals with herpes simplex virus type 2, but virus antigens were not demonstrated in these tumours (Nahmias *et al.*, 1970[217]). The transformation of hamster embryo fibroblasts in culture on exposure to herpes simplex virus type 2 inactivated with ultra-violet light has been reported; these transformed cells produced tumours on injection into new-born hamsters. No infectious virus was recovered from the cells but herpes simplex viral antigens were detected in the transformed cells by the indirect immunofluorescence technique (Duff and Rapp, 1971*a*[218]; 1971*b*[219]). Herpes simplex type 2 antigens have been observed in cells from patients in the early stages of cervical carcinoma (Aurelian *et al.*, 1970[220]) but tumour cells can acquire viral antigens from viruses which were not responsible for the original transformation. The role of herpes simplex virus type 2 in carcinoma of the cervix remains to be determined but the epidemiology of the tumour suggests that it is probably related to an infectious agent; the type 2 virus seems to be the most likely agent (see review by Nahmias, 1971[221]).

Most experiments designed to demonstrate viruses in human tumours directly have involved either the electron-microscopic examination of tumour cells or plasma for virus particles, or in the inoculation of animals with cell-free preparations of leukaemic or tumour tissue. Both these procedures have given positive results; but the presence of virus particles does not prove that the tumour is caused by the virus, nor does the isolation of a tumour-producing virus by the inoculation of an experimental animal prove that the virus was in the original inoculum. An increasing number of non-pathogenic viruses are being discovered which make the origin and significance of a newly-discovered virus very difficult to determine.

Ever since the discovery of the mouse mammary tumour virus, repeated attempts have been made to demonstrate a similar virus in human milk and mammary tissue. No convincing evidence of the presence of a virus was forthcoming until Moore and his colleagues (1969)[222], using improved concentrating and staining methods, demonstrated particles identical to the mouse mammary tumour virus in five of seventy-five samples of milk from normal women. In milk samples from women with a family history of breast cancer a higher proportion was positive. The Parsees living in Bombay form an isolated community separate from the Hindus, Moslems and Christians and they have a very high incidence of breast cancer. In forty-six milk samples from Parsee women, virus particles were present in eighteen (39 %) (Moore *et al.*, 1971[223]). Evidence that the virus particles seen in milk samples are tumour viruses is indirect. The virus particles are associated with an enzyme activity, RNA dependent DNA polymerase or reverse transcriptase (Schlom *et al.*, 1971[224]), which has been found in all RNA tumour viruses so far tested. This enzyme uses the single-stranded RNA genome of the tumour virus as a template for the synthesis of a double-stranded DNA which could be integrated into the genetic apparatus of the cell. In human mammary tumour extracts, RNA sequences have been detected which are homologous to RNA in mouse mammary tumour virus (Axel *et al.*, 1972[225]). The mouse virus was used as the human virus was not available in sufficient quantities. Mouse leukaemia virus and extracts of other human tumours acted as controls, but hybridization only occurred in significant degree between the malignant mammary tumour cell RNA and the DNA complementary to the mouse mammary tumour viral RNA. Thus there is evidence that the mammary tumour cells contain a virus with sequences complementary to those in a known mammary tumour virus. The human disease is in some respects similar to that in mice and it seems likely that the production of mammary tumours in the human will involve genetic factors and hormones as well as the virus.

Addendum

There have been three recent symposia published on the oncogenic herpes viruses (Biggs, de Thé and Payne, 1972[226]); Pathology Society Symposium 1972[227] and National Cancer Institute Symposium 1974[228]) and their role in human cancer has been reviewed by Klein (1972)[228a] and Rapp (1973)[229]. New evidence for the viral oncogene theory has been presented by Todaro and Huebner (1972)[230]. This theory would predict that the hamster cells transformed by herpes simplex virus type 2 would contain a C type RNA virus but Rapp, Conner, Glaser and Duff (1972)[231] could find no leukosis viruses or their antigens in such transformed cells. Glaser, Duff and Rapp (1972[232]) have reported on the ultrastructural morphology of hamster cells transformed by herpes simplex type 2. In some degenerating cells there were small numbers of virus-like particles similar in size and morphology to non-enveloped herpes viruses. The hamster transformed cells have been reported (Collard *et al.*, 1973[233]) to transcribe herpes simplex virus type 2 RNA sequences derived from a small portion of the viral genome which is present in both type 1 and type 2 virus. The cross hybridization of virus specific RNA from transformed cells with both type 1 and type 2 viral DNA is consistent with data showing that type 1 and type 2 viral DNA shares 35–39 per cent of their base sequences and with the reported transformation of hamster cells by type 1 virus. The transformed hamster cells would be expected to have a virus coded antigen but Duff, Doller and Rapp (1973)[234] found that preimmunization of hamsters with herpes simplex virus type 1 or 2 or simian virus forty did not produce resistance to transplantation of the transformed cells. However, immunization with herpes virus increased the incidence of lung metastases.

Herpes simplex virus infected cells are reported to contain a non-virion viral antigen (Tarro and Sabin 1973)[235]; this antigen is reported to be present in human cervical tumour cells (Holinshead *et al.*, 1972 and 1973[236, 237]) but this finding has not yet been confirmed by other workers. A fragment of DNA comprising 39 per cent of the viral genome has been found in cells of one human cervical tumour (Frankel *et al.*, 1972[238]) but other cervical tumours have been negative. However at least 10 per cent of the viral genome would have to have been incorporated in the cells for it to have been detected, and this is more of the viral genome than is possibly required for transformation. The demonstration of viral genetic material, if any, in the tumour cells must await a more sensitive test. Human cells showing some of the properties of transformed cells have been obtained by exposing human embryo lung cells in culture to herpes simplex virus type 2. Inhibition of the lytic infection was obtained by maintaining the cells at 42° C for eight days, (Darai and Munk, 1973[239]). A further study of the incidence of herpes simplex virus antibodies in patients with carcinoma of the cervix has been reported by Adam, Kaufman, Melnick, Levy and Rawls (1972)[240].

The biology of the mouse mammary tumour virus has been reviewed by Bentvelzen (1972)[241]. In human milk Sarkar and Moore (1972)[242] have observed three types of virus particles. Typical B-type particles were infrequently found. (These are generally associated with the mouse mammary tumour virus and have regular spikes on their membrane which make them easily identifiable). Another type of particle with surface projections different from the B-type particle, and C-type particles with no surface projections were more commonly found. Chopra *et al*, (1973)[243] detected no B-type particles in 460 milk samples but C-type particles were present in fifty. They were found in virtually the same proportion of milk specimens from donors irrespective of a family history of cancer and there was no consistent correlation between the finding of particles and the presence of an RNA-directed DNA polymerase. The difficulty in differentiating C-type particles from cell fragments is pointed out by Calafat and Hageman (1973)[244]. The significance of the particles found in human milk is difficult to assess but the particles are similar to the simian agent (Masan-Pfizer monkey virus) (Chopra and Oie, 1972[245]). Other methods of searching for the human mammary tumour viruses may resolve the problem. Schlom and his colleagues (1973)[246] report the quantitation of RNA tumour virus in human milk by hybridization to polyadenylic acid sequences. Müller and Grossmann (1973)[247], using the micro-double-diffusion technique, have found in the sera of women with breast cancer antigens which cross-react with rabbit anti-mouse mammary tumour virus sera. The sera of thirty-five healthy women were negative whereas the sera from ten of thirty-six women with breast cancer were positive. Keydar and his colleagues (1973)[248] have isolated an oncornavirus from milk and tumour tissue from four patients with breast cancer using human embryo tissue cultures grown in the presence of insulin and hydrocortisone hemisuccinate. The virus producing cultures have continued to produce virus in low concentration for 11 months. Another approach to the search for human tumour viruses is suggested by the observation of Závada (1972)[249] that cells simultaneously infected by vesicular stomatitis virus and an avian or murine leukaemia virus produce vesicular stomatitis virus with an envelope whose antigens are specified by the leukaemia virus. Using this technique Závada and his colleagues (1972)[250] have obtained a virus particle from a line of cells derived from a mammary tumour which may have an envelope specified by a virus latent in the cell line.

The RD 114 virus obtained from human cells passaged in kittens is under consideration as a human C-type virus. Its major internal proteins are distinct from other C-type viruses both antigenically and by virtue of a unique iso-electric point (McAllister *et al.,* 1972[251]; Oroszlan *et al.,* 1972[252]). The reverse transriptase of RD 114 is antigenically different from the feline, murine, avian and viper enzymes (Long *et al.,* 1973)[253]. In order to show that the unique properties of RD 114 virus are not due to passage in RD cells, McAllister and his colleagues (1972)[251] have passaged feline leukaemia virus and Kirsten mouse sarcoma virus in RD cells and examined the properties of these viruses after passage. The mouse and feline viruses were both apparently unchanged by passage in RD cells. Todaro, Fischinger and Sarma (reported by McAllister *et al.*[251]) have found a C-type virus with antigenic properties similar to RD 114 in a line of cat cells and it may be that RD 114 is a feline virus after all. Further support for this view comes in a paper by Ruprecht, Goodman and Spiegelman (1973)[254]. Lysogenic bacteria and tumour viruses, which have the ability to add their genetic information to the genome of their host cell, both have nucleic acid with some homology for the host cell DNA. The RD 114 virus hybridized to normal cat DNA but not to human DNA.

The presence of a reverse transcriptase in the white blood cells of human leukaemic patients is reported by Sarngadharan *et al.* (1972)[255], Baxt *et al.* (1972)[256] and Todaro and Gallo (1973)[256a]. Baxt and his colleagues found in the cells of twenty-three of the twenty-four patients they examined evidence of a reverse transcriptase associated with a seventy S RNA that was used as a template to generate DNA complements. In all thirteen cases where it was possible to test, the synthesized DNA hybridized specifically to RNA of the mouse leukaemia virus. The white blood cells of eighteen non-leukeamic patients, nine of whom had high white blood cell counts, were negative.

The human papova virus isolated from the brain in cases of progressive multifocal leukoencephalopathy has been shown to have DNA very similar to simian virus 40 (Sack *et al.,* 1973[257]). This close relationship between the two viruses suggests the possibility that the human virus may be oncogenic.

Volume 18 of Progress in Experimental Tumour Research is devoted to the oncogenic adenoviruses and contains reviews on most of the oncogenic adenoviruses. The structure and serological aspects of the oncornaviruses are reviewed by Nowinski, Fleissner and Sarkar (1973)[258].

References

1. Rowson, K. E. K. and Mahy, B. W. J. *Bact. Rev.*, **31,** 110 (1967).
2. Roe, F. J. C. and Rowson, K. E. K. *Int. Rev. Exp. Path.*, **6,** 181 (1968).
3. Southam, C. M., Tanaka, S., Arata, T., Simkovic, D., Mivra, M., and Peptiopules, S. F., *Prog. Exp. Tumour Res.*, **11,** 194 (1969).
4. Ellerman, V. and Bang, O. *Zbl. Bakt. I. Abt. Orig.*, **46,** 595 (1908).
5. Rous, P. *J. exp. Med.,* **12,** 696 (1910).
6. Rous, P. *J. exp. Med.,* **13,** 397 (1911).
7. Rous, P. *J. exp. Med.*, **19,** 570 (1914).
8. Wile, U. J. and Kingery, L. B. *J. Am. med. Ass.*, **73,** 970 (1919).
9. Shope, R. E. *J. exp. Med.*, **56,** 803 (1932).
10. Shope, R. E. *J. exp. Med.,* **58,** 607 (1933).
11. Bittner, J. J. *Science*, **84,** 162 (1936).
12. Bittner, J. J. *Am. J. Cancer*, **36,** 90 (1939).
13. Bittner, J. J. *J. Nat. Cancer Inst.*, **1,** 155 (1940).
14. Bittner, J. J. *Science*, **95,** 462 (1942).
15. Lucké, B. *J. exp. Med.*, **68,** 457 (1938).
16. Duryee, W. R. *J. Franklin Inst.*, **261,** 377 (1956).
17. Furth, J., Ferris, H. W. and Reznikoff, P. *J. Am. med. Ass.*, **105,** 1824 (1935).
18. Gross, L. *Proc. Soc. exp. Biol. Med. N.Y.*, **76,** 27 (1951).
19. Dmochowski, L. *Prog. med. Virol.*, **3,** 363 (1960).
20. Gross, L. *Adv. Cancer Res.*, **6,** 149 (1961).
21. Miller, J. F. A. P. *Adv. Cancer Res.*, **6,** 291 (1961).
22. Sinkovics, J. G., *A. Rev. Microbiol.*, **16,** 75 (1962).
23. Stansley, P. G. *Prog. exp. Tumour Res.*, **3,** 216 (1963).
24. Moloney, J. B. *Ann. Rev. Med.*, **15,** 383 (1964).
25. Gross, L. *Acta Haemat*, **32,** 44 (1964).
26. Gross, L. *Acta. Haemat.*, **32,** 81, (1964).
27. Gross, L. *Oncogenic Viruses*, second edition. Pub. Pergamon Press.
28. Boiron, M., Lévy, J. P. and Périès, J., *Prog. med. Virol*, **9,** 341 (1967).
29. Dougherty, R. M. and Di Stefano, H. S., *Prog. med. Virol.,* **11,** 154 (1969).
30. Pasternak, G. *Advances Cancer Res.*, **12,** 1 (1969).
31. Gross, L. *Proc. Soc. exp. Biol. Med. N.Y.*, **83,** 414 (1953).
32. Stewart, S. E. *Anat. Rec.*, **117,** 532 (1953).
33. McCulloch, E. A., Howatson, A. F., Siminovitch, L., Axelrad, A. A., and Ham, A. W., *Nature*, **183,** 1535 (1959).
34. Huebner, R. J., Rowe, W. P., Hartley, H. W. and Lane, W. T. *Ciba Foundation Symposium on Tumour Viruses of Murine Origin*, p. 314, Churchill, London (1962).
35. Stewart, S. E., Eddy, B. E. and Borgese, N., *J. natn. Cancer Inst.*, **20,** 1223 (1958).
36. Sachs, L., Fogel, M. and Winocour, E. *Nature*, **183,** 663 (1959).
37. Hartley, J. W., Rowe, W. P., Chanock, R. M. and Andrews, B. E. *J. exp. Med.*, **110,** 81 (1959).
38. Rowe, W. P. *Bact. Rev.*, **25,** 18 (1961).
39. Eddy, B. E., Borman, G. S., Berkeley, W. H. and Young, R. D. *Proc. Soc. exp. Biol. Med. N.Y.*, **107,** 191 (1961).
40. Sweet, B. H. and Hilleman, M. R. *Proc. Soc. exp. Med. N.Y.*, **105,** 420 (1960).
41. Eddy, B. E., Borman, G. S., Grubbs, G. E. and Young, R. D. *Virology*, **17,** 65 (1962).

42. Girardi, A. J., Sweet, B. H., Slotnick, V. B. and Hilleman, M. R. *Proc. Soc. exp. Biol. Med. N.Y.,* **109,** 649 (1962).
43. Gerber, P. and Kirschstein, R. L. *Virology*, **18,** 582 (1962).
44. Rabson, A. S., O'Conor, G. T., Kirschstein, R. L. and Branigan, W. J. *J. nat. Cancer Inst.*, **29,** 765 (1962).
45. Eddy, B. E. *Fed. Proc.*, **21,** 930 (1962).
46. Eddy, B. E. *prog. exp. Tumor Res.*, **4,** 1 (1964).
47. Gerber, P., Hottle, G. A. and Grubbs, R. E. *Proc. Soc. exp. Biol. Med. N.Y.,* **108,** 205 (1961).
48. Morris, J. A., Johnson, K. M., Ausilio, C. G., Chanock, R. M. and Knight, V. *Proc. Soc. exp. Biol. N.Y.*, **108,** 56 (1961).
49. Melnick, J. L. and Stinebaugh, S. *Proc. Soc. exp. Biol. N.Y.*, **109,** 965 (1962).
50. Shein, H. M. and Enders, J. F. *Proc. natn. Acad. Sci* (*U.S.A.*), **48,** 1164 (1962).
51. Shein, H. M. and Enders, J. F. *Proc. natn. Acad. Sci.* (*U.S.A.*), **48,** 1350 (1962).
52. Koprowski, H., Ponten, J. A., Jensen, F., Ravdin, R. G. Moorhead, P. and Saksela, E. *J. cel. Comp. Physiol*, **59,** 281 (1962).
53. Jensen, F., Koprowski, H. and Ponten, J. A. *Proc. natn. Acad. Sci.* (*U.S.A.*), **50,** 343 (1963).
54. Shein, H. M., Enders, J. F., Palmer, L. and Grogan, E. *Proc. Soc. exp. Biol. N.Y.*, **115,** 618 (1964).
55. Jensen, F., Koprowski, H., Pagano, J. S., Ponten, J. A. and Ravdin, R. G. P. *natn. Cancer Inst.*, **32,** 917 (1964).
56. Fraumeni, J. F., Ederer, F. and Miller, R. W. *Amer. med. Ass.*, **185,** 713 (1963).
57. Trentin, J. J., Yabe, Y. and Taylor, G. *Science*, **137,** 835 (1962).
58. Huebner, R. J., Rowe, W. P. and Lane, W. T., *Proc. natn. Acad. Sci.* (*U.S.A.*), **48,** 2051 (1962).
59. Trentin, J. J., Van Hoosier, G. L. and Samper, L. *Proc. Soc. exp. Biol. Med.*, **127,** 683 (1968).
60. McAllister, R. M., Nicolson, M. O., Reed, G., Kern, J., Gilden, R. V. and Huebner, R. J. *J. Nat. Cancer Inst.*, **43,** 917 (1969).
61. Huebner, R. J., Rowe, W. P., Turner, H. C. and Lane, W. T. *Proc. natn. Acad. Sci.* (*U.S.A.*), **50,** 379 (1963).
62. Yabe, Y., Samper, L., Bryan, E., Taylor, G. and Trentin, J. J. *Science*, **143,** 46 (1964).
63. Rabson, A. S., Kirschstein, R. L. and Paul, F. J. *J. natn. Cancer Inst.*, **32,** 77 (1964).
64. Huebner, R. J., Pereira, H. G., Allison, A. C., Hollinshead, A. C. and Turner, H. C. *Proc. natn. Acad. Sci.* (*U.S.A.*), **51,** 432 (1964).
65. Huebner, R. J. *Perspective in Virology V* (1967), Chapter 7, p. 147, Ed. Pollard Pub. Academic Press, N.Y.
66. Gilden, R. V., Kern, J., Lee, Y. K., Rapp, F., Melnick, J. L. Riggs, J. L., Lennette, E. H., Zbar, B., Rapp, H. J., Turner, H. C. and Hubner, R. J. *Amer. J. Epidemiology*, **91,** 500 (1970).
67. Shaw, G. J. and McFarlane, E. S. *Canad. J. Microbiol.*, **15,** 811 (1969).
68. Anderson, J., Yates, V. J., Jasty, V. and Mancini, O. *J. Nat. Cancer Inst.*, **43,** 575 (1969).
69. Hull, R. N., Culbertson, C. G., Reimer, C. B. and Wright, H. F. *Science*, **150,** 1044 (1965).
70. Darbyshire, J. H. *Nature*, **211,** 102 (1966).

71. Sarma, P. S., Huebner, R. J. and Lane, W. T. *Science*, **149,** 1108 (1965).
72. Sarma, P. S., Vass, W., Huebner, R. J., Igel, H., Lane, W. T. and Turner, H. C. *Nature*, **215,** 293 (1967).
73. Dulac, G. C., Swango, L. J., and Burnstein, T. *Canad. J. Microbiol.*, **16,** 391 (1969).
74. Rowe, W. P. *Perspectives in Virology*, **5,** 123 (1967) Ed. Pollard M. Pub. Academic Press.
75. Rapp, F. *Ann. Rev. Microbiol.*, **23,** 293 (1969).
76. Hoggan, M. D. *Prog. in med. Virol.*, **12,** 211 (1970).
77. Sprecher-Goldberger, S., Dekegel, D., Otten, J. and Thiry, L. *Arch. ges. Virusforschung*, **30,** 16 (1970).
78. Rapp, F. and Melnick, J. L. *Prog. med. Virol.*, **8,** 349 (1966).
79. Jarrett, O. *Advances in Cancer Research*, **13,** 39 (1970).
80. Harvey, J. J. *Nature*, **204,** 1104 (1964).
81. Aaronson, S. A., Jainchill, J. L. and Todaro, G. J. *Proc. natn. Acad. Sci.* (*U.S.A.*), **66,** 1236 (1970).
82. Harvey, J. J. and East, J. *Int. Rev. exp. Path,* **10,** 266 (1971).
83. Snyder, S. P. and Theilen, G. H. *Nature*, **221,** 1074 (1969).
84. Sarma, P. S., Log, T. and Huebner, R. J. *Proc. natn. Acad. Sci.* (*U.S.A.*), **65,** 81 (1970).
85. Steeves, R. A., Fjelde, A. and Mirand, E. A. *Proc. natn. Acad. Sci.* (*U.S.A.*), **68,** 2391 (1971).
86. Mizell, M., Toplin, I. and Isaacs, J. J. *Science*, **165,** 1134 (1969).
87. Churchill, A. E. *J. Nat. Cancer Inst.*, **41,** 939 (1968).
88. Epstein, M. A., Achong, B. G., Churchill, A. E. and Biggs, P. M. *J. Nat. Cancer Inst.*, **41,** 805 (1968).
89. Meléndez, L. V., Hunt, R. D., Daniel, M. D., Garcia, F. G. and Fraser, C. E. O. *Lab. Anim. Care*, **19,** 378 (1969).
90. Meléndez, L. V., Hunt, R. D., Daniel, M. D., Blake, B. J. and Garcia, F. G. *Science*, **171,** 1161 (1971).
91. Nayak, D. P., *J. Virol.*, **8,** 579 (1971).
92. Epstein, M. A. *Adv. in Cancer Res.*, **13,** 383 (1970).
93. Feldman, D. G. and Gross, L. *Cancer Res.*, **30,** 2702 (1970).
94. Carter, R. L. and Penman, H. G. *Infectious mononucleosis*, Blackwell Scientific Publications. Oxford. (1969).
95. Epstein, M. A. *Lancet*, p. 1344 (1971).
96. Huebner, R. J. and Todaro, G. J. *Proc. natn. Acad. Sci.*, **64,** 1087 (1969).
97. Meier, H. and Huebner, R. J. *Proc. natn. Acad. Sci.*, **68,** 2664 (1971).
98. Gardner, M. B., Officer, J. E., Rongey, R. W., Estes, J. D. Turner, H. C. and Huebner, R. J. *Nature*, **232,** 617 (1971).
99. Beard, J. W. *Ann. N.Y. Acad. Sci.*, **68,** 473 (1957).
100. Campbell, J. G. *Br. vet. J.*, **117,** 316 (1961).
101. Weiss, R. A., Friis, R. R., Katz, E. and Vogt, P. K. *Virology*. **46,** 920 (1971).
102. Gross, L. *Proc. Soc. exp. Biol. N.Y.*, **78,** 342 (1951).
103. Krischke, W. and Graffi, A. Unpublished, see Moloney (24).
104. Mirand, E. A. and Grace, J. T. *Virology*, **16,** 344 (1962).
105. Salaman, M. H. and Harvey, J. J. *Nature*, **191,** 509 (1961).
106. Salaman, M. H. and Harvey, J. J. *Nature*, **196,** 283 (1962).
107. Dawe, C. J., Law, L. W., Morgan, W. D. and Shaw, M. G. *Fed. Proc.* **21,** 5 (1962).
108. Law, L. W *Proc. Soc. exp. Biol. N.Y.*, **111,** 615 (1962).
109. Rowe, W. P., Hartley, J. W., Lander, M. R., Pugh, W. E. and Teich, N. *Virology*, **46,** 866 (1971).

109a. Gaugas, J. M., Chesterman, F. C., Hirsch, M. S., Rees, R. J. W., Harvey, J. J. and Hilchrist, C. *Nature*, **221**, 1633 (1969).
110. Law, L. W., Rowe, W. P., Hartley, J. W. and Dawe, C. J. *J. natn. Cancer Inst.*, **28**, 629 (1962).
111. Biggs, P. M., Churchill, A. E., Rootes, D. G. and Chubb, R. C. *Perspectives in Virology*, **VI**, p. 211 (1968).
112. Calnek, P. W., Adldinger, H. K. and Kahn, D. E. *Avian Dis.*, **14**, 219 (1970).
113. Nazerian, K. and Witter, R. L. *J. Virol.*, **5**, 388 (1970).
114. Burmester, B. R. and Fontes, W. G. *J. nat. Cancer Inst.*, **25**, 307 (1960).
115. Salaman, M. H. and Rowson, K. E. K. *Lab. Anim. Cent. Coll. Pap.* **9**, 61 (1960).
116. Stoker, M. *Br. J. Cancer*, **14**, 679 (1960).
117. Stewart, S. E., Eddy, B. E. and Stanton, M. F. *Canad. Cancer Conf.*, **3**, 287 (1959).
118. Habel, K. and Silverberg, R. J. *Virology*, **12**, 463 (1960).
119. Stanton, M. F. *Cancer Res.*, **20**, 487 (1960).
120. Meyer, G. *Advances in Cancer Res.*, **14**, 71 (1971).
121. Melnick, J. L. *In Vitro*, **6**, 335 (1971).
122. Paul, J. *Cancer Res.*, **22**, 431 (1962).
123. Macpherson, I. A. *Proc. Roy. Soc. Lond. B.*, **177**, 41 (1971).
124. Stoker, M. and Macpherson, I. *Virology*, **14**, 359 (1961).
125. Macpherson, I. and Stoker, M. *Virology*, **16**, 147 (1961).
126. Fraser, K. B. and Gharpure, M. *Virology*, **18**, 505 (1962).
127. Macpherson, I. A. and Montagnier, L. *Virology*, **22**, 291 (1964).
128. Stoker, M. G. P. *Lancet*, **1**, 362 (1969).
129. Stanners, C. P., Till, J. E. and Siminovitch, L. *Virology*, **21**, 448 (1963).
130. Stoker, M. and Abel, P. *Cold Spring Harb. Symp. quant. Biol.*, **27**, 375 (1962).
131. Medina, D. and Sachs, L. *Virology*, **19**, 127 (1963).
132. Kisch, A. L. and Fraser, K. B. *Virology*, **24**, 186 (1964).
133. Stoker, M. *Nature*, **200**, 756 (1963).
134. Stoker, M. *Virology*, **24**, 123 (1964).
135. Stoker, M. *Virology*, **24**, 165 (1964).
136. Stoker, M. *Virology*, **20**, 366 (1963).
137. Abel, P. and Crawford, L. V. *Virology*, **19**, 470 (1963).
138. Temin, H. M. and Rubin, H. *Virology*, **6**, 669 (1958).
139. Vogt, M. and Dulbecco, T. *Virology*, **16**, 41 (1962).
140. Winocour, E. and Sachs, L. *Virology*, **13**, 207 (1961).
141. Fogel, M. and Sachs, L. *Virology*, **37**, 327 (1969).
142. Fogel, M. and Sachs, L. *Virology*, **40**, 174 (1970).
143. Vogt, M. *J. Mol. Biol.*, **47**, 307 (1970).
144. Sabin, A. B. and Koch, M. A. *Proc. natn. Acad. Sci. U.S.A.*, **50**, 407 (1963).
145. Gerber, P. *Science*, **140**, 889 (1963).
146. Watkins, J. F. and Dulbecco, R. *Proc. natn. Acad. Sci. (U.S.A.)*, **58**, 1396 (1967).
147. Gerber, P. *Science*, **145**, 833 (1964).
148. Hanafusa, H., Hanafusa, T. and Rubin, H. *Proc. natn. Acad. Sci. (U.S.A.)*, **49**, 572 (1963).
149. Hanafusa, H., Hanafusa, T. and Rubin, H. *Virology*, **22**, 591 (1964).
150. Hanafusa, H., Hanafusa, T. and Rubin, H. *Proc. natn. Acad. Sci. (U.S.A.)*, **51**, 41 (1964).
151. Hanafusa, T., Hanafusa, H. and Rubin, H. *Virology*, **22**, 643 (1964).
152. Rubin, H. and Vogt, P. K. *Virology*, **17**, 194 (1962).

153. Hellström, I. and Hellström, K. E. *J. natn. Cancer Inst.*, **31**, 1525 (1963).
154. Habel, K. *Cancer Res.*, **26**, 2018 (1966).
155. Law, L. W. *Cancer Res.*, **29**, 1 (1969).
156. Habel, K. *Proc. Soc. exp. Biol. N.Y.* **106**, 722 (1961).
157. Sjögren, H. O., Hellström, I. and Klein, G. *Expl. Cell,* **23**, 204 (1961).
158. Sjögren, H. O. *Virology*, **15**, 214 (1961).
159. Habel, K. *J. exp. Med.*, **115**, 181 (1962).
160. Hellström, I., Hellström, K. E. and Sjögren, H. O. *Virology*, **16**, 282 (1962).
161. Dulbecco, R. *Science N.Y.*, **166**, 962 (1969).
162. Winocour, E. *Advances in Cancer Research*, **14**, 37 (1971).
163. Temin, H. M. and Mizutani, S. *Nature*, **226**, 1211 (1970).
164. Rowson, K. E. K., Roe, F. J. C., Ball, J. K. and Salaman, M. H. *Nature*, **191**, 893 (1961).
165. Malmgren, R. A., Bennison, B. E. and McKinley, J. W. *Proc. Soc. exp. Biol. N.Y.*, **79**, 484 (1952).
166. Prehn, R. T., *J. nat. Cancer Inst.*, **31**, 791 (1963).
167. Duran-Reynals, M. L. *Prog. exp. Tumour Res.*, **3**, 148 (1963).
168. Salaman, M. H. and Roe, F. J. C. *Br. med. Bull.*, **20**, 139 (1964).
169. Salaman, M. H. *Antibiotica et Chemotherapia*, **15**, 393 (1969).
170. Salaman, M. H. *Proc. Roy. Soc. Med.*, **63**, 11 (1970).
171. Law, L. W. and Chang, S. S. *Proc. Soc. exp. Biol. Med.*, **136**, 420 (1971).
172. Wooley, G. W. and Small, M. C. *Ann. N.Y. Acad. Sci.*, **68**, 533 (1967).
173. Law, L. W. and Dawe, C. J. *Proc. Soc. exp. Biol. N.Y.*, **105**, 414 (1960).
174. Law, L. W. *Science*, **147**, 164 (1965)
175. Chang, S-S and Rasmussen, A. F. *Nature*, **205**, 623 (1965).
176. Friedman, R. M. and Rabson, A. S. *J. exp. Med.*, **119**, 71 (1964).
177. Gresser, I., Bourali, C., Lévy, J. P., Fontaine-Brouty-Boyé, D. and Thomas, M.T. *Proc. Natn. Acad. Sci.* (*U.S.A.*), **63**, 51 (1969).
178. Gresser, I., Thomas, M. T. and Brouty-Boyé, D. *Nature New Biol.*, **231**, 20 (1971).
179. Weinstein, A. J. Gazdar, A. F., Sims, H. L. and Levy, H. B. *Nature New Biol.*, **231**, 53 (1971).
180. Walder, B. K., Robertson, M. R. and Jeremy, D. *Lancet*, **2**, 1282 (1971).
180a. Hoover, R. and Fraumeni, J. F. *Lancet*, **ll**, 55 (1973).
181. Hellström, I., Hellström, K. E., Sjögren, H. O. and Warner, G. A. *Int. J. Cancer*, **8**, 185 (1971).
182. Hilleman, M. R. in, *Viruses, Nucleic Acids and Cancer*, p. 580, Williams and Wilkins, Baltimore (1963).
183. Glass, A. G., Mantel, N., Gunz, F. W. and Spears, G. F. S. *J. Nat. Cancer Inst.*, **47**, 329 (1971).
184. Kessler, I. I. and Lilienfeld, A. M. *Advances Cancer Res.*, **12**, 225 (1969).
185. Burkitt, D. *Br. J. Surg.*, **46**, 218 (1958).
186. Burkitt, D. In *Viruses, Nucleic Acids and Cancer*, p. 615 Williams and Wilkins, Baltimore (1963).
187. Burkitt, D. P. *J. Nat. Cancer Inst.*, **42**, 19 (1969).
187a. Burkitt, D. P., and Wright, D. H. *Burkitts Lymphoma*, E. and S. Livingstone, Edinburgh and London (1970).
188. Epstein, M. A., Henle, G., Achong, B. G. and Barr, Y. M. *J. exp. Med.* 121, 761 (1965).
189. Public Health Laboratory Report. *Brit. med. J.*, **4**, 643 (1971).
190. Henle, G. and Henle, W. *J. Bact.*, **91**, 1248 (1966).
191. Pereira, M. S., Blake, J. M. and Macrae, A. D. *Brit. med. J.*, **4**, 526 (1969).

192. Niederman, J. C., Evans, A. S., Subrahmanyan, L. and McCallum, R. W. *New Eng. J. med.*, **282,** 361 (1970).
193. Klein, G., Clifford, P., Klein, E., Smith, R. T. Minowada, J. Kovrilsky, F. M. and Burchenal, J. H. *J. Nat. Cancer Inst.,* **39,** 1027 (1967).
194. Klein, E., Bollettino dell' *Instituto Sicroterapico Milanese*, **50,** 140 (1971).
195. Henle, W., Henle, G., HO, H. C., Burtin, P., Cachin, Y., Clifford, P., de Schryver, A., de The, G., Diehl, V. and Klein, G. *J. Nat. Cancer Inst.*, **44,** 225 (1970).
196. Gerber, P., Whang-peng, J. and Monroe, J. H. *Proc. natn. Acad. Sci.* (*U.S.A.*), **63,** 740 (1969).
197. Kafuko, G. W. and Burkitt, D. P. *Int. J. Cancer*, **6,** 1 (1970).
198. Pike. M. C., Morrow, R. H., Kisuule, A. and Mafigiri, J. *Brit. J. Preventive Med.*, **24,** 39 (1970).
199. Wedderburn, N. *Lancet*, **2,** p. 1114 (1970).
200. Johansson, B., Klein, G., Henle, G., Henle, W. *Int. J. Cancer*, **6,** 450 (1970).
201. Levin , P. H., Ablashi, D. V., Berard, C. W., Carbone, P. P. Waggoner, D. E. and Malan, L. Cancer 27, 416 (1971).
201a. Goldman, J. M. and Aisenberg, A. C. *Cancer*, **26,** 327 (1970).
202. Hirshaut, Y., Glade, P., Vieira, L. O. B. D., Ainbender, E., Dvorak, B., and Siltzbach, L. E. *New Eng. J. Med.*, **283,** 502.
203. Wahren, B., Carlens, E., Espmark, H., Lundbeck, S., Lofgren, S., Madar, E., Henle, G. and Henle, W. *J. Nat. Cancer Inst.*, **47,** 747 (1971).
204. Evans, A. S., Rothfield, N. F. and Niederman, J. C. *Lancet*, **1,** 167 (1971).
205. Josey, W. E., Nahmias, A. J., Naib, Z. H., Utley, P. M., McKenzie, and Coleman, M. T. *Amer. J. Obstet & Gynec.*, **96,** 493 (1966).
206. Nahmias, A. J., Naib, Z. H., Josey, W. E. and Clepper, A. C. *Obstet. & Gynecol.*, **29,** 395 (1967).
207. Dowdle, W. R., Nahmias, A. J., Harwell, R. W., and Paul, F. P. *J. Immunol.*, **99,** 974 (1967).
208. Plummer, G. *Brit. J. exp. Path.*, **45,** 135 (1964).
209. Schneweis, K. E. *Z. Immunitätsforsch*, **124,** 24 (1962).
210. Rawls, W. E., Tompkins, W. A. F. and Melnick, J. L. *Amer. J. Epid.*, **89,** 547 (1969).
211. Sprecher-Goldberger, S., Thiry, L., Cattoor, J. P., Hooghe, R. and Pastiau, J. *Lancet*, **3,** 266 (1970),
212. Nahmias, A. J., Josey, W. E., Naib, Z. M., Luce, C. F. and Duffey, A. *Amer. J. Epidem*, **91,** 547 (1970).
213. Royston, I. and Aurelian, L. *Amer. J. Epidem.*, **91,** 531 (1970).
214. Catalano, L. W. and Johnson, L. D. *J. Amer. Med. Ass.*, **217,** 447 (1971).
215. Rowson, K. E. K. and Jones H. M. In *Oncogenis and herpestype viruses*, Ed. Biggs, P. J., de-Thé, G. and Payne, L. M. IARC Scientific Publications No. 2 Lyon (1972).
216. London, W. T., Catalano, L. W., Nahmias, A. J., Fucillo, D. A. and Sever, J. L. *Obstet. Gynec.* **37,** 501 (1971).
217. Nahmias, A. J., Naib, Z. M., Josey, W. E., Murphy, F. A. and Luce, C. D. *Proc. Soc. exp. Biol. Med.*, **134,** 1065 (1970).
218. Duff, R. and Rapp, F. *J. Virol.*, **8,** 469 (1971).
219. Duff, R. and Rapp, F. *Nature New Biol.*, **233,** 48 (1971).
220. Aurelian, L., Royston, I. and Davis, H. J. *J. Nat. Cancer Inst.*, **45,** 455 (1970).
221. Nahmias, A. J. *Perspectives in Virology*, **7,** 73
222. Moore, D. H., Sarkar, N. H., Kelly, C. E., Pillsbury, N. and Charney, J. *Texas Rep. Biol. Med.*, **27,** 1027 (1969).

223. Moore, D. H., Charney, J. Kramarsky, B., Lasforgues, E. Y., Sarkar, N. H., Brennan, M. J., Burrows, J. H., Sirsat, S. M., Paymaster, J. C. and Vaidya, A. B. *Nature*, **229,** 611 (1971).
224. Schlom, J., Spiegelman, S. and Moore, D. *Nature*, **231,** 97 (1971).
225. Axel, R., Schlom, J. and Spiegelman, S. *Nature*, **235,** 32 (1972).
226. Biggs, P. J., de-Thé, G. and Payne, L. N. *Oncogenesis and Herpesviruses*, Pub. W.H.O. I.A.R.C. Scientific Publications No. 2, Lyons (1972).
227. *Pathology Society Symposium Fed. Proc.*, **31,** 1625 (1972).
228. 'International Symposium on Human Tumors Associated with Herpesviruses', *Cancer Research*, **34,** 1083 ((1974).
228a. Klien, G. *Proc. Nat. Acad. Sci.* (*U.S.A.*), **69,** 1056 (1972).
229. Rapp, F. *J. Nat. Cancer Inst.*, **50,** 825 (1973).
230. Todaro, G. J. and Huebner, R. J. *Proc. Nat. Acd. Scia.* (*U.S.A.*), **69,** 1009 (1972).
231. Rapp, F., Conner, R., Glaser, R. and Duff, R. *J. Virol.*, **9,** 1059 (1972).
232. Glaser, R., Duff, R. G. and Rapp, F. *Cancer Res.*, **32,** 2803 (1972).
233. Collard, W., Thornton, H. and Green, M. *Nature New iBol.*, **243,** 264 (1973).
234. Duff, R., Doller, E. and Rapp, F. *Science*, **180,** 79 (1973).
235. Tarro, G. and Sabin, A. B. *Proc. Nat. Acad. Sci.* (*U.S.A.*), **70,** 1032 (1973).
236. Hollinshead, A. Lee, O. B., McKelway, W., Melnick, J. L. and Rawls, W. E. *Proc. Soc. exp. Biol. Med.*, **141,** 688 (1972).
237. Hollinshead, A. C. and Tarro, G. *Science*, **179,** 698 (1973).
238. Frankel, N., Roizman, B., Cassai, E. and Nahmias, A. *Proc. Nat. Acad. Sci.* (*U.S.A.*), **69,** 3784 (1972). m
239. Darai, G. and Munk, K. *Nature New Biol.*, **241,** 268 (1973).
240. Adam, E., Kaufman, R. H., Melnick, J. L., Levy, A. H. and Rawls, W. E. *Am. J. Epid.*, **96,** 427 (1972).
241. Bentvelzen, P. *Int. Rev. exp. Path.*, **11,** 259 (1972).
242. Sarkar, N. H. and Moore, D. H. *Nature,* **236,** 103 (1972).
243. Chopra, H., Ebert, P., Woodside, N., Kredar, J., Albert, S. and Brennan, M. *Nature New Biol.*, **243,** 159 (1973).
244. Calafat, J. and Hageman, P. C. *Nature*, **242,** 260 (1973)
245. Chopra, H. C. and Oie, H. K. *J. Nat. Cancer Inst.*, **48,** 1059 (1972).
246. Schlom, J., Colcher, D., Spiegelman, S., Gillespie, S., and Gillespie, D. *Science*, **179,** 696 (1973).
247. Müller, M. and Grossmann, H. *Nature New Biol.*, **237,** 116 (1972).
248. Keydar, J., Gilhead, Z., Karby, S. and Harel, E. *Nature New Biol.*, **241,** 49 (1973).
249. Zavada, J. *Nature New Biol.*, **240,** 122 (1972).
250. Zavada, J., Zavadova, Z., Malir, A. and Kocent, A. *Nature New Biol.*, **240,** 124 (1972).
251. McAllister, R. M., Nicolson, J., Gardner, M. B., Rongey, R. W., Rasheed, S., Sarma, P. S., Huebner, R. J., Hatanaka, M., Oroszlan, S., Gilden, R. V., Cabigting, A. and Vernon, L. *Nature*, **235,** 3 (1972).
252. Oroszlan, S., Bova, D., White, M. H., Toni, R., Forman, C., and Gilden, R. V. *Proc. Nat. Acad. Sci.* (*U.S.A.*), **69,** 1211 (1972).
253. Long, C., Sachs, R., Norvell, J., Huebner, V., Hatanaka, M., and Gilden, R. *Nature New Biol.*, **241,** 147 (1973).
254. Ruprecht, R. M., Goodman, N. C. and Spiegelman, S. *Proc. Nat. Acad. Sci.* (*U.S.A.*), **70,** 1437 (1973).
255. Sarngadharan, M. G., Sarin, P. S., Reitz, M. S. and Gallo, R. C. *Nature New Biol.*, **240,** 67 (1972).

256. Baxt, W., Hehlmann, R. and Spiegelman, S. *Nature New Biol.*, **240,** 98 (1972).
256a. Todaro, G. J., and Gallo, R. C. *Nature*, **294,** 206 (1973).
257. Sack, G. H., Narayan, O., Danna, K. J., Weiner, L. P. and Nathans, D. *Virology*, **51,** 345 (1973).
258. Nowinski, R. C., Fleissner, E. and Sarkar, N. H. Perspectives in Virology, Virology, VIII, p. 31 (1973).

Chapter 12

MECHANISMS OF ESCAPE OF ANTIGENIC TUMOURS FROM HOST CONTROL

P. ALEXANDER, Ph.D., D.Sc.
Professor of Radiobiology, Chester Beatty Research Institute, Institute of Cancer Research, London

---

The concept of immunological surveillance—'I am convinced that during development and growth malignant cells arise extremely frequently but that in the majority of people they remain latent due to the protective action of the host. I am also convinced that this natural immunity is not due to the presence of anti-microbial bodies but is determined purely by cellular factors. These may be weakened in the older age groups in which cancer is more prevalent.'

Paul Ehrlich, (1909). From *Collected Papers Vol. II.* p. 561. Editor Sir Henry Dale. Pergamon Press, 1957.

Since the first edition of this book was written there has been a dramatic increase in research into all aspects of tumour immunology. Any comprehensive review of this subject would now require a separate monograph and, in view of the speed with which the subject is advancing, such a summary would rapidly become out of date. I have, therefore, chosen to concentrate on two aspects: (1) the properties of tumour antigens, and (2) the mechanisms whereby an antigenic tumour grows, metastasizes and kills in the face of an active host resistance.

Nature of tumour antigens

TUMOUR ANTIGENS AND TUMOUR-ASSOCIATED MACROMOLECULES

Some introductory comments and definitions concerning the antigens which evoke the host reactions are needed. The term 'tumour antigen' has been used to describe two entirely different classes of macromolecule. In this review we are concerned with those substances present in tumours which the syngeneic or autochthonous host recognizes as foreign and to which it reacts immunologically by producing humoral and cell-mediated responses that are directed specifically against these substances and which can, therefore, be truly called 'tumour-specific antigens'. Such tumour-specific antigens may be present both on the surface as well as in the interior of the tumour cells. In this review we are not concerned with the latter since an antigen which is not on the cell surface cannot provide a target by which immunological host reactions can destroy living tumour cells. On the other hand, an immunological reaction directed against antigens on the cell surface is likely to interfere with the growth of the tumour. Antibodies may bind to the surface and cause complement components to be fixed which lyse the cell membrane; immunologically specific cytotoxic lymphoid cells or macrophages may bind to surface antigens and destroy the tumour cells or inhibit their growth. For this reason such antigens are referred to as 'transplantation-type tumour specific antigens' (TSTAs) since they mimic in a qualitative way the histocompatibility antigens that are responsible for the rejection of foreign tissue grafts.

The same term 'tumour antigen' has also been used to describe tumour-associated macromolecules which are identified and measured by means of an antiserum raised in a foreign species. Such tumour-associated products are not antigenic in the tumour-bearing host and should not, therefore, strictly be called 'tumour antigens'. They certainly cannot form a point of attack for any immunologically-mediated reaction directed against the tumour cells. The misnomer 'tumour antigen' has arisen out of purely operational considerations, since antisera are used for their detection. Tumour-associated products which are not antigenic in the tumour-bearing host are frequently of embryonic or foetal origin—i.e. substances which are present normally during development but which disappear in the adult animal and reappear in the tumour (Alexander, 1972[1]). Such products are extremely useful for diagnostic purposes, since they provide a chemical marker for the presence of tumour. Typical examples are the carcinoembryonic antigen (CEA), found associated with many types of carcinoma, and α-foetoprotein which is associated with primary hepatomas and some teratomas (see Chapter 7). In principle, these tumour-associated embryonic macromolecules do not differ from other tumour products, such as hormones which may be made by the tumour and not by the corresponding normal adult tissue; a familiar example of this type of hormone is choriogonatrophin which, normally present during pregnancy, is synthesized by choriocarcinomas and some teratomas.

ORIGINS OF TRANSPLANTATION TYPE TUMOUR SPECIFIC ANTIGENS

Macromolecules having the properties of TSTAs may also be of embryonic origin and Table 12.1 summarizes the biological properties of different embryonic materials which recur during tumour growth. These have been referred to as oncofoetal antigens (OFAs). Thomson *et al.* (1973)[2] were able to demonstrate the presence of three embryonic components in chemically induced sarcomas in rats: two of these components were not antigenic, the third was antigenic and thus had the properties of a TSTA. In addition, such a chemically-induced sarcoma also contained a TSTA which did not appear to be of embryonic origin (see Table 2). Little progress has been made in identifying the chemical nature or physiological function (e.g. possible enzymatic activities) of TSTAs; but this situation is likely to change quickly now that techniques for the isolation and purification of TSTAs from both animal and human tumours have been developed (cf. Thomson, Steele and Alexander, 1973[3]).

While little is known of the origin of TSTAs in human neoplasms, three quite different types of TSTA can be distinguished in animal tumours on the basis of their origin. These are:

(1) Macromolecules, present at an early stage of embryonic development, which disappear during ontogeny before the immune system has developed; tolerance to such macromolecules is not developed. The control of the genome into malignant cell is less perfect than in normal cells and hitherto 'silent' genes may be switched on and untoward gene products—such as macromolecules only made in early embryonal growth—are produced.

(2) Products coded for by the nucleic acids (RNA or DNA) of oncogenic viruses that caused the tumour. It is not, of course, necessary for such viruses to persist in the cell of the tumour since the genetic information carried by the virus can be incorporated into the genome of the tumour cells.

(3) Macromolecules which appear to be completely novel (i.e. no counterpart being found in embryonic tissues) to the animal in which the tumour has arisen. These may have been produced as the result of a mutation induced by the carcinogenic agents used, but the alternative possibility that they rise by de-repression of 'silent' genes cannot be excluded. The first TSTAs to be unambiguously identified as such belong to this class and were found in chemically-induced sarcomas of mice (Foley, 1953[4]); they have now been demonstrated in all chemically and physically induced neoplasms of

Table 12.1. Classification of cross-reacting antigenic substances in tumours and in foetal (embryonic) tissues

Macromolecules present in tumours and foetus	*Immunogenic in*		*Causes cytotoxic reaction in tumour-bearing host*	*Suggested name*
	heterologous host	*autologous or syngeneic host*		
1. but also found in some normal adult tissues	Yes	No	No	Onco-foetal associated antigen (OFA-associated)
2. absent from all normal adult tissue but occurs late in foetal life and induces tolerance	Yes	No	No	Onco-foetal specific hetero antigen (OFA-specific)
3. adult recognizes as foreign because they only occur in early foetal life or are present in a cryptic form				
(*a*) found in interior of tumour cell	Yes	Yes	No	Onco-foetal specific auto-antigen (OFA-auto)
(*b*) associated with plasma membrane of tumour cell	Yes	Yes	Yes	Onco-foetal transplantation-type antigen (OFA-transplantation)

experimental animals. They are characterized by a great diversity of type and give rise to the antigenic uniqueness of chemically-induced tumours. For example, fifteen sarcomas induced in mice by 3-methylcholanthrene were all shown by transplantation tests to have TSTAs (see *Fig. 1*), yet none of them cross-reacted with each other (Klein and Klein, 1962)[5]. The individuality of the TSTAs of chemically-induced sarcomas is emphasized by an experiment (Globerson and Feldman, 1964[6]) in which two sarcomas were induced at different sites in the same rat by the same chemical carcinogen; both sarcomas were antigenic but their TSTAs did not cross-react with one another. In sharp contrast, all tumours induced by the same virus share common TSTAs (see (2) above), even when produced in different species. Different viruses produce tumours with different TSTAs (Old and Boyse, 1964[7]).

NATURE OF HOST REACTIONS TO TSTAS

TSTAs of types 2 and 3, constitute an effective target for the destruction of tumour cells by immunological defences of the host: antibodies and cytotoxic cells directed against such TSTAs will kill the cells on the surface of which they are found. On the other hand the role of the TSTAs of embryonic origin (e.g. OEA.1; see Table 12.2) is less clear. A variety of *in vitro* tests[2] (Cf.

Table 12.2. (From Thomson and Alexander, 1973[2]). Properties of four different tumour associated antigens found in the membrane of cells from a rat sarcoma (the MC-1 tumour)

Antigen	*Found in*	*Antigenic in syngeneic host*	*Molecular weight*
TSTA	MC-I only and not in embryonic tissue	Yes	40–50,000
OEA I	Many rat sarcomas and in early but not in late embryos	Yes	Unknown
OEA II	Perchloric acid soluble extract of all rat tumours, in embryos and in low concentration in adult tissue	No	40,000
OEA III	Early embryos, all rat tumours and adult skin	No	67–70,000

Thomson and Alexander, 1973, Baldwin *et al.*, 1972[8, 9]) showed that the host mounts both a humoral and cell-mediated response against TSTAs of this type. Moreover, there appears to be considerable cross-reactivity and different tumours appear to have the same TSTAs of embryonic origin. Yet tumours sharing such OFAs do not give rise to detectable cross-immunity—in the type of experiment illustrated in *Fig. 12.1*, for example, resistance induced to subsequent tumour grafts can be induced by TSTAs of Type 3 (as defined above) but not apparently by embryonic TSTAs. Numerous possibilities for the failure of the host reaction to embryonic TSTAs to induce detectable immunity to a subsequent innoculum of tumour cells can be suggested, such as low densities of these antigens on the tumour cell surface or perhaps their ready release from the membranes; but this phenomenon requires more

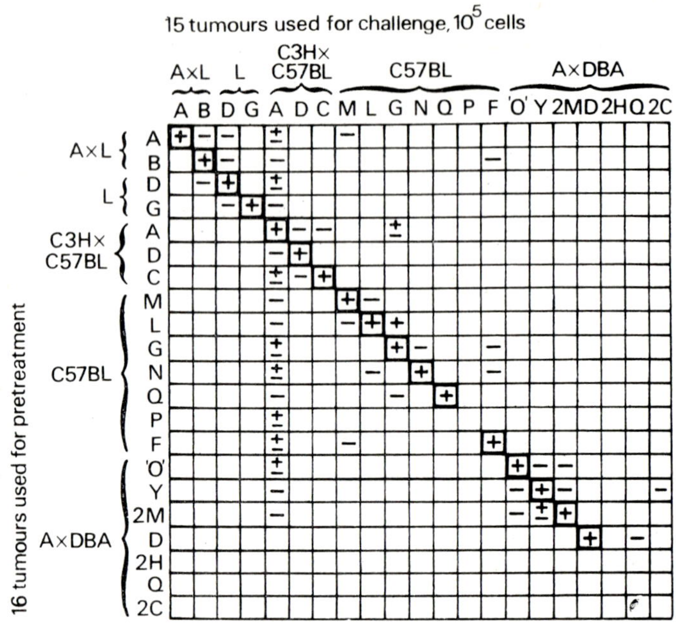

Fig. 12.1. Schematic summary of cross-resistance tests between different methylcholanthrene-induced sarcomas. The + sign indicates the existence of resistance produced by heavily-irradiated cells of the tumours indicated by strain and serial symbols on the ordinate. Each line corresponds to a different tumour. The symbols on the abscissa designate the tumours that have been used for the challenge with viable cells. The—sign indicates a clearcut absence of cross-reactivity while ± corresponds to slight usually expressed in the form of delayed growth curves. The significance of the latter groups is dubious[5].

detailed study since TSTAs of this type appear to predominate in human malignant disease.

TSTAS IN HUMAN TUMOURS

Very much less is known of the TSTAs on the membranes of human tumour cells. Inevitably there is no direct evidence that TSTAs of human tumours can evoke true immunity by inducing the rejection of a second tumour challenge, because the decisive type of experiment illustrated in *Fig. 12.1* can only be made in experimental animals. Evidence for the existence of TSTAs in human tumour cells comes from *in vitro* experiments showing that patients with tumours had circulating antibodies and mononuclear cells which were capable of combining with or killing their own tumour cells cultured *in vitro* (Hellström *et al.*, 1971[9]).

As yet, nothing is known of the origin of the TSTAs detected by these tests. They show a cross-reactivity of a type which has not so far been encountered in animal tumours. For example, the TSTAs of all melanomas appear to cross-react but are distinct from the TSTAs of different types of carcinoma. Carcinoma of different histogenic origins have different TSTA, but those of the same histogenic origin share TSTAs. Thus, all carcinomas of the bladder which have been examined appear to have TSTAs that cross-react, but they are different from the TSTAs of renal carcinomas. This cross-reactivity of TSTAs has a formal similarity with the cross-reactivities of the TSTAs of tumours induced by the same virus in experimental animals. But to sustain this analogy one would have to postulate that a different virus is responsible for all tumours of the same histogenic origin, i.e. that there is one virus that produces all bladder tumours and another virus which produces all kidney tumours and so on. There is no experimental evidence to support such a hypothesis.

It seems more likely that the TSTA of human tumours detected by the *in vitro* tests currently available may reveal an organ-specific embryonic antigen which recurs during carcinogenesis. It is certainly very surprising that TSTAs of type 2 and 3, which induce such powerful immunity in experimental systems have not been found in human tumours. There is as yet no evidence for any tumour individual TSTAs in, for example, bladder carcinomas which one might expect to be chemically-induced. On the other hand, no cross-reactivity has been detected between histogenically different childhood tumours, some of which one might anticipate (by analogy with the animal data) to be induced by the same virus.

The fact remains, however, that most human tumours evoke in the host, when adequately studied, an immune reaction which can be recognized by the presence of lymphoid cells in a specific way. Presumably their activity is directed against a component in the membrane of the tumour cell which appears to be absent from or obscured in the membrane of normal cells of the same host. Antibodies to these membrane determinants have, in general, only been noted in early disease or following surgical removal of the tumour (see later).

Escape from immunological host control

By definition TSTAs are formally related to the normal histocompatibility antigens carried by all cells. In a quantitative sense, however, there is a marked difference. Grafts of normal tissues are almost invariably rejected and transplantation of organs is only possible by prolonged immunosuppression of the recipient. On the other hand, most tumours grow progressively; spontaneous regressions of malignant neoplasms are exceedingly rare. One of the key questions of current cancer research concerns the mechanisms by which cancer cells escape from the immunological defence mechanisms of the host which are so effective in rejecting allogeneic normal tissues.

The first point to stress is that the question of escape is not unique to tumours. It is a phenomenon which characterizes many infectious diseases. Tuberculosis, for example, may progress relentlessly in the face of an active host response and cell mediated immunity to the disease only disappears when the disease is far advanced. Current investigations in the field of tumour immunology and earlier studies from the field of infectious diseases have shown that escape from host defence is a complex process involving many factors.

IMMUNE TOLERANCE AND PARALYSIS

At one time it had been postulated that the success of an antigenic tumour was due to the fact that the tumour-bearing host was unable to mount an effective immune response. In animals with spontaneous tumours it had been alleged that the animals had become truly tolerant to TSTAs. In particular, tolerance was claimed to be established for tumours resulting from the vertical transmission of mouse mammary tumour virus and by the mouse leukaemia viruses. It is now known that the claims that such animals had developed tolerance were due to methodological errors; tumour-bearing animals *do* recognize TSTAs induced by these viruses on the surface of the tumour cells.

It had also been claimed that a reason why antigenic tumours are successful was that the tumour-bearing host was immunologically 'paralysed'. This concept came from clinical studies in which it was found that patients with advanced malignant disease were immunologically anergic and unable to respond to many types of immunological challenge. For example, such patients frequently give little or no tuberculin reaction or failed to react to microbial antigens to which normal people respond powerfully. This anergy, was, however, soon shown to be a consequence of cancer and not a cause of it. If patients with advanced cancer were treated by extensive surgery or aggressive chemotherapy such that their total tumour burden was greatly reduced, they quickly recovered normal immunolgical responsiveness. Again, studies made on patients with early malignant disease revealed that such individuals were not initially anergic but only became so as their disease progressed. Clearly, the hypothesis that escape is due to an inherent failure of the patient to mount a competent immune response is not generally applicable.

ANATOMICAL LIMITATIONS OF THE VARIOUS EFFECTOR ARMS

Anatomical considerations are of great importance when considering escape, because all sites at the body are not equally accessible to the different effector mechanisms of the immune response. It is here that analogy with bacterial diseases is particularly informative. For example, the streptococcus which causes puerperal fever thrives in the post-partum uterus even though these same organisms do not grow elsewhere. The anatomical limitations of the immune response become apparent when the individual effector arms are examined in detail.

(*a*) *Antibodies*

Antibodies are molecules of high molecular weight; and cytotoxic IgM antibodies, in particular, find great difficulty in extravasating from the bloodstream into extracellular spaces. *Fig. 12.2* shows an experiment in which the level of IgM antibodies in a sheep were measured simultaneously in blood and lymph (Hall *et al.*, 1969[10]). It will be seen that the levels in lymph are very much lower than in blood. Not only is the activity of antibody directed to a tumour limited by its relatively low concentration in extracellular fluid, but to gain access to the tumour it has to diffuse from the extracellular fluid into the tumour mass itself. Here again the rate of diffusion of a high molecular

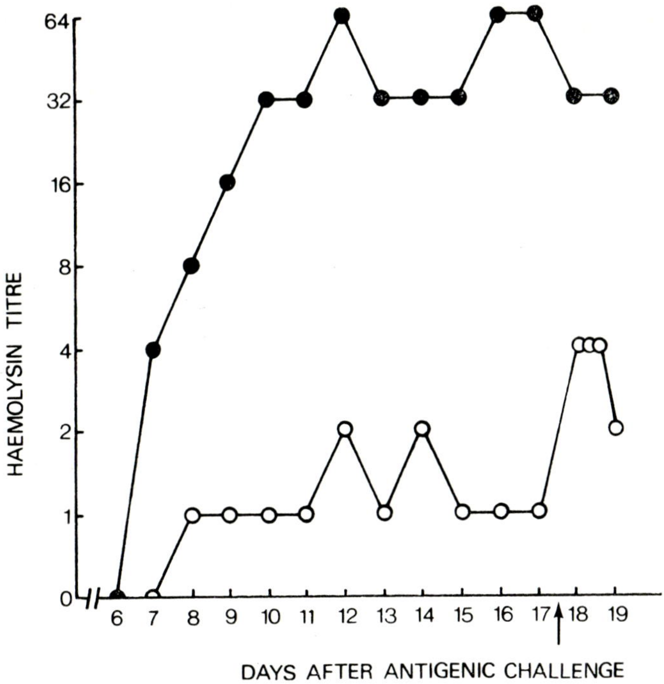

Fig. 12.2. The appearance of mercaptoethanol-sensitive haemolysins in the blood plasma (●) and peripheral lymph (○) of a sheep that had been challenged with goat red cells. The arrow denotes the time at which a solution of fluoro-dinitrobenzene was painted on the leg to induce inflammation in the area drained by the lymphatic fistula[10].

Table 12.3. Effect of immune serum given to DBA/2 mice one day after inoculation with 1000 syngeneic leukaemic cells (L51787)

0.5ml Serum administered intravenously	*Tumour free survivors at 35 days following leukaemic cells given* (*a*) *i.p.*	(*b*) *subcut*
None	0%	0%
From CBA strain mice hyper-immunized with the leukaemic cells which do not grow in this strain	12/15	3/10
From CBA mice hyper immunized with spleen cells from DBA/2 mice	0/10	—
From rats hyper-immunized with leukaemic cells and absorbed with normal spleen cells from DBA/2 mice	8/10	2/10

weight substance will be extremely slow. The effectiveness of antibody to protect the vascular space and the relative ineffectiveness of antibody to protect extravascular sites has been well demonstrated in experiments in which passively injected antibody was used to protect animals against bacterial infection. Following the injection of potent antisera, guinea pigs were well protected when the micro-organism was injected intravenously but were not at all protected if the micro-organism was injected intramuscularly. The same pattern is also seen with tumours. Table 12.3 shows an experiment in which the intravenous injection of an antibody specifically directed against a lymphoma was able to eradicate this lymphoma if it was growing intraperitoneally but had almost no effect if the lymphoma was growing subcutaneously (Alexander, 1967[11]).

(*b*) *Immunoblasts*

By contrast lymphocytes pass readily through capillary walls and gain access to extravascular sites. One of the most effective arms of the cell-mediated response is provided by immunoblasts (Alexander and Hall, 1970[12]). These are pyroninophilic lymphoid cells which are released from the draining node within three to ten days after antigen has reached this node. The immunoblasts can be readily identified in efferent lymph and Table 12.4 and *Fig. 12.3*

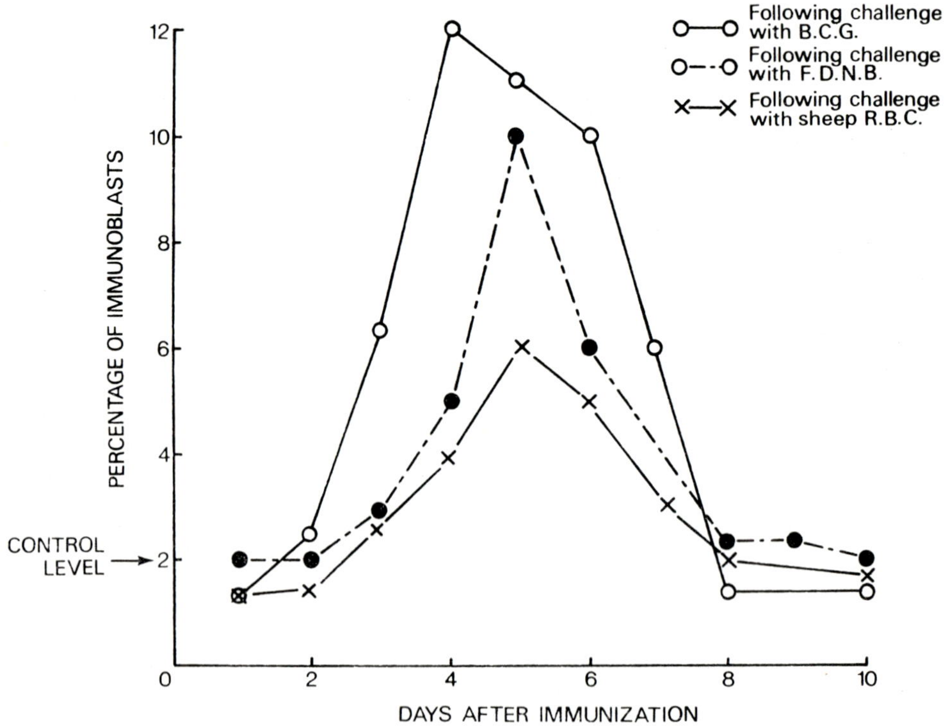

Fig. 12.3. Appearance in rat thoracic duct lymph of immunoblasts following antigenic stimulation. The antigens were injected at multiple sites below the diaphragm[12].

Table 12.4.[12] **Some properties of immunoblasts**

Immunological	*Cytological*	*Physiological*
B-immunoblasts contain and secrete specific antibody Timmunoblasts kill target cells in the absence of complement	They are large lymphoid cells which often display prominent nucleoli, negative Golgi effects, and mitotic figures	Immunoblasts arise in lymph nodes from the transformation of recirculating small lymphocytes; they are discharged into the efferent lymph between 70 and 140 hr after antigenic stimulation
Some of them are capable of transforming into plasma cells *in vivo*	Their cytoplasm is strongly basophilic and pyroninophilic owing to the high concentration of RNA	Because they leave the bloodstream very rapidly, very few of them are present in the blood at any one time.
Following their injection into syngeneic recipients, a high titer of specific antibody appears in the blood	Electron microscopy shows RNA to be in the form of polyribosomes which are not attached to membranes; true endoplasmic reticulum is typically scanty	They do not preferentially enter lymphoid organs as such and for this reason very few recirculate from blood to lymph. They enter the extravasular tissues generally but are particularly numerous in the lamina propria of the gut
They are capable of entering homografts	They incorporate nucleic acid precursors and amino acids with avidity	They are motile cells and when viable they show bizarre, serpentine configurations and pseudopodia

show respectively their cytology and the kinetics of their appearance in the lymph following antigenic stimulation. Immunoblasts formed in response to transplantation antigens and TSTAs are cytotoxic effector cells. There are B- and T- classes of immunoblasts. B-type immunoblasts exert their immunologically specific cytotoxic action mainly through complement binding antibodies present on the surface but also through free antibodies. T-immunoblasts kill by a complement-independent process requiring cell-to-cell contact with immunoblasts derived from T-lymphocytes. Both types of cytotoxic immunoblasts appear at approximately the same time following antigenic stimulation.

The distribution of immunoblasts of both types within the body can be followed relatively easily since many of the immunoblasts leaving lymph nodes in the efferent lymph synthesize DNA and can therefore be labelled with a radioactive marker. Where labelled immunoblasts obtained from lymph are injected into syngeneic animals they rapidly leave the bloodstream and distribute themselves as shown in *Fig. 12.4*. Virtually all of the labelled immunoblasts are eventually localized either to the small gut or to lymphoid organs. (Hall and Smith, 1970[13]). In experiments in which the recipient of labelled immunoblasts bore a tumour, immunoblasts directed specifically against this tumour did not migrate to the tumour but still homed to the small gut and the lymph nodes, spleen and liver (Alexander and Hall, 1970[12]) This predilection of immunoblasts for certain sites in the body constitute a severe anatomical limitation of an immune response directed against the

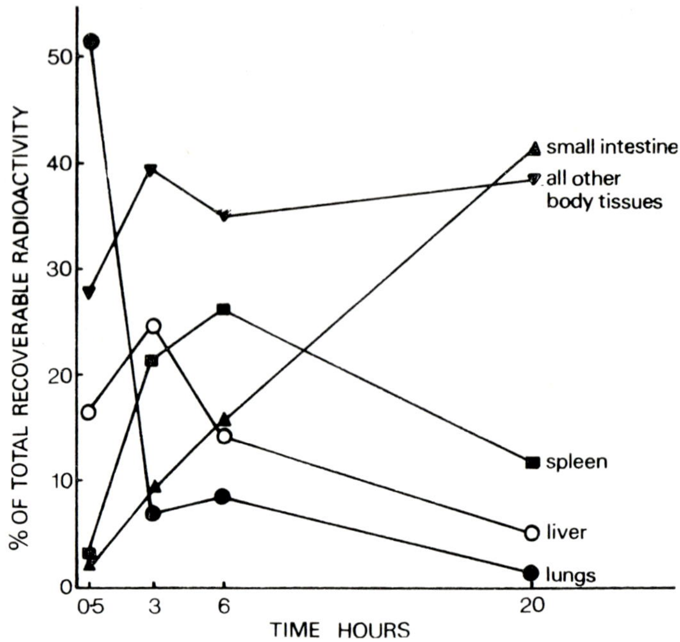

Fig. 12.4. Homing of immunoblasts derived from thoracic duct of stimulated rats to the small intestine. Distribution of radioactivity in syngeneic recipients in the 20 hour period after intravenous injection of[125] I.U.D.R. Labelled thoracic duct cells. Data expressed as % of the total radioactivity recovered.

tumour since immunoblasts formed in response to TSTAs migrate predominantly to other sites in the body. All attempts to divert the traffic of the immunoblasts from the small gut towards the tumour have so far been unsuccessful.

(c) The 'contact activated' lymphoid cells

The lymphoid organs of animals with growing tumours or from animals that had been immunized against the tumour also contain cells, derived from T-lymphocytes, which have the inherent capacity to recognize target cells in an immunologically specific way but which need to be 'contact activated' before they actually kill the target cell (Denham *et al.*, 1970; Alexander *et al.*, 1972[14, 15]). This transformation from a potential to an active cytotoxic cell occurs within a few hours of contact with the specific target cell; it is associated with various changes, the one most easy to measure being an increase in resistance to X-rays (see Tables 12.5, 12.6).

In the early stages of the immune response the immunoblasts are probably the most important cells in lymphoid tissue; later, the 'contact activated' lymphoid cells appear to constitute the major cytotoxic potential in lymph nodes and sphere. These cells, which morphologically are small lymphocytes, do not circulate in blood and lymph and they appear to be sessile in lymphoid organs. They cannot, therefore, contribute to systemic protection but they

Table 12.5. Effector mechanisms of cell mediated immunity

	Persistance after Antigenic stimulus	*Mechanism of cytotoxic action*
(*a*) *Directly cytotoxic lymphoid cells* 1. Antibody secreting immunoblasts 2. Cytotoxic immunoblasts	4–14 days	Specific; Rapid; Do not undergo further transformation on contact with antigen
(*b*) *Contact activated lymphoid cells* 1. Directly cytotoxic 2. Release antigen specific factors which arm macrophages	> 14 days	Specific; Transform on coming into contact with specific antigen and only then become capable of killing or arming.
(*c*) *Monocytes and Macrophages*		Armed by immuno lymphoid cells; Kill relatively slowly by direct contact with target cells. Phagocytosis occurs after cell death.

Table 12.6(a) Properties of directly cytotoxic lymphoid cells

	Antibody secreting immunoblasts	*Cytotoxic immunoblasts*
Radioresistance†	> 10,000r	<1000r
Inhibited by puromycin	Yes	Yes
Complement needed	Yes	No
Supernatant cytotoxic	Yes*	No
Need to be in contact with target	No	Yes
Inhibited by rabbit anti γ globulin	Yes	Yes
Present in spleen	Yes	Yes
thoracic duct lymph	Yes	Yes
thymus	No	No

Table 12.6.(b) Properties of contact activated lymphoid cells

	*Directly cytotoxic**		*Arming of macrophages*†	
	Before contact with antigen	*After contact with antigen*	*Before contact with antigen*	*After contact with antigen*
Radioresistance†	200r	1000r	200r	1000r
Inhibited by anti γ globulin	No	Yes	No	No
Mechanism of kill	lysis by direct contact with target cell		supernatant 'arms' macrophage	
Need for Complement	No		No	
Present in spleen	Yes		Yes	
thymus	No		Yes	
blood and lymph	No		Yes	
Target cells killed	both lymphoma and sarcoma cells			

*Transformation by contact with target cells requires >4 and <8 hours.
†Dose needed to abolish 90 per cent of specific cytotoxicity.

may, of course, be of great importance locally—e.g. in responding to tumour cells newly metastasized to the draining lymph nodes. 'Contact-activated' lymphocytes which 'arm' either cells can be found in the circulation.

(d) Macrophages

Another important effector arm of the immune response is provided by cytotoxic macrophages (cf. Alexander *et al.*, 1972[15]). In animals bearing a subcutaneous tumour macrophages can be found in the peritoneal cavity which kill tumour cells in an immunologically specific way (Alexander *et al.*, 1973[17]). This explains why concomitant immunity is so powerfully expressed in the peritoneal cavity. Thus an animal with a subcutaneous tumour which grows progressively and is lethal if not treated, is able to resist a challenge of tumour cells injected intraperitoneally. Here is a situation where to one anatomical site (the peritoneal cavity) there is a superfluity of effector cells capable of destroying tumour; yet at another site (the subcutaneous tissues), the tumour grows apparently unopposed. Presumably, macrophages in the peritoneal cavity cannot gain access to a tumour growing subcutaneously.

(e) Concomitant immunity

This phenomenon provides one of the most effective means for studying escape mechanisms. It has been known for a long time that tumour-bearing animals are able to reject to some extent a further challenge of tumour cells given at a site distant to the growing tumour (Gershon *et al.*, 1967[16a]). The resistance to challenge of the tumour-bearing animal is generally less than that of an animal that has been deliberately immunized (as in the experiment previously illustrated in *Fig. 12.1*). It has, however, recently become apparent (Alexander *et al.*, 1973[17]) that the expression of concomitant immunity is closely dependent on anatomical site. Thus concomitant immunity may appear relatively weak when the challenge with tumour is made subcutaneously, but very strong when the challenge is given intravenously or intraperitoneally. The phenomenon of concomitant immunity clearly illustrates the importance of anatomical location in relation to the efficiency of the expression of the host immune defences; and it also indicates that escape cannot be attributed to some systemic failure, irrrespective of whether such escape is due to a hypothetical blocking factor (see p 00) or to a generalized paralysis of the host's immune response. The fact that an animal bearing a tumour which grows relentlessly is able to reject tumour cells when injected at a different site, and that the capacity to reject such a second challenge depends on where the tumour cells are given, illustrates the complexity of the escape phenomenon and the need to consider it in relation to anatomical and physiological factors.

(f) Paralysis of draining lymph nodes by overloading with antigen

Antigen introduced into the drainage area of a lymph node leads to the appearance of specific immunoblasts in the efferent lymph. These cells first appear approximately 70 hours after antigenic stimulation and continue for about five or six days, when the production of these cells in the nodes ceases. As shown in *Fig. 12.3*, such an immunoblast response occurs in response to

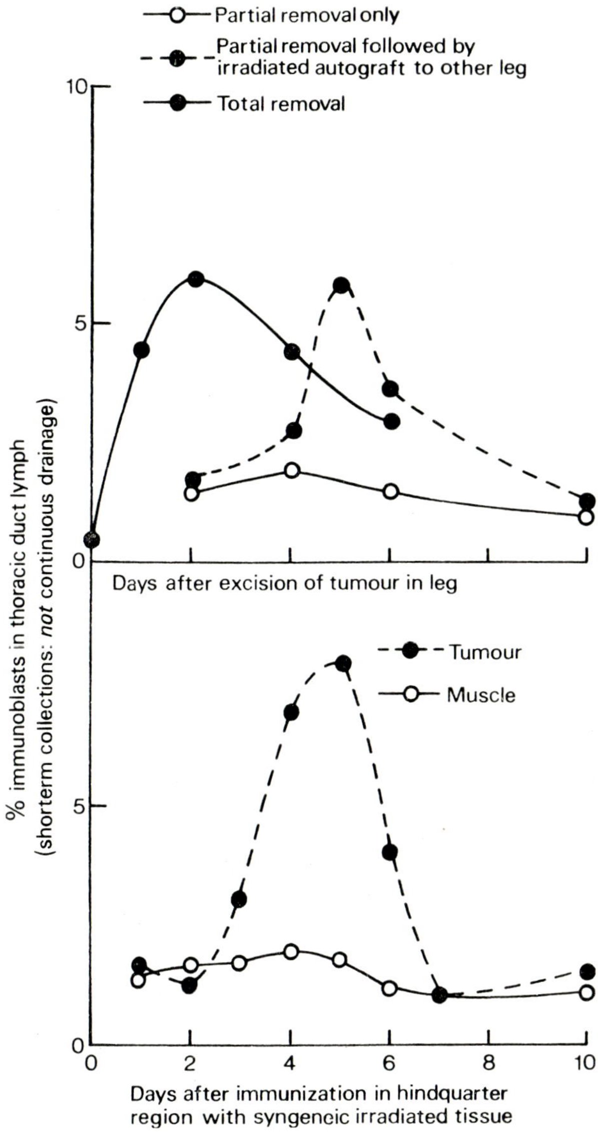

Fig. 12.5. The bottom diagram shows a typical immunoblast response provoked by the tumour-specific antigens of a rat sarcoma which had been rendered non-viable by irradiation prior to being used for immunization. Animals with a growing sarcoma do not have anti-tumour immunoblasts in the thoracic duct. The top diagram shows that after total removal—but not after partial removal—immunoblasts rapidly appear. This shows that the 'block' in the immunoblast release is due to the presence of tumour. This block is confined to the draining node because as shown in the top diagram an autograft of tumour placed in the non-tumour-bearing leg gives rise to a typical immunoblast response[18].

every type of antigenic stimulus including that induced by TSTAs following immunization with irradiated syngeneic tumour (see *Fig. 12.5*).

If a graft of living tumour is innoculated instead of irradiated tumour (which does not grow), there is an initial immunoblast response but this does not persist as the tumour grows. Detailed experiments (Alexander *et al.*, 1969[18]) showed that the failure of nodes draining a growing tumour to continue to discharge immunoblasts is due to antigen overload. The node is flooded with TSTA and the immunoblasts directed against the TSTAs remain fixed in the nodes. The overall effect is that antibody production continues normally from plasma cells in the nodes but that dissemination of an important class of effector cells is prevented. This effect is immunologically specific and the nodes draining a tumour respond quite normally to other unrelated antigens. Within 24 hours of surgically removing the tumour the specific paralysis due to excess TSTA disappears and immunoblasts once again leave the node (see *Fig. 12.5*). This type of paralysis clearly constitutes an important escape mechanism for a growing antigenic tumour and may also explain (see below) why immunization at distant sites of a tumour bearing animal may be therapeutically effective: such immunization causes the appearance of immunoblasts directed against TSTA in rats with growing tumours (see *Fig. 12.5*).

Serum factors which facilitate escape

'INHIBITION' VERSUS 'BLOCKING'

Hellström *et al.* (1969)[19] studied the host reaction to tumours in man using an *in vitro* test in which the effect of mononuclear cells from the blood (referred to as 'lymphocytes' though monocytes or monocyte precursors may also have been present) was measured on the patient's own tumour cells *in vitro*. In nearly every case in man and in a few instances also in experimental animals, the authors found that the patients had lymphocytes in their blood which were capable of killing their own tumour cells *in vitro*.

Furthermore, they claimed that if the patient's tumour cells were first exposed to the patient's own serum they were then protected against the cytotoxic action of the peripheral blood lymphocytes. This protective action was referred to as 'blocking' and was attributed to the presence of a special antibody; this antibody bound to the surface of the tumour cells but did not bind complement. Thus, the antibody was not cytotoxic but, by coating the tumour cells, it rendered them inaccessible to the cytotoxic action of circulating lymphoid cells. The Hellströms proposed that this blocking antibody played a predominant role in the escape mechanism of tumours and much speculation was provoked concerning the opposing effects of a *humoral* response to the tumour antigens which, through its blocking activities protected the tumour and a *cell-mediated* response which was cytotoxic and would destroy the tumour. It was, in fact, proposed that a useful therapeutic effect might be achieved by selective suppression of functioning B-cells, which are concerned with antibody production, leaving the T-cell-derived cytotoxic cells intact.

While this hypothesis seemed plausible no evidence was produced that the protective blocking factor in the serum was, indeed, antibody. In many laboratories experiments had been made in which target cells had been deliberately coated with antibody and then exposed to cytotoxic lymphocytes; but in none of these experiments was a protecting (or blocking) effect seen (e.g. Alexander *et al.*, 1966[20]). An exception was provided by the studies of Brunner and Serottini (1968)[21] who found that by adding a very high concentration of serum to the mixture of target cells and cytotoxic lymphocytes a protecting effect of the antibody could be observed. When the Hellströms' group set out to determine the exact nature of the blocking factor in the serum, they subsequently discovered that it was an antibody-antigen complex; pure antibody did not block in their systems (Sjögren *et al.*, 1971[22]).

The need to have an antigen-antibody complex, immediately resolved one of the paradoxes of the Hellströms' original experiments, namely that blocking activity was only found in sera of tumour-bearing hosts and not after the tumour had been removed—this applied both to human and animal situations—yet after tumour removal antibody levels in general were high.

Meanwhile, in our laboratory evidence began to accumulate that tumour-specific antigens are released from the tumour cells into the circulation and that these circulating antigens are capable of interfering with the host's immune reaction (Currie and Basham, 1972[23], Thomson *et al.*, 1973[29]). To avoid confusion a new terminology has to be introduced and this is shown in Table 12.7. The term 'blocking' had been used indiscriminately to describe

Table 12.7.[24] Serum factors which interfere with the destruction in vitro of target cells by immune lymphocytes

	Blocking factor	*Inhibitor*
Definition:	Specifically absorbed from serum by target cells (Hellström *et al.* 1972[25])	Does *not* act on target cells (Currie & Basham 1972[23])
Postulated mode of action:	Combines with target cells and shields these against cell-mediated attack	Combines with 'aggressor cells' and renders them non-cytotoxic
Nature:	(*a*) Non-complement binding antibody (Hellström *et al.* 1969[18]) (*b*) Antibody-antigen complex (Sjögren *et al.* 1971[22])	Soluble tumour-specific antigens

all situations where the addition of serum reduced the cytotoxicity of mononuclear cells to tumours as assayed by *in vitro* tests. We propose that the term 'blocking' is used to describe the situation as defined by Hellström and Hellström (1972)[25] where the serum component is added to the target cells and presumably binds to these because the blocking effect persists after the target cells have been washed. Secondly, we propose that the term 'inhibition' be used where the active serum components interact with the aggressor cells but not with the target cells. In our experiments, both in man and in rats, we failed to find any evidence that blocking as defined above plays a role in the tumour-host relationship. Certainly the appearance of circulating antibody has not accelerated tumour growth or dissemination. Indeed, there is much indirect evidence to indicate that the presence of circulting antibody is a favourable prognostic sign (see 'Effects of autoimmunization' on p. 274). Consequently, we cannot subscribe to the familiar proposition that humoral responses favour tumour growth and that cell-mediated responses tend to suppress it.

CIRCULATING SOLUBLE TSTA IN THE SERUM AND LYMPH OF RATS

In experimental animals with growing syngeneic or autochthonous tumours, antibodies directed against TSTA on the tumour cells can be detected in the serum within a few days after removal of the tumour; but such antibodies are rarely demonstrable while the tumour is *in situ* (Pilch and Riggins 1966, Baldwin and Baker, 1967, Thomson Steele and Alexander, 1973[26–28]). The

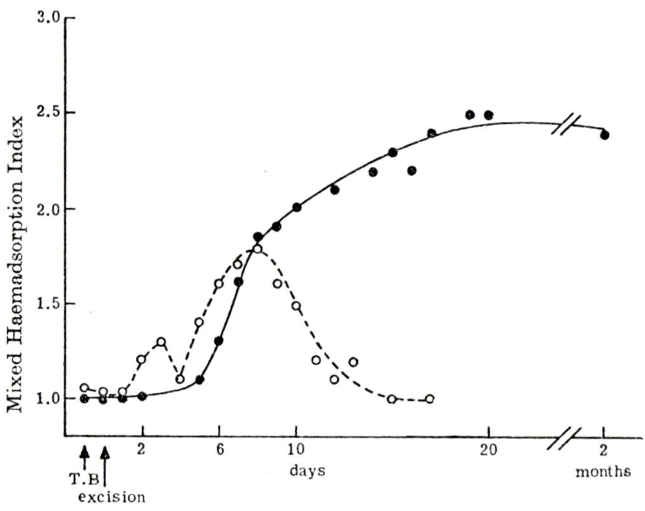

Fig. 12.6. Time sequence of the appearance of anti MC-I tumour-specific antibody in the serum (●———●) and lymph (O———O) of animals after excision of their MC-I sarcoma. Serum and lymph were tested at 1:3·5 and 1:4 dilution respectively by ^{51}Cr-labelled mixed haemadsorption test. Each point represents the average of 3 rats per group on day indicated[23].

explanation that the antibody was absorbed *in vivo* by the tumour was shown not to be an important factor by Thomson Eccles and Alexander (1973)[29] who demonstrated that the level of antibody in the thoracic duct lymph of rats with tumours growing in the leg was also very low and rose after the tumour was excised. The nodes draining such tumours are intensely stimulated and contain many plasma cells, and antibody produced in these nodes must pass through the thoracic duct before entering the blood. Thus the level of antibody in the thoracic duct lymph cannot be influenced by absorption of the antibody by the tumour. However, *Fig. 12.6* shows that in rats with sarcomas the antibody levels in both blood and lymph are very low but both rise sharply after excision of the tumour.

Thomson, Steele and Alexander (1973)[28] therefore set out to test whether TSTA is released by the tumour into the blood and lymph, whether released TSTA combines with circulating antibody, and whether, in the presence of a growing tumour, there is an excess of antigen over antibody in the tissue fluids. Two types of experiments provided direct support for this hypothesis. Anti-TSTA antibodies found in the serum of rats from which the tumour had been excised could be neutralized specifically by serum from rats with a growing tumour. Secondly, increased levels of antigen were found after splitting antigen-antibody complexes in the serum from tumour-bearing animals.

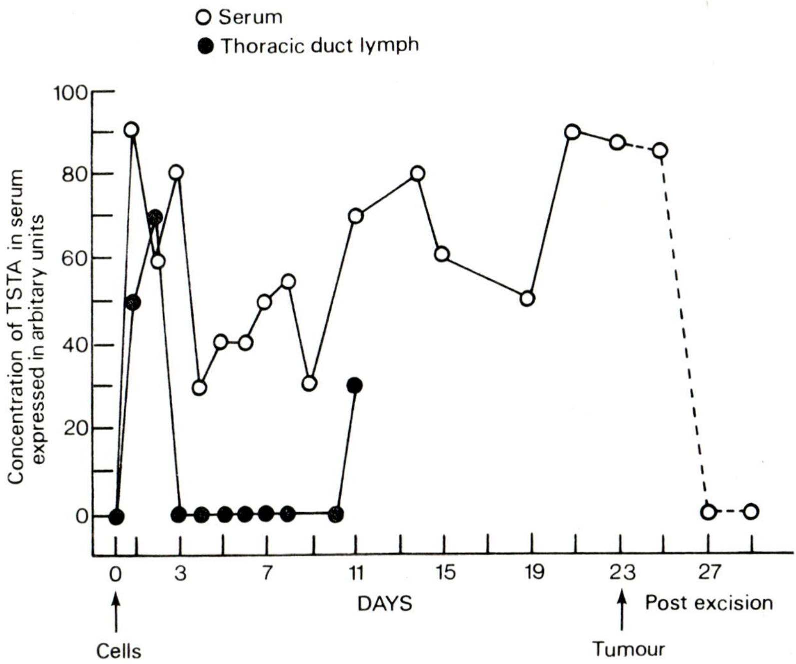

Fig. 12.7. Estimation by radioimmunoassay of TSTA in serum of rats bearing MC-1 sarcoma.[24].

A radioimmunoassay has now been developed which measures the level of circulating TSTA in the serum (Thomson *et al.*, 1973[3]). TSTA was directly purified by affinity chromatography, in which the absorbent was antiserum directed to the TSTA. The radioimmunoassay uses this purified antigen and the antiserum, and was used to measure TSTA in tissue fluids. In rats with a growing sarcoma there are considerable amounts of TSTA in the serum, but these disappear within three days after excision of the tumour (see *Fig. 12.7*).

EVIDENCE FOR SOLUBLE TSTA IN THE SERA OF PATIENTS WITH MALIGNANT MELANOMAS AND CARCINOMAS

Evidence for the presence of such antigens in the serum of cancer patients was obtained from studies in which the capacity of carefully separated blood lymphocytes to destroy tumour cells *in vitro* was measured (Currie and Basham, 1972[23]). Only patients with small localized tumours were found to have blood cells capable of killing cells derived from a tumour of the same

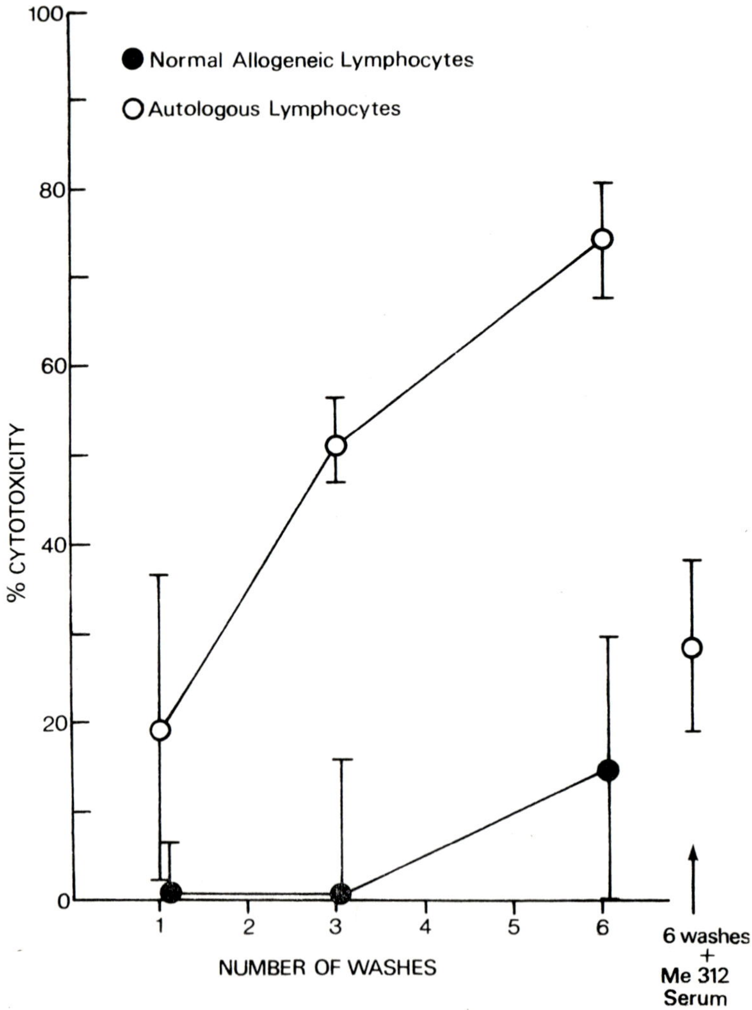

Fig. 12.8. Effect of increasing number of washes on cytotoxicity of lymphocytes from a patient with extensive malignant melanoma tested on his autologous tumour cells (Me 312). The cytotoxic effect increases with washing and this increase is abolished by the addition of autologous serum[23].

histogenic type; patients with advanced malignant disease did not have such cells. However, when the lymphocytes of patients with advanced disease were washed extensively, they showed powerful cytotoxicity towards cells from their own tumour or other tumours of the same origin (see *Fig. 12.8*). Furthermore, the serum from patients with advanced disease inhibited the cytotoxicity of the well-washed autologous lymphocytes; the serum from patients with early disease did not inhibit the cytotoxicity of lymphocytes which was, of course, already manifested prior to washing. The inhibitory factor in the serum has an affinity for the lymphocytes, and pre-treatment of the tumour cells with the inhibitory serum does not protect them against the cytotoxic action of the washed lymphocytes. The available data is consistent with the hypothesis that the inhibitory action is due to antigen, either free or present in excess in a complex with antibodies or other proteins, which combines with the cytotoxic leukocytes and thus pre-empts their reaction with the same antigen on the target cells (cf. Alexander *et al.*, 1973[24]). The inhibitor clearly binds firmly to the lymphocytes since extensive washing is required before they regain cytotoxicity.

The inhibitory activity of the serum of patients with advanced cancer is specific for tumours of the same histogenic type: thus serum from patients with malignant melanoma will inhibit the cytotoxic action of lymphocytes from all melanoma patients but it does not affect the cytotoxicity of lymphocytes from patients with bladder carcinoma which (of course), is in turn directed only against cells derived from bladder carcinomas). Fractionation of sera with immunologically specific inhibitory properties shows that the inhibitor is a molecule of less than 100,000 molecular weight; inhibitory activity can also occasionally be found in fractions of molecular weight higher than 100,000 (Alexander *et al.*, 1973[24]). It would appear, therefore, that both free antigen and some antigen-antibody complexes can inhibit the cytotoxicity of human blood lymphocytes.

Table 12.8.

	Localized disease	*Disseminated disease*
Specifically cytotoxic leukocytes		
(*a*) Before 'washing'	Yes	No
(*b*) After 'washing'	Yes	Yes
Inhibitor in serum	No	Yes
Tumour-specific antibody	Yes	No

The cytotoxic properties of the lymphocytes and the inhibition of this reaction by the patients' serum have now been studied in a large number of patients with early and advanced malignant disease of different types (Currie, 1973[30]). On the basis of the immunological reactions *in vitro* of serum and blood lymphocytes to tumour target cells almost all of the patients studied fall into one or other of the two categories shown in Table 12.8. There is an apparent correlation between the clinical staging of the patients and these laboratory tests. Early disease being associated with Category A and advanced disease with Category B.

MECHANISMS OF THE RELEASE OF TSTAS

Preliminary experiments (Thomson *et al.*, 1973[3,29]) suggest that there are several mechanisms by which the TSTAs of tumour cells reach the circulation as soluble macromolecules. In rats with chemically-induced sarcomas circulating antigen cannot be detected if the rats have been exposed to whole-body irradiation and sufficiently immuno-suppressed so as not to form antibody. This suggests that the release of the TSTAs occurs as a by-product of an immune reaction.

The recent demonstration that antibody does not remain for long periods on the surface of tumour cells maintained in tissue culture, suggests that TSTA may be taken out of the cell membrane by antibody. This mechanism cannot, however, give rise to the excess of TSTA over antibody that is observed in tumour-bearing rats. A precipitous fall in antibody levels is seen in immune animals (i.e. in animals from which the growing tumour has been surgically removed) following the injection of tumour cells which are rejected (see *Fig. 12.9*). This aberration is most readily explained by the release of

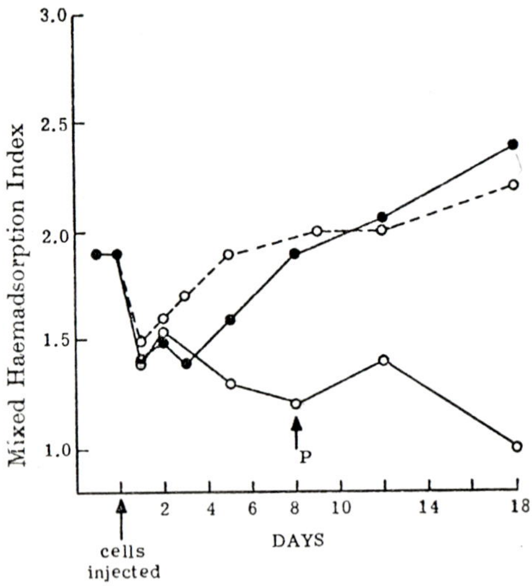

Fig. 12.9. The effect of injecting MC-I cells on the levels of antibody to MC-I in rats that had been immunized by a growing tumour which was excised 14 days earlier. 1 × 10⁶ MC-I cells (O———O), 2 × 10⁷ cells without progressive tumour growth (●———●) and with progressive tumour growth (O———O). 'P' indicates the time when the tumour was first detectable by palpation of the hind limb[29].

soluble antigen into the circulation from tumour cells that have been destroyed at the site of inoculation. In addition, there is a third mechanism for the release of tumour-specific antigen which we have observed in sarcomas which spontaneously metastasize. Such sarcomas give rise to soluble TSTA in the circulation even when immuno-suppressed and also release TSTA spontaneously into the culture fluid when maintained *in vitro* (Thomson *et al,* 1973[3]; Currie and Alexander, 1974[41]).

We conclude that there are at least three mechanisms by which TSTAs are released from the membrane of tumour cells into the circulation; (i) during the course of tumour necrosis; (ii) as a by-product of an immune reaction directed against the tumour; (iii) by spontaneous release from the tumour cells. This third mechanism is not seen with sarcomas which *in vivo* give rise to local tumours and do not metastasize. It may be that tumours which readily release TSTA may metastasize more readily than those which do not produce directly soluble TSTAs in the absence of an immune response of the host or of tumour necrosis.

THE ROLE OF CIRCULATING TSTA IN ESCAPE

Soluble antigen in the serum may not be important in facilitating tumour growth, and the demonstration of soluble TSTA in the serum may merely indicate that the disease has now overwhelmed the immune response. In other words, high levels of circulating TSTA are a consequence but not the cause of advanced malignant disease. We speculate that the biologically important role of soluble TSTAs may be at local sites where they may permit a small number of malignant cells to become established. The release from the tumour cell of soluble antigen may permit locally the escape from immune attack of micro foci of tumour cells, whether they be primary or secondary lesions.

The effect on tumour growth of injecting irradiated tumour cells—therapy or facilitation

The administration of irradiated tumour cells prevented local recurrence of radiation-treated primary sarcomas in rats—but such treatment was ineffectual if a large amount of tumour remained to be treated (Haddow and Alexander, 1964[31]). Similarly, an inoculum of 10^3 lymphoma cells was prevented from growing in mice by a subsequent injection at distant sites of irradiated tumour cells. A possible rationale for this type of 'immunotherapy' is the stimulation of lymphoid tissue distant from the primary tumour since the functioning of the draining nodes is impaired by antigen overload (see p. 264). However, in experiments designed to test if 'active immunization' can affect the growth of distant metastases (Vanwijek, Godrick, Smith, Goldweits and Wilson, 1971[32]; Godrick, Michaelson, Vanwijek and Wilson, 1972[33]) therapy was shown to be dependent upon a precise titration of the number of irradiated cells: If too many cells were injected then metastatic spread was facilitated rather than hindered. With rat tumours which metastasize spontaneously to the lung from a primary implant in the leg, Proctor *et al.* (1973)[34] also found (see Table 12.9) that a high dose of irradiated cells given to these rats increased the incidence of lung metastases. In somewhat related experiments, Vaage (1972)[35] found that injection of irradiated tumour cells into animals that were immune, following surgical excision of a non-metastasizing tumour, lowered the capacity of such animals to reject a second tumour challenge. These

Table 12.9. Effect of immunization with irradiated syngeneic tumour cells on metastatic spread of transplantable hepatomas

Day	0	7 14 21	34	86
	↑ tumour implant in leg	↑ immunization	↑ primary excised	↑ rats killed and autopsied

Tumour used	*Immunization*	*Number of rats with lung metastases*	*Average number of lung metastases per rat*
Late passage high incidence of spontaneous metastases	None (Controls)	8/9	22 (range 0 → 78)
	10^6 irradiated tumour cells	9/10	6 (range 0 → 13)
	10^9 irradiated tumour cells	8/9	34 (range 0 → 121)
Early passage lower incidence of metastases	None	2/5	—
	10^9 irradiated cells	5/5	—

observations indicate that under certain conditions, immune reactivity to the tumour may be impaired by injection of irradiated tumour cells.

That this phenomenon may be caused by the release from the injected cells of soluble TSTA into the circulation is suggested by the experiments shown in *Fig. 12.9* in which the level of circulating antibody to TSTA in immunized rats initially fell after injection of tumour cells. Consequently when considering immunotherapy with irradiated tumour cells one is faced with the possibility that harm could result from raising the level of circulating TSTAs. The hazard is probably small when there is a significant amount of residual tumour which is already contributing a great deal of circulating TSTAs, but it may be serious in situations of minimal residual disease where the level of circulating TSTA is undetectable.

Proctor *et al.* (1973)[34] found that the facilitation of metastatic spread following auto-immunization could be prevented by sumultaneously stimulating the reticulo-endothelial system (RES) with agents such as BCG or *corynebacterium parvum*. The most characteristic biological action of such agents is that they increase the rate at which colloids are removed from the blood. Consequently if administered with RES stimulants, the harmful effects of treatment with irradiated cells may be minimized, and the beneficial effect predominate. Furthermore, the striking reduction in the number of lung metastases which is found if *C. parvum* only is given after surgical removal of the primary implant (Proctor *et al.*, 1973[34])—and the failure of this treatment when given when the original tumour is still *in situ*—can also be interpreted in terms of accelerated clearance of soluble tumour-specific antigens.

DISAPPEARANCE OF SOLUBLE ANTIGEN FROM THE BLOOD FOLLOWING AUTO-IMMUNIZATION

Extensive clinical investigations carried out in our laboratory on patients with malignant melanoma have shown that auto-immunization results in the temporary appearance of circulating antibodies to tumour antigens (Ikonopisov *et al.*, 1970[36]). In patients with advanced disease no circulating antibody to melanoma cells could be detected but, following auto-immunization with at least 10^8 irradiated autologous melanoma cells, antibodies appeared transiently. In such patients auto-immunization also causes the temporary appearance in the blood of lymphocytes that are cytotoxic without excessive washing.

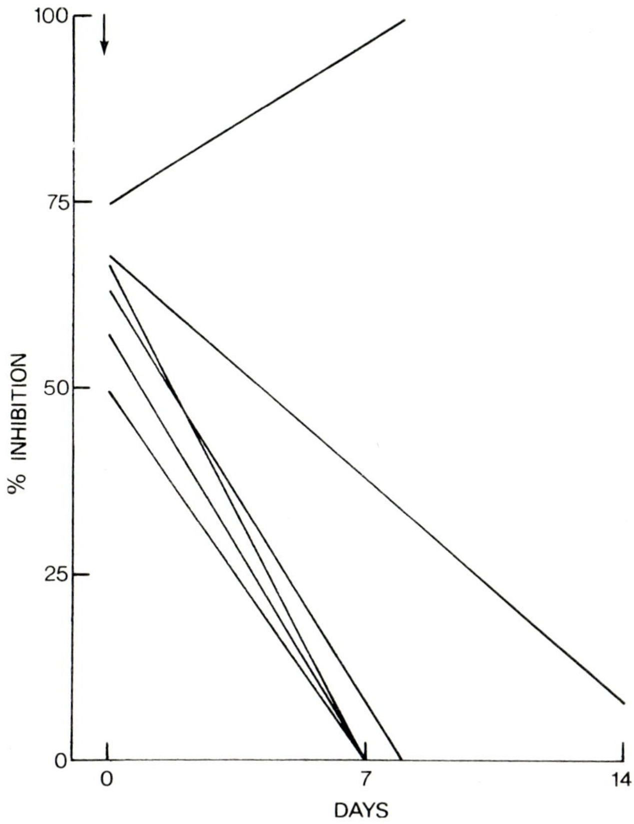

Fig. 12.10. Effect of autografting on the level of inhibitor found in the sera of 5 patients with advanced malignant melanoma and one patient with renal carcinoma. The serum was tested against autologous lymphocytes which had been extensively washed and which were highly cytotoxic to autologous tumour cells. There was an appreciable level of inhibitor present prior to autoimmunization. However, following autoimmunization with irradiated tumour cells the level of the inhibitor decreased in the sera of 5 of the 6 patients tested. For each of the cases reported measurements were made at two times, at Day-0, that is before immunization, and at either Day-7, 8 or 14 as indicated on the diagram (Currie, 1973[39]).

(Currie, Lejeune and Fairley, 1971[37]). An effect of autoimmunization on cell-mediated immunity has also been observed in patients with acute leukaemia (Powles, Blachin, Fairley and Alexander, 1971[38]).

Reference has been made previously to the failure to find antibodies to

TSTAs in patients with advanced disease; these individuals also lack lymphocytes which are cytotoxic without being extensively washed (see Table 12.8. In patients with disseminated cancer the capacity of serum to inhibit cytotoxic lymphocytes frequently disappeared after auto-immunization (see *Fig. 12.10*). It has already been noted that, in our view, the inhibitory action of serum is due to circulating TSTA which combines with the cytotoxic lymphocytes.

The changes in the immunological parameters of patients with advanced disease induced by auto-immunization are summarized in Table 12.10. But

Table 12.10. Effect of auto-immunization with irradiated autologous tumour cells in patients with advanced disease

	Before auto-immunization	*After auto-immunization*
Cytotoxicity of blood lymphocytes		
Before washing	−ve	+ve
After washing	+ve	+ve
Circulating antibody	−ve	+ve
Inhibitor of cytotoxic lymphocytes in serum	+ve	−ve

it must be stressed that in the majority of cases these effects are only transient within a few weeks after immunization the patient reverts to his original status as far as these tests are concerned. The simplest mechanism to explain the effects following auto-immunization with killed tumour cells is that the formation of antibody has been stimulated so that there is a temporary change in the serum from antigen excess to antibody excess. Under these conditions the lymphocytes will be cytotoxic without having to be washed as there is no free TSTA in the circulation.

Depending on conditions, therefore, autoimmunization can cause either an increase or a decrease in circulating TSTA. Whether the therapeutic effects of immunization with irradiated cells that have been observed in animal systems (and possibly in cases of acute leukaemia in man) can be attributed to either reduction of circulating TSTA, or a raised level of immune reactivity—cellular and/or humoral—remains to be established.

This interpretation for the changes that occur following auto-immunization with tumour rests on the following assumption: that although soluble TSTA is capable of combining with the effector arms of the immune response (and thereby neutralizing them), that it is essentially non-immunogenic. To induce an effective immune response the TSTA must be presented in a particulate form (e.g. attached to a plasma membrane). The non-immunogenicity of soluble antigens has frequently been encountered with proteins, and both Wolf (1969)[39] and Baldwin and Glaves (1972)[40] have been unable to immunize rodents to tumours with solubilized preparations isolated from tumour cells; fractions containing membranes were immunogenic.

References

1. Alexander, P. *Nature*, **235,** 137 (1972).
2. Thomson, D. M. P. and Alexander, P. *Br. J. Cancer*, **27,** 35 (1973).
3. Thomson, D. M. P., Sellens, V., Eccles, S. and Alexander, P. *Br. J. Cancer*, **28,** 377 (1973).
4. Foley, E. J. *Cancer Res.*, **13,** 578 (1953).
5. Klein, G. and Klein, E. *Cold Spring Harbor Symp. Quant. Biol.*, **27,** 463 (1962).
6. Globerson, A. and Feldman, M. *J. nat. Cancer Inst.*, **32,** 1229 (1964).
7. Old, L. J. and Boyse, E. A. *Ann Rev. Med.*, **15,** 167 (1964).
8. Baldwin, R. W., Glaves, D., and Pimm, M. In *Progress in Immunology*, publ. Acad. Press, editor Amos, p. 907 (1971).
9. Hellström, I., Hellström, K. E., Sjögren, H. O. and Warner, G. A. *Int. J. Cancer*, **7,** 1 (1971).
10. Hall, J. G., Smith, M. E., Edwards, P. A. and Shooter, K. V. *Immunology*, **16,** 773 (1969).
11. Alexander, P. *Cancer Res.*, **27,** 2521 (1967).
12. Alexander, P. and Hall, J. G. *Adv. Cancer Res.*, **13,** 1 (1970).
13. Hall, J. G. and Smith, M. E. *Nature*, **226,** 262 (1970).
14. Denham, S., Grant, C. K., Hall, J. G. and Alexander, P. *Transplantation*, **9,** 366 (1970).
15. Alexander, P., Evans, R. and Grant, C. *Ann. Inst. Pasteur*, **122,** 645 (1972).
16. Gershon, R. K., Carter, R. L. and Kondo, K. *Nature*, **213,** 674 (1967).
17. Alexander, P., Evans, R. and Mikulska, Z. B. In *Chemotherapy of Cancer Dissemination and Metastasis*, pp. 177–185. Eds. S. Garattini and G. Franchi, Raven Press, New York, 1973.
18. Alexander, P., Bensted, J., Delorme, E. J., Hall, J. G. and Hodgett, J. *Proc. R. Soc.* (*Lond.*), **B174,** 237 (1969).
19. Hellström, I., Hellström, K. E., Evans, C. A., Heppner, G. H., Pierce, G. E. and Yang, J. P. S. *Proc. Nat. Acad. Sci.*, **62,** 362 (1969).
20. Alexander, P., Connell, D. and Mikulska, Z. B. *Cancer Res.*, **26,** 1508 (1966).
21. Brunner, K. T., Maud, J. and Schindler, R. *Nature*, **213,** 1246 (1967).
22. Sjögren, H. O., Hellström, I., Bansal, S. C. and Hellström, K. E. *Proc. Nat. Acad. Sci.*, **68,** 1372 (1971).
23. Currie, G. A. and Basham, C. *Br. J. Cancer*, **26,** 472 (1972).
24. Alexander, P., Currie, G. A. and Thomson, D. M. P. 27th Ann. Symp.—*Fundamental Cancer Res. Univ. of Texas, M. D. Anderson Hospital, publ.* Williams and Wilkins, Baltimore (1973).
25. Hellström, I. and Hellström, K. E. *Nature*, **240,** 471 (1972).
26. Pilch, Y. H. and Riggins, R. S. *Cancer Res.*, **26,** 871 (1966).
27. Baldwin, R. W. and Baker, C. R. *Br. J. Cancer*, **21,** 793 (1967).
28. Thomson, D. M. P., Steele, K. and Alexander, P. *Br. J. Cancer*, **27,** 27 (1973).
29. Thomson, D. M. P., Eccles, S. and Alexander, P. *Br. J. Cancer,* **28,** 6 (1973).
30. Currie, G. A. *Br. J. Cancer*, **28,** 25 (1973).
31. Haddow, A. and Alexander, P. *Lancet*, **i,** 452 (1964).
32. Vanwijek, R. R., Godrick, E. A., Smith, H. G., Goldweitz, J. and Wilson, R. E. *Cancer Res.*, **31,** 1559 (1971).
33. Godrick, E. A., Michaelson, J. S., Vanwijek, R. R. and Wilson, R. E. *Ann. of Surgery*, **176,** 544 (1972).
34. Proctor, J., Rudenstam, C-M. and Alexander, P. *Biomedicine Express*, **19,** 248 (1973).
35. Vaage, J. *Cancer Res.*, **32,** 193 (1972).

36. Ikonopisov, R. L., Lewis, M. G., Hunter-Craig, I. D., Bodenham, D. C., Phillips, T. M., Cooling, C. I., Proctor, J., Hamilton Fairley, G. and Alexander, P. *Brit. Med. J.*, **2,** 752 (1970).
37. Currie, G. A., Lejeune F. and Hamilton Fairley, G. *Brit. Med. J.*, **2,** 305 (1971).
38. Powles, R. L., Balchin, L., Hamilton Fairley, G. and Alexander, P. *Brit. Med. J.*, **1,** 486 (1971).
39. Wolf, A. *Transplantation*, **7,** 49 (1969).
40. Baldwin, R. W. and Glaves, D. *Clin. Exp. Immunology*, **11,** 51 (1972).
41. Currie, G. A. and Alexander, P. *Br. J. Cancer*, **29,** 72 (1974).

Chapter 13

CHEMOTHERAPY OF CANCER

J. A. STOCK, Ph.D., F.R.I.C.

Senior Lecturer, Department of Chemistry, Chester Beatty Research Institute, Institute of Cancer Research, London

---

The search for chemical means of eradicating cancer has been long, sporadic and, until the middle of this century, almost fruitless. About twenty-five years ago, activity in the field began to grow and in a few years reached a high level which has been sustained ever since. Various agents have now been produced that are strikingly successful in the treatment of a few kinds of human malignancy (Table 13.1). In addition, more effective ways of administering

Table 13.1. Agents generally accepted as clinically effective[1]

Alkylating agents	*Anti-metabolites*	*Antibiotics*	*Plant products*	*Hormones*	*Miscellaneous*
BCNU	6-Azauridine triacetate	Actinomycin D	Vinblastine	*Adrenocorticoids*	L-Asparaginase
Busulphan	Cytosine arabinoside	Adriamycin	Vincristine	Cortisone	o, p^1-DDD
CCNU	5-Flourouracil	Daunorubicin		Hydrocortisone	DIC
Chlorambucil	6-Mercaptopurine	Mithramycin		Prednisolone	Hydroxyurea
Cyclophosphamide	Methotrexate	Streptonigrin		Prednisone	Procarbazine
Degranol	6-Thioguanine	Streptozotocin		*Androgens*	
Dibromomannitol (DBM)				Fluoxymesterone	
Melphalan				Testosterone	
Merophan				*Oestrogens*	
Nitrogen mustard (HN2)				Diethylstilboestrol	
Sarcolysine				Ethinyl oestradiol	
Thiotepa				*Other*	
Trenimon				ACTH	
Triethylenemelamine (TEM)				Progesterone	

[1]Based on official National Cancer Institute list (Wood, 1971)[1].

cytotoxic drugs have been introduced and some of the major chemotherapeutic advances seen in the last ten years have been in the use of multiple drugs—combination chemotherapy. It is also true to add that the most dramatic and encouraging episode in recent years has been the success of chemotherapy—with no particular dose regimens—against Burkitt's lymphoma, a disease occurring mainly among children in certain areas of tropical Africa where it is the commonest form of childhood cancer. Surgical excision of tumour masses used to be performed in this disease but with little success; radiotherapy is not available in most parts of tropical Africa and its value is in any event limited because of the disseminated nature of the malignancy. But this gloomy picture has now changed enormously: treatment with a cytotoxic drug—merophan, for example—usually causes prompt regressions which may be prolonged or even permanent (Burkitt, 1970[2]; Clifford, 1970[3]).

Choriocarcinoma, a tumour of the trophoblast, was almost invariably fatal in the past. This rare disease can now usually be eliminated by intensive chemotherapy (Bagshawe, 1969[4]), and it was indeed 'the first of the regularly metastasizing lethal cancers to be rationally and predictably curable' (Park, 1971[5]).

It is arguable that in these two types of tumours the therapeutic success may reflect a rather special immunological situation (Klein, 1970[6]; Bagshawe, 1969[4]); but this does not alter the fact that they may be cured by the use of chemical agents alone.

Chemotherapy is now the generally preferred form of treatment in the leukaemias, and it is an alternative to radiotherapy in Hodgkin's disease and other lymphomas. A number of other malignancies are susceptible to chemotherapy. It has been estimated that 10 to 15 per cent of all cancer in the United States responds well to this form of treatment, and that about half of the treated patients in this group can expect to live a normal life span (Zubrod, 1972[7]).

Nevertheless, for the great bulk of cancers—gastrointestinal, bronchial, mammary—surgery is commonly the primary method of attack, with radiation as a fairly frequent alternative. Chemotherapy is sometimes used as an adjunct, or occasionally as primary treatment, in a proportion of cases. Both surgery and radiotherapy have obvious limitations and neither can be used in disseminated disease, and it is here that chemotherapy may have its greatest potential, despite the serious limitations seen in the agents in current use. Various experimental and clinical aspects of cancer chemotherapy are discussed in a recent multi-author review (Elderbout *et al.*, 1971[8]).

Problems in cancer chemotherapy

DRUG SPECIFICITY

The first major problem is to find agents selective against cancer. This difficulty is hardly surprising because neoplastic diseases, whatever their causes, arise from normal tissues and remain very much like them in many ways. One is not attacking a pathogen having some clear qualitative and exploitable biochemical difference from the host cells. It is to be hoped that much more selective agents will be found, but with the exception of hormonal agents which are relatively non-toxic, drugs available at the present time for cancer treatment are highly toxic. Most of them affect DNA synthesis or DNA function (*Fig. 13.1*). There has, however, been a considerable improvement in the efficacy of these agents, particularly in the acute leukaemias, by using them in combination—a manoeuvre which enables the clinician to achieve a greater degree of specificity. Specificity only within a tissue type may be inadequate.

For example, an agent might be developed which destroyed lung cancer cells without harming normal lung tissue. This would be a very considerable achievement; but if the drug damaged the bone marrow or intestinal mucosa—tissues which are very sensitive to our present range of cytotoxic agents—its clinical potential would be undermined.

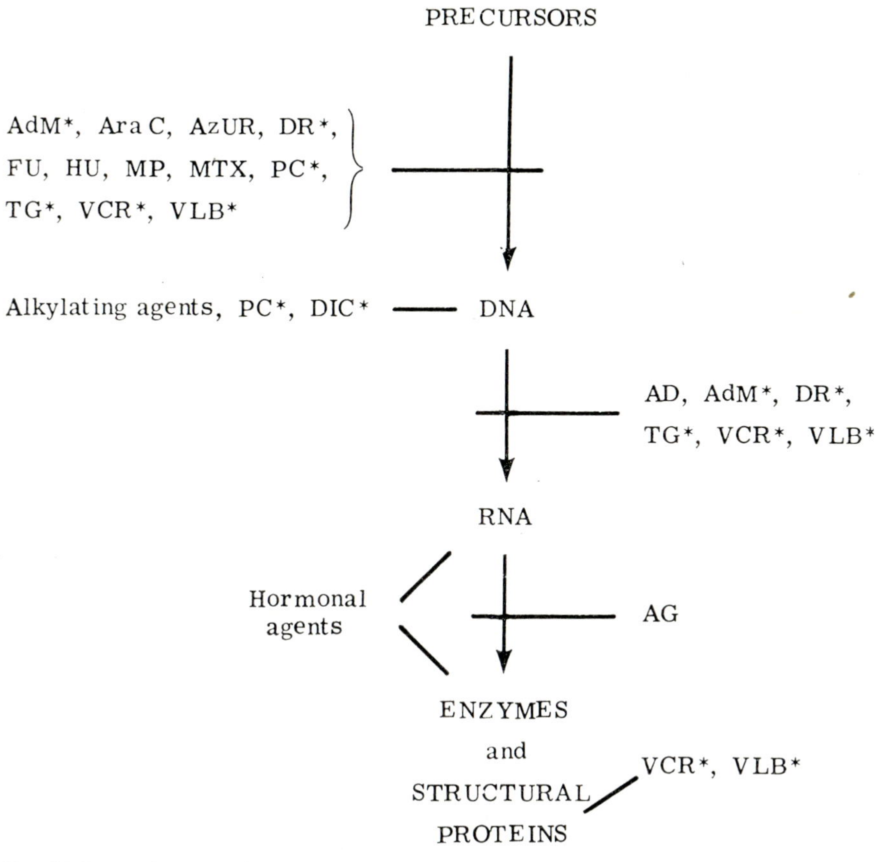

Fig. 13.1. Probable major significant biochemical sites of action of antitumour agents. AdM—adriamycin; AG—L-asparaginase; AD—actinomycin D; Ara C—cytosine arabinoside; AzUR—6-azauridine (base or triacetate); DR—daunorubicin; FU—5-fluorouracil; HU—hydroxyurea; MP—6-mercaptopurine; MTX—methotrexate; PC—procarbazine; TG—6-thioguanine; VCR—vincristine; VLB—vinblastine.

*Relative importance of sites of action less well established.

It is perhaps appropriate to raise here the question of tissue-specific chemotherapy, applicable to tumours arising from organs not essential for survival such as pancreas, ovary and prostate (Cobb, 1970)[9]. It is assumed that malignant cells retain certain exploitable characteristics of the tissue of origin. This approach has been used in the treatment of carcinoma of the thyroid, but has not been generally explored.

Other methods have been devised to achieve a greater selectivity of drug action. An example is regional perfusion, explored extensively a decade or more ago (Creech and Krementz, 1961[10]; Garai *et al.*, 1962[11]): some successes were seen but the overall results were not encouraging. Another approach is to use fast-reacting alkylating agents to contain drug action within the tumor area—see p. 298.

DRUG RESISTANCE

Another major difficulty is drug resistance, a common problem in cancer chemotherapy. A tumour may be resistant from the outset. Quite often, however, treatment causes an initial remission lasting weeks or months; but the disease begins to progress again and renewed administration of the original

Table 13.2. Mechanisms of resistance to anti-cancer drugs in mammalian cells

Factors associated with resistance	*Exemplified by*	*References*
1. Reduced uptake of drug	Alkylating agents	Ball, 1969[14]; Wolpert and Ruddon, 1969[15]; Hill *et al.*, 1971[16]; Inaba *et al.*, 1972[17].
	Methotrexate	Blakley, 1969[18]; Ball, 1969[14].
	6-Mercaptopurine	Paterson and Hori, 1962[19].
	Actinomycin D	Kessel and Bosmann, 1970[20].
	Daunorubicin	Riehm and Biedler, 1971[21].
2. Reduced activation of drug	Purine and pyrimidine antagonists[1]	Stock, 1966[22].
3. Increased catabolism of drug	6-Thioguanine	Sartorelli *et al.*, 1958[23].
	Cytosine arabinoside	Steuart and Burke, 1971[24].
	Alkylating agents	Harrap and Hill, 1970[25].
	Actinomycin D[2]	Simard and Cassingena, 1969[26].
4. Increased catabolism of drug metabolite	6-Thioguanine	Bieber and Sartorelli, 1964[27]; Wolpert *et al.*, 1971[28].
5. Increased production of target molecule	Methotrexate	Blakley, 1969[18]; Ball, 1969[14].
	Asparaginase	Canellos and Haskell, 1970[29].
6. Increased intracellular concentration of agent-neutralizing molecules	Alkylating agents[3].	Calcutt and Connors, 1963[30].
7. Reduced sensitivity of target enzyme	5-Fluorouracil[4]	Heidelberger *et al.*, 1960[31].
8. Alternative metabolic pathway or site	6-Thioguanine[5]	LePage, 1971[32].
	Actinomycin D[2]	Simard and Cassingena, 1969[26].
9. Increase in rate of repair of drug-induced lesions	Alkylating agents	Ball, 1969[14].
10. Defect in receptor site	Steroid hormones	Rosenau *et al.*, 1972[33].

[1]Common and best-established effect is reduced conversion of drug to its ribonucleotide; in one case (5-fluorouracil; see Sköld, 1963[21a]), reduced efficiency of uridine kinase observed.
[2]Factor 3 and/or 8 indicated.
[3]Increase in ratio free SH/bound SH.
[4]Thymidylate synthetase.
[5]Reduced ability of resistant cells to use preformed purines; cells therefore more dependent upon *de novo* purine synthesis.

drug is found to be ineffective. The clinician may then turn to agents of another type, but this cycle is likely to be repeated and, in any case, the choice of drugs available is limited. In consequence, an increased understanding of the development of drug resistance and the discovery of ways either of overcoming it or, perhaps, of turning it to therapeutic advantage could contribute markedly to cancer therapy. For example, one way by which tumour cells become resistant to alkylating agents may be through an improved capacity to repair their own agent-damaged DNA. Better therapeutic effects in experimental animals have been reported when substances which inhibit DNA repair mechanisms (e.g. caffeine or chloroquin) were given with the alkylating agent (Gaudin and Yielding 1969[12]; Cohen, 1972[13]). Again, if a tumour cell becomes resistant by enzyme deletion to a drug requiring activation by that enzyme, this commonly means that part of the cell's normal anabolic equipment is deleted or reduced so that collateral sensitivity may arise (Hutchinson, 1963[13a]). An attack on a second biosynthetic pathway may then have a greater effect on the resistant cell than on the corresponding sensitive line since the latter has an extra anabolic option open to it.

These examples are only two of a number of ways in which drug resistance might to some extent be countered. In general, it seems reasonable to assume that a combination of several drugs acting at different biochemical sites is more likely to delay the emergence of resistant cells than a single drug. There is, however, a danger that some combinations can produce antagonisms (see below).

Factors associated with the development of resistance are listed in Table 13.2 and the onset of drug resistance is represented diagrammatically in *Fig. 13.2* (lower section).

DRUG ACCESS

The question of access of drug to tumour is difficult to appraise but there is no doubt that many tumours are poorly vascularized (Willis, 1967[34]). The vascular stroma of tumours was discussed in Chapter 5 and it is merely noted here that penetration of drugs and other materials into a large tumour mass is often limited (Goldacre and Sylven, 1962[35]; Griffiths, 1965[36]).

SCREENING OF ANTI-TUMOUR DRUGS

The problems of selecting anti-tumour agents likely to be of clinical value are formidable. The animal transplantable tumour systems, though far from ideal, have proved practicable and useful and other selection systems are generally less predictive (Connors and Roe (1964)[37]; Rosenoer (1966)[38]). The Drug Research and Development branch of the National Cancer Institute (formerly the Cancer Chemotherapy National Service Centre) now employs mouse leukaemias L1210 and P388 (the latter having recently replaced the Walker rat carcinosarcoma 256) as its major primary screens (Goldin *et al.*, 1971[39]; Zubrod, 1972[7]). At the Chester Beatty Research Institute, the Walker 256 and L1210 tumours have been used for many years. The European Organization for Research and Treatment in Cancer (EORTC) employs the

L1210 and the Ehrlich ascites mouse tumour as primary screens (EORTC Screening Group, 1972[40]) while in the Soviet Union a number of mouse tumours are commonly used (Larionov, 1970)[41]. Other tumour lines may be used as alternatives in primary screening and for more detailed studies.

The animal tumour screens are valuable in selecting agents active against certain kinds of leukaemia. A recent survey indicates that the Walker 256 and P1798 systems are useful for detecting drugs for inducing remissions in acute lymphoblastic leukaemia in children. Agents useful in acute myeloblastic leukaemia can be selected satisfactorily with the L1210 tumour screen (Goldin *et al.,* 1971[39]). It is arguable whether useful agents of a different kind would be revealed in these systems; certainly, L-asparaginase would have been rejected had only these screens been available. For the commoner forms of cancer, it is unfortunately still true to say that there are no reliable screening models: experimentally active agents are assessed empirically. It is, however, becoming possible to test drugs directly against human tumour biopsies growing as xenografts in thymectomized animals treated with antilymphocyte serum (ALS)—a technique that may provide a valuable extension of present methods (Cobb, 1972[42]; Berenbaum and Sheard, 1972[43]; *Lancet* editorial, 1972[44].)

In vitro screens have provided useful preliminary or additional data (Foley and Epstein, 1964[45]; Thayer *et al.,* 1971[46]). They are not regarded as satisfactory susbstitutes for *in vivo* tests at the present time though recent developments may markedly extend their potential (Tanneberger, 1971[47]; Mitchell *et al.,* 1972[48]; Hudson, 1972[49]).

New drugs should receive intensive toxicological and pharmacological assessment (Dixon, 1971[50]; Oliverio, 1971[51]) before they are given to patients in any clinical trials.

DRUGS, SCHEDULES AND CELL KINETICS

The antitumour agents fall into several groups: alkylating agents, antimetabolites, antibiotics, plant products, hormones and miscellaneous compounds. Table 13.1 lists the main substances currently used in clinical practice.

As mentioned earlier, the normal tissues most sensitive to (non-hormonal) anti-tumour agents are bone marrow and intestinal mucosa—sites with a high rate of cell division. Similarly, the malignancies that respond most satisfactorily to chemotherapy tend to be those with a high mitotic rate with doubling times of one to four days; Burkitt's lymphoma, choriocarcinoma, acute lymphoblastic leukaemia, Hodgkin's disease, lymphosarcoma, reticulum cell sarcoma, testicular tumours, Wilms' tumour, Ewing's sarcoma and retinoblastoma (Skipper, 1971[52]; Zubrod, 1972[7]).

It should not, however, be concluded that the response to a given drug is determined solely by the rate of cell proliferation in the tumour. An agent may completely inhibit one kind of experimental tumour and have no effect on another, even though the mitotic activities are closely similar (Ball *et al.,* 1967[53]). It has also been reported that an experimental transplantable osteosarcoma responds well to BCNU*, CCNU and isophosphamide (a

*BCNU is bis-chloroethylnitrosourea, CCNU is chloroethylcyclohexylnitrosourea.

cyclophosphamide analogue) but not to chlorambucil or HN2 and only moderately to melphalan; yet the more effective agents showed relatively little increase in activity *in vivo* against rapidly proliferating, compared to resting, haemopoietic stem cells (Van Putten, 1972).[54] It should be noted that the more effective drugs in this experiment require activation whilst the others do not, and that this fact may have affected the result in some way. Investigations in other laboratories have, however, also shown that in certain circumstances the extent of depression of bone marrow stem cells by nitrogen mustards in rats and mice may not be dependent upon proliferation rate (Dunn, 1972*a*, *b*[55,56]; Blackett and Adams, 1972[56a] see also below). A similar conclusion was reached in work with experimental myelomas (Ogawa *et al.*, 1973[56b]). Two closely related bone marrow cell lines showed different sensitivities towards the sulphonic ester alkylating agent, busulphan, not related to proliferation rate. (Beckett and Millard, 1973[56c]). Furthermore, prolonged therapy with the same agent in experimental animals and in man sometimes damages tissues with a low mitotic activity (Koss, 1969[57]) but this may be because the agent is exceptional (Dunn, 1972*c*[58]). However, despite these various exceptions it is broadly true that the rate at which the cells in a tissue are dividing is directly related to the sensitivity of that tissue to chemotherapeutic agents.

Most of the initial quantitative studies on the effects of agents in tumour cell populations *in vivo* were carried out by Skipper and his colleagues, who used the L1210 ascites tumour in mice. They first showed that the survival time of mice inoculated with this tumour was related logarithmically to the number of cells in the inoculum (Skipper *et al.*, 1964). The survival time of a group of mice thus enabled an estimate to be made of the number of viable tumour cells remaining after drug treatment. The important conclusion was that a given dose of an antimetabolite killed a constant *fraction* of the tumour cells, whatever the *size* of the original inoculum (*Fig. 13.2*). This conclusion was only valid if the initial number of tumour cells was not excessive (i.e. not more than about 10^6 cells per mouse). At the other end of the scale, it was recognized that one leukaemic cell may eventually cause the death of an animal. Most tumour-inhibitory antimetabolites act only on processes concerned in DNA synthesis—that is, they are phase specific. It was therefore reasoned that tumour cells could be completely eliminated only if all of them were exposed to an adequate drug concentration during the sensitive S (synthetic) phase. The effectiveness of the treatment would, however, depend upon the degree of selectivity of drug action. It had already been demonstrated that the value of a drug could be markedly affected by the dosage regimen. For example, large doses of methotrexate given every four days increased the survival time of leukaemic mice much more than smaller daily doses (Goldin *et al.*, 1956[60]). The same was true of weekly, as opposed to daily, treatment with cyclophosphamide (Lane, 1959[61]). An important finding was that these larger, more widely spaced, doses were less toxic than daily doses. In other words, the host recovered between doses more quickly than the tumour regrew.

In the later, quantitative work, groups of multiple doses of the phase-specific agent cytosine arabinoside, given at appropriate intervals to allow recovery of the host, cured leukaemic mice of their disease; the only proviso was that the burden of L1210 cells prior to treatment did not exceed about 10^6 cells per mouse (Skipper *et al.*, 1967)[62]; Kline *et al.*, 1966[63]). In confirmation of the earlier work, the action of other phase-specific agents (methotrexate; 6MP) was also greatly improved by spaced intensive treatment, though cures were not seen in the L1210 system because toxicity to the host was limiting (Skipper, 1971[64]; Straus *et al.*, 1971[65]).

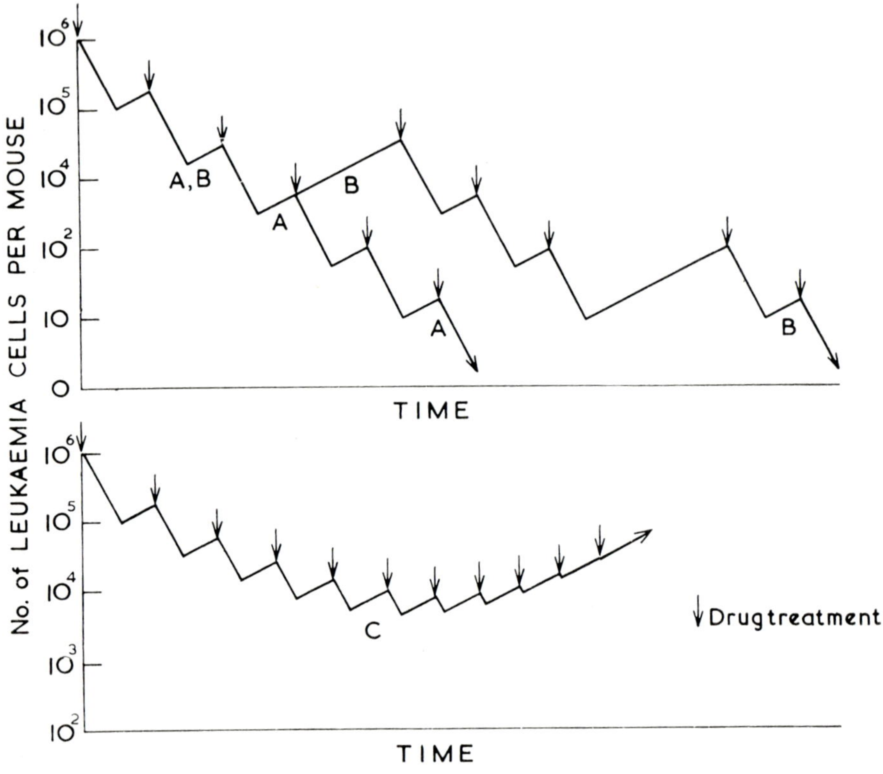

Fig. 13.2 Idealized growth curves of experimental leukaemia in mice treated with multiple doses of a tumour-inhibitory drug.
Curve A: Each successive dose kills constant proportion (90%) of residual viable cells; tumour cured if sufficient doses given.
Curve B: As A, but drug toxicity necessitates breaks in treatment to allow host to recover. Tumour growth occurring during these periods lengthens time required for cure to be achieved.
Curve C: Tumour developing resistance to drug.

A different picture emerges when treatment is delayed so that the number of L1210 cells per mouse rises to 10^7–10^8. Cytosine arabinoside is not curative under these circumstances but, surprisingly, the increase in median survival time is substantially greater with two treatments per day than with eight. Moreover, the more effective schedule used a much smaller total daily dose (Venditti, 1971[66]). Clearly, the response of an advanced tumour to chemotherapy is complex.

In some circumstances, treatment schedules based on the concept of a significant resting (G_0) tumour cell population can lead to cure. An example is the use of successive courses each consisting of a single dose of cyclophosphamide (toxic both to proliferating and G_0 cells, though less toxic to the latter), follosed by two doses of 6-mercaptopurine (toxic only to proliferating cells). The tumour system used here was the established adenocarcinoma 755 in mice; treatment was begun seven days after implant. The alkylating agent was given first in order to reduce the total viable (cycling and non-cyling) cell population so that the remaining G_0 cells would be called into cycle and become sensitive to the antimetabolite (Schabel, 1969[67]).

A study of the relative effects of agents on normal haematopoietic tissue and tumour cells *in vivo* was made by assessing the spleen colony-forming ability of bone marrow stem cells and of AKR lymphoma cells taken from animals which had been treated with the agents (Bruce *et al.,* 1966[68]). This initial work placed agents in three classes (*Fig. 13.3*). In class I belonged agents (only HN2 at first) whose toxic action was independent of cell proliferation rate. Subsequent studies with haematopoietic colony-forming cells in different proliferative states showed that the situation is more complex. (Dunn, 1972*a*, *b*[55,56]; van Putten and Lelieveld, 1971[69]; Valeriote and Tolen, 1972[70]—see also discussion earlier in this section). Whether or not HN2 and other nitrogen mustards fall into class I or class III (see below) depends on the species (mouse or rat), the timing of the assay (i.e. the interval between drug treatment and the removal of cells from the treated animal), and the assay system (colony-forming ability or erythroid repopulating ability). It is probable that all the nitrogen mustards are basically class III (i.e. proliferation-rate dependent) agents, and that class I represents an artificial situation arising from the timing of the assay, in which other factors, perhaps immunological, come into play and modify the response (Dunn, 1972*d*[17]). A fourth class of agents (*Fig. 13.3*), established thus far only for busulphan in rats, is now recognized (Dunn, 1972*c*[58]). Here, bone marrow cells are more resistant when they are proliferating faster as judged by tritiated thymidine cell-suicide curves. Busulphan in the rat is called 'phase resistant', because it appears to be without effect on colony-forming rat bone marrow cells during their S phase. The plateaux seen in class II and IV show that beyond a certain point, an increase of dose does not increase cell kill, reflecting the fact that agents in these groups are effective only during part of the cell cycle. In class II, the plateau levels show that the lymphoma cells are reduced to around 0·05 per cent or less whereas about 20 per cent of the bone marrow colony forming units survive at high doses. In class III the cell kill for both kinds of cells increases with dose throughout the dose range. The much steeper slope in the lymphomadose response curve again reveals a considerable degree of selective toxicity. Normally, the fraction of haematopoietic colony-forming cells in DNA synthesis is very low, but if their numbers are depleted (such as by drug action), the generation time of the remainder shortens, so that they proliferate rapidly to make up the loss (Becker *et al.,* 1965[71a]). The rapid proliferation renders them very much more sensitive to class II and class III drugs (Valeriote and Bruce, 1967[72]; Bruce and Meeker, 1967[73]).

Experimental studies of the kinds discussed above have helped to establish

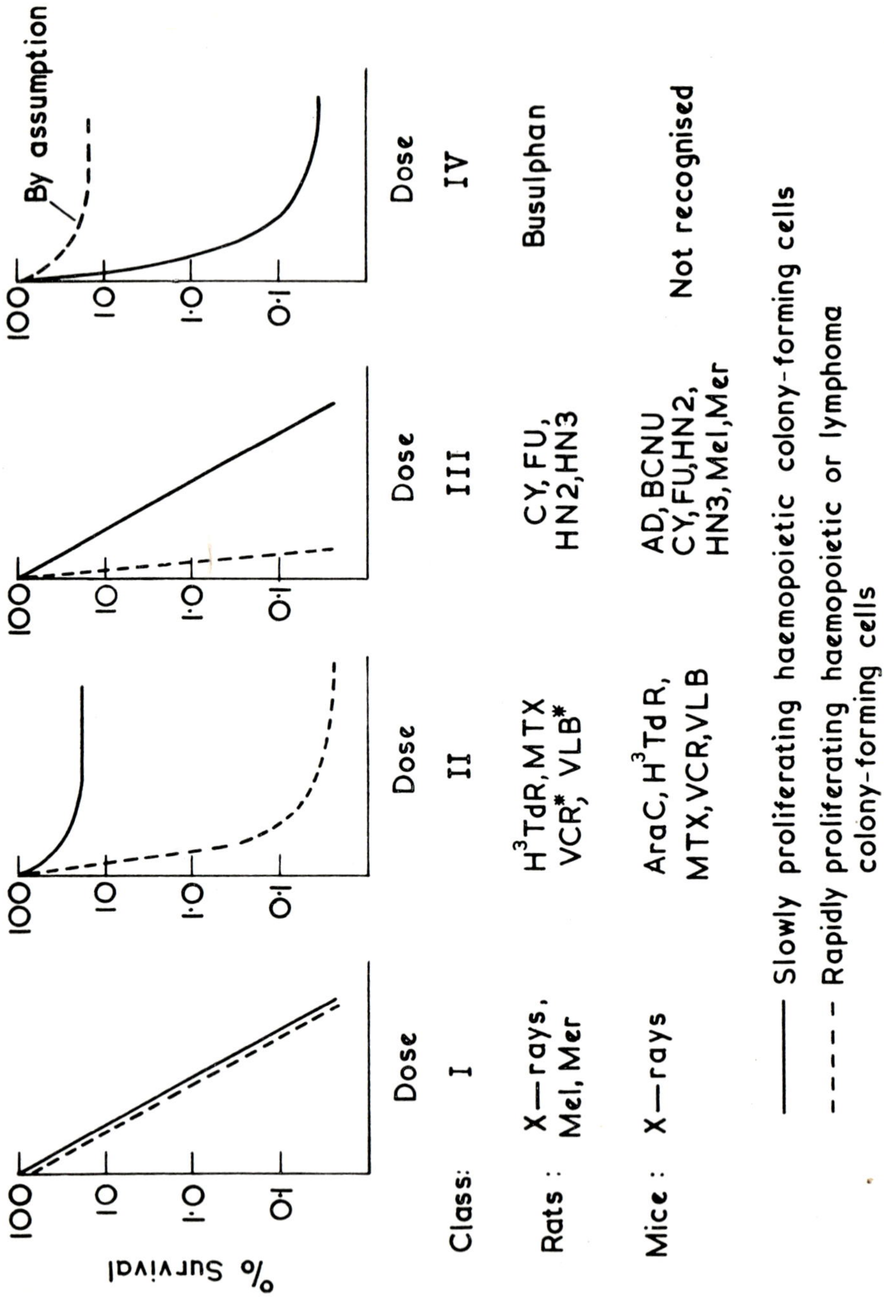

Fig. 13.3. Functional classification of cytotoxic agents. Class I, non-specific; II, phase specific; III, cycle specific; IV, phase resistant. BCNU—bischloroethylnitrosourea; CY—cyclophosphamide; HN2—nitrogen mustard; HN3—trischloroethylamine; H^{3}TdR—tritiated thymidine; Mel—melphalan; Mer—merophan; Other abbreviations as in Fig. 1.

*Probably Class II but CNS toxicity in rats precludes use of doses at plateau level in this species (Dunn, 1972d[71]).

new patterns of drug treatment in clinical cancer, particularly those where repeated intensive courses of therapy are used with intervals to allow haematopoietic recovery. The clinical results with a drug-sensitive tumour sometimes resemble the experimental situation with early leukaemia in mice. For example the dose-response curves in the present-day treatment of choriocarcinoma are reminiscent of those seen with the L1210 mouse leukaemia (cf. *Fig. 13.2*), indicating a contant fractional kill per dose (Bagshawe, 1969[4]).

There are, however, many complicating factors in most human tumours. The effects of cellular crowding, for instance, may lead to a decreasing growth fraction with a higher proportion of cells out of the S phase (cf. Tannock, 1968[74]). Again, the true cell population doubling time is rarely known for human tumours. Even volume doubling times vary widely, from a few days to a year or more. From a study of 175 published cases, the median volume doubling time was assessed at sixty or seventy days (Steel, 1969[75]). Volume doubling time does not necessarily give an indication of the kinetics of the dividing cell population. A tumour may be slow-growing even though the proliferating cells are dividing rapidly, because of extensive cell losses or a large proportion of non-dividing cells. In another tumour, a low growth rate may be due not to a low growth fraction or large cell loss, but to a long cell cycle time (Steel, 1969[75]). Because of such differences, the results of treatment of two superficially similar tumours could be entirely different.

The chemotherapy of human tumours including combination chemotherapy

Table 13.3 lists drugs which have been used with some degree of success against various malignant conditions. The categories that generally respond best are indicated; the table is based on recent reviews on the observed clinical responses to drugs in current use (Livingston and Carter, 1970[76]; Carter, 1971[77]). Although therapy with a single agent is still preferred in some malignancies, the combination of two or more drugs has become common clinical practice during recent years. The general rationale is that a combination of drugs having different biochemical properties may enable the toxic effects to be spread; at the same time (given favourable circumstances) the action against the tumour will be additive or synergistic. An example is the combination of vincristine, whose major toxic effects are neurological, with methotrexate which shows haematological toxicity. The scheme may be roughly regarded as equivalent to giving a bigger dose of antitumour drug safely. Additionally, it is reasonable to suppose that the emergence of drug resistance is likely to be delayed under such circumstances.

Most of the experience in drug combination therapy has been acquired in the field of acute lymphoblastic leukaemia (ALL) in children (Goldin *et al.*, 1971[39]). Careful studies of the induction and subsequent maintenance of remissions have resulted in the development of certain drug combinations and schedules which represent a considerable advance over earlier treatment. Median survival times of children with ALL are now measured in years rather than months (Holland, 1969[82]; Carter, 1971[77]; Goldin *et al.*, 1971[39]; Galton and Spiers, 1971[83]; Henderson and Samaha, 1969[83a]).

The aim of therapy in ALL is to induce a prompt and complete remission,

Table 13.3. Response of human cancers to single agents[1]

Agent	*Neoplasms most likely to respond*
BCNU	Hodgkin's disease; ALL (meningeal); brain
Busulphan	CGL; polycythaemia vera
Chlorambucil	CLL; ovary; Hodgkin's disease; CGL; macroglobulinaemia
Cyclophosphamide	Breast; melanoma; lung; Hodgkin's disease; lymphosarcoma; reticulum cell sarcoma; ALL; AGL; ovary; rhabdomyosarcoma; neuroblastoma; Ewing's sarcoma
Degranol[2]	Hodgkin's disease; CLL
Dibromomannitol	CGL
Melphalan[3]	Multiple myeloma
Merophan	Burkitt's lymphoma
Nitrogen mustard (HN2)	Hodgkin's disease, lymphosarcoma
Sarcolysine[3,4]	Seminoma; multiple myeloma; Ewing's sarcoma
Trenimon[5]	Polycythaemia vera
Cytosine arabinoside	AGL
5-Fluorouracil	Gastro-intestinal tract; breast; pancreas; cervix; uterus
6-Mercaptopurine	ALL
Methotrexate	ALL esp. meningeal; head and neck; choriocarcinoma; breast
Actinomycin D	Testicular tumours; Wilms' tumour; choriocarcinoma; rhabdomyosarcoma
Daunorubicin	ALL, AGL
Streptozotocin	Pancreas
Vinblastine	Hodgkin's disease
Vincristine	ALL; AGL (children); Hodgkin's disease; lymphosarcoma; reticulum cell sarcoma; neuroblastoma; Wilms' tumour; rhabdomyosarcoma; Ewing's sarcoma; retinoblastoma; brain; cervix
Prednisone/prednisolone	ALL; CLL; Hodgkin's disease; lymphosarcoma; breast; multiple myeloma
Androgens	Breast
Oestrogens	Breast; prostate
Progesterone	Uterus
L-Asparaginase	ALL
o, p'-DDD[6]	Adrenal
DIC	Melanoma
Hydroxyurea	Melanoma
Procarbazine	Hodgkin's disease

[1]Based largely on survey by Livingston and Carter (1970)[76]; results of combination therapy are not included.

[2]Kelner *et al.*, (1955)[78].

[3]Melphalan and Sarcolysine are the L and DL isomers respectively of *para*-phenylalanine mustard.

[4]Larionov (1965)[75].

[5]Gerhartz (1964)[80].

[6]Hutter and Kayhoe (1966)[81].

ALL—acute lymphoblastic and undifferentiated leukaemias; AGL—acute granulocytic leukaemia; CLL—chronic lymphocytic leukaemia; CGL—chronic granulocytic leukaemia.

and then to maintain it. An agent useful in the former phase is not necessarily of value in the second.

A combination of prednisone and vincristine is commonly given to induce a rapid remission. Sometimes other agents are also administered in this phasee; a much used combination is POMP [prednisone oncovorin (vincristine), methotrexate and purinethiol (6-mercaptopurine)], often continued to maintain the remission. Methotrexate has usually been employed in recent trials with childhood ALL for maintenance of remission, either alone or in combination with, for example, mercaptopurine and cyclophosphamide. More recently, asparaginase and daunorubicin have been included in some protocols for treating childhood ALL, both in the induction and maintenance phases. In a study with POMP therapy, BCNU is given at the end of a long course of treatment to destroy if possible the remaining leukaemia cells which may be out of cycle (Carter, 1971[77]).

The assessment of the numerous combinations and schedules in use takes years to complete, but progress continues. In one of the best series to date, twenty-six children with ALL were given prednisone and vincristine for induction, then a one-week intensive course of mercaptopurine, methotrexate and cyclophosphamide followed by daily mercaptopurine and weekly methotrexate, cyclophosphamide and vincristine. In addition, the cerebrospinal axis—where leukaemic cells may be present but inaccessible to most systemic drugs—was irradiated (Cobalt-60). The median survival time of the group was thirty-five months, and five of the twenty-six patients were reported as '5-year cures'—i.e. free of all evidence of acute leukaemia for five years (Pinkel, 1971[84]).

Acute granulocytic leukaemia (AGL, comprising myeloblastic, myelomonocytic and monocytic acute leukaemias—see Galton and Spiers, 1971[83]) is more difficult to treat successfully. It is the predominant form of adult leukaemia. Although high remission rates can now be obtained, subsequent relapse rates are equally high (Galton and Spiers, 1971[83]). Cytosine arabinoside is probably the most active drug used singly in the treatment of AGL, but in most current therapy it is used in combination. Currently favoured regimens which are being assessed include: cytosine arabinoside and thioguanine or daunorubicin; cytosine arabinoside, thioguanine and prednisone; cytosine arabinoside, thioguanine and vincristine; COAP [cyclophosphamide, vincristine (oncovorin), cytosine arabinoside (aracine), and prednisone]; 5-component mixtures which go under the name of PRAVDA and POMPA (Carter, 1971[77]; Goldin *et al.*, 1971[39]; Galton and Spiers, 1971[83]; Freireich *et al.*, 1971[85]); and an 8-component mixture, TRAMPCOL (Spiers, 1972[86]). A recent study suggests that daunorubicin alone may be superior to POMP therapy (Wiernick and Serpick, 1972[87]). But, whichever treatment is used the results are far less satisfactory than those regularly obtained in ALL; only about one-fifth of AGL patients survive one year from diagnosis. An initial trial of chemotherapy plus immunotherapy has, however, given greatly improved results (Powles, 1972[88]).

Considerable success has been achieved in Hodgkin's disease with combination chemotherapy. In one study, the use of MOPP (nitrogen mustard, vincristine, procarbazine and prednisone) gave a complete remission rate of 81 per cent, and the median value of unmaintained remission calculated from the end of therapy was over two years (DeVita *et al.,* 1970[89]). The value of MOPP in Hodgkin's disease has been confirmed (Rubens *et al.,* 1972[90]).

Drug combination therapy is now also common in cancer chemotherapy outside the leukaemias and lymphomas. The field is too extensive to review here, but mention may be made of valuable studies being made in the therapy of advanced breast cancer. It appears that combination therapy in this disease can lead to objective responses in over 50 per cent of the patients treated, a better over-all result than hormonal therapy (Carter, 1972[91]).

The clinical assessment of the value of one combination of drugs against another can be arduous. Even experimentally, and with only two drugs, the situation is complex because of such factors as frequency and timing of administration and of relative doses. When five or more drugs are given sequentially, or together, the system almost defies analysis. It is also becoming clear that drug antagonism is to be anticipated (see below). Nevertheless, carefully planned clinical trials can give substantial guidance as to the value of one regimen compared with another.

Patient-isolation procedures (barrier nursing) are often used with intensive drug treatment because the reduction in immunological competence caused by the agents may be of such a degree as to render the patient highly susceptible to fatal infection (Mathé, 1971[92]). Isolation is not, however, universally approved. The patient himself is not pathogen-free and the relative risk of lethal infection is arguable. In addition, hindrance to close contact between doctor or nurse and patient is a disadvantage.

DECREASED HOST TOXICITY WITHOUT LOSS OF TUMOUR INHIBITORY EFFECT

Therapeutic synergism can sometimes be achieved by giving, at an appropriate time, a second substance to reduce toxicity to the host selectively. An example is the use of citrovorum factor (folinic acid), a natural folate metabolite, following methotrexate treatment of leukaemic mice (Goldin *et al.,* 1955[93]). This experimental work was followed by clinical applications of folinic acid rescue (Djerassi, 1967[94]; Mitchell *et al.,* 1968[95]; Hryniuk and Bertino 1969[96]; Goldie *et al.,* 1972[97]).

Another recent experimental example is the administration of isophosphamide in combination with *N*-acetylcysteine to leukaemic (L1210) mice. The host is thereby selectively protected against the toxic effects of the antitumour agent, so that larger doses of the latter can be used; a marked therapeutic advantage was gained (Kline *et al.,* 1972[98]). Similarly the compound ICRF 159 protected mice against the toxicity of daunorubicin but did not reduce the antitumour activity of the antibiotic; with multiple dosage, therapeutic synergism was seen (Woodman *et al.,* 1972[99]; Herman *et al.,* 1972[100]).

DRUG ANTAGONISM AND AUTO-ANTAGONISM

Multiple drug therapy in the clinic has outstripped experimental investigation, and it is therefore important for the clinician to be aware of the possibility of unexpected antagonisms between agents which could negate the value of certain drug combinations. It is true that a less efficacious regimen may eventually be discarded as a result of clinical trials, but the experimental establishment of antagonistic behaviour can indicate which combinations or schedules of drugs are best avoided. Antagonism has been demonstrated *in vitro* and *in vivo* between methotrexate and L-asparaginase, but timing is important (Capizzi *et al.,* 1970[101]; Connors and Jones, 1970[102]). Arabinosyl cytosine also antagonizes methotrexate *in vitro* and *in vivo*; the sequence of drug administration is important here as well (Grindey and Nichol, 1972[103]; Tattersall *et al.,* 1972[104]). The situation is made more complex by tissue differences. For example, necrosis induced in intestinal crypt cells by cytosine arabinoside or HN2 is prevented by the administration of cycloheximide which inhibits protein synthesis. In lymphoid tissue, however, the cylcoheximide enhanced the damaging action of the other agents (Lieberman *et al.,* 1970[105]).

A drug which interrupts more than one biochemical pathway may be less efficient as a result of its own multiple action. Methotrexate provides an illustration of such 'autoantagonism'. This agent kills cells primarily by inhibiting the synthesis of thymidylate from deoxyuridylate during the S phase of the cell cycle. But methotrexate also suppresses *de novo* purine synthesis, and such suppression may *reduce* the killing effect of thymidylate inhibition by preventing the cells from reaching or progressing through the sensitive S phase. The addition of purine ribosides or deoxyribosides to L cells *in vitro* increased the killing effect of methotrexate. It has been proposed that the added purines enable the cells to progress into the S phase of the cycle where they die a 'thymineless death' (Borsa and Whitmore, 1969[106]). [This kind of effect is not, however, always observed. The addition of purines to L5178Y cells *in vitro lessened* the killing action of methotrexate (Hrynink *et al.*, 1969[106a]). This discrepancy may indicate that mechanisms of drug action vary from one system to another (Borsa, 1971[106b])]. Similarly, the compound ICRF 159 is less lethal to a mammalian cell line *in vitro* in certain higher concentrations than in lower, as judged by subsequent plating efficiency. If the drug concentration is high enough, the cells do not progress through the cycle, but enzymic repair may proceed so that a high proportion of the cells can then begin to grow again when transferred to fresh medium. When the drug concentration inhibits DNA synthesis but is inadequate to arrest the cells in cycle, the eventual metabolic imbalance leads to a relatively high cell kill (Creighton, 1972[107]).

IMMUNOTHERAPY AND IMMUNOCHEMOTHERAPY

The ability of tumours to evoke a host response and the possible therapeutic application of this ability are considered in Chapter 12 and in a recent review (Currie, 1972[108]). It may be that the success of chemotherapy against Burkitt's lymphoma and choriocarcinoma is in part due to an effective immunological reaction by the host. Although there is some experimental evidence for this view (Carter *et al.*, 1973; Moore and Whithams, 1973[108a, b]), attempts to utilize or stimulate host immune reactions against tumours in man have been disappointing—the more so because the fruitful harnessing of immunological reactions against tumours could be expected to provide a degree of specificity far beyond that seen with current drugs. There may, however, be a more immediate place for immunotherapy combined with chemotherapy. The administration of heat-killed *Corynebacterium parvum* as a non-specific immunostimulant potentiated the antitumour action of cyclophosphamide in an experimental animal tumour system, but the timing of its administration was vital (Currie and Bagshawe, 1970[109]). Interest in this kind of active immunization stemmed from clinical work in which the combination of BCG (Bacillus Calmette-Guèrin, an attenuated strain of *M. tuberculosis*) with chemotherapy appeared to be advantageous in the treatment of acute lymphoblastic leukaemia (Mathé *et al.,* 1969[110]). It seemed possible that stimulation of the immune system after intensive chemotherapy might result in the destruction of all or nearly all of the relatively few remaining leukaemic cells, with consequent cure or prolonged remission. A subsequent Medical Research Council trial did not, however, confirm that BCG increases the duration of remission when given after multiple drug treatment (MRC Leukaemia Committee and Working Party on Leukaemia in Childhood, 1971[111]). As mentioned earlier, however, treatment of acute granulocytic leukaemia patients with cytotoxic drugs plus immunostimulants was much more effective in terms of median survival times than was chemotherapy alone (Powles, 1972[88]).

The idea of attaching a cytotoxic group to tumour-specific antibodies is not new, but a successful exploitation has recently been reported. The nitrogen mustard drug, chlorambucil, was complexed with antibodies against a human melanoma. Subsequent administration of the complex led to regression of the patient's metastases. The method was also effective experimentally (Ghose *et al.,* 1972[112]).

Notes on chemotherapeutic agents and their mechanisms of action

No attempt will be made here to discuss in detail the chemical, biological and biochemical aspects of antitumour agents. A few review references are given, together with some general comments and a brief consideration of specific areas of current interest. Structures of most of the agents previously listed in Table 13.1 are given in *Figs. 13.4, 13.5* and *13.6*; excluded are ACTH (adrenocorticotrophic hormone) which is a linear polypeptide containing thirty-nine amino acid residues, and L-asparaginase, a protein.

Biological alkylating agents

The alkylating agents have been discussed in detail elsewhere (Ross, 1962[113]; Ochoa and Hirschberg, 1967[114]; Stock, 1971[115]; Connors, 1973[116]). Their antitumour activity depends upon their ability to enter into chemical reaction under physiological conditions.

The great majority of agents in current use fall into four classes: (*a*) *N*-haloethylamines, usually *N*, *N*-di(2-chloroethyl)amines (nitrogen mustards); (*b*) ethyleneimines and ethyleneimides; (*c*) epoxides; (*d*) sulphonic acid esters. The presence of at least two reactive centres in the alkylating molecule is

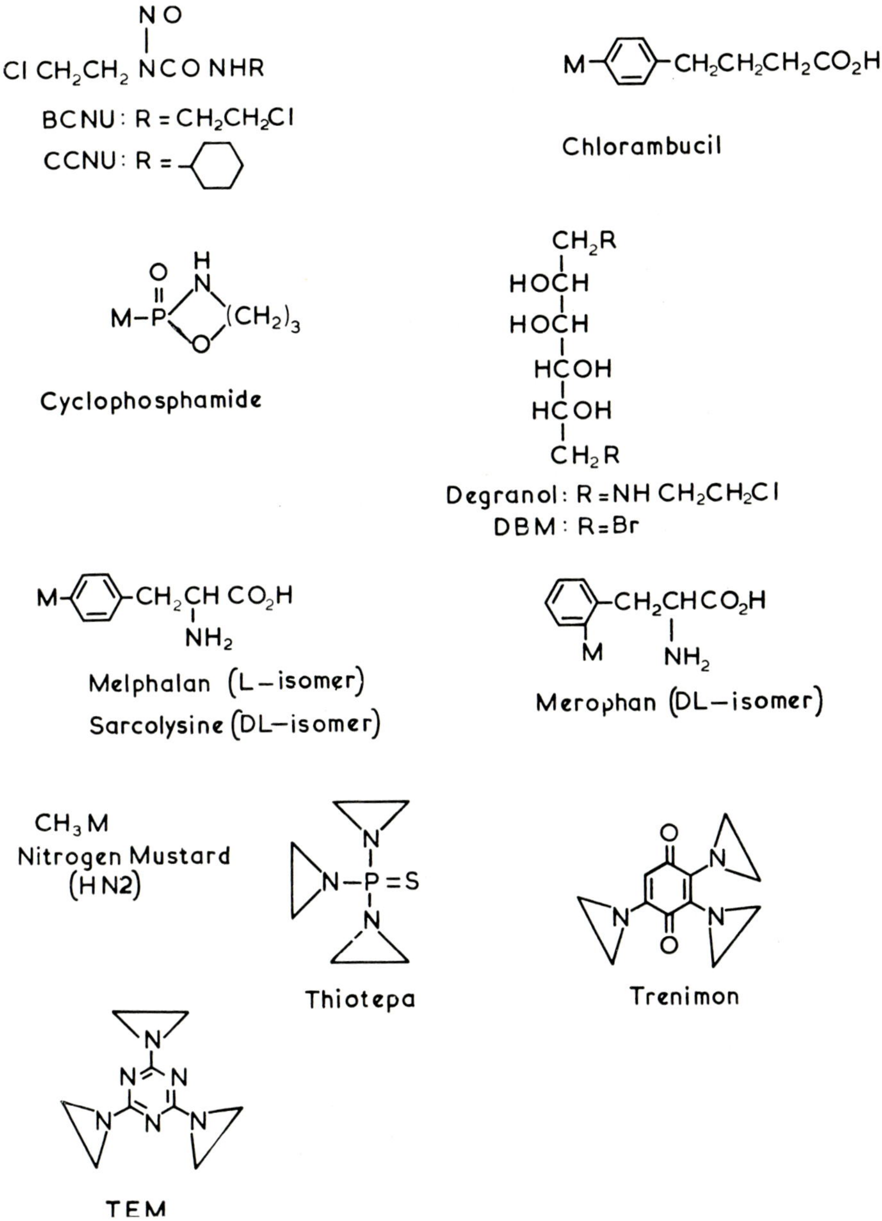

Fig. 13.4. Structures of alkylating agents; M = $(ClCH_2CH_2)_2N$–

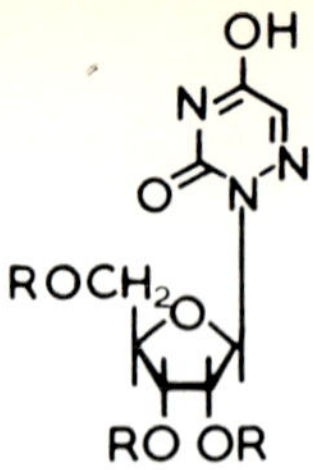

6-Azauridine : R = H

6-Azauridine triacetate : R = CH_3CO

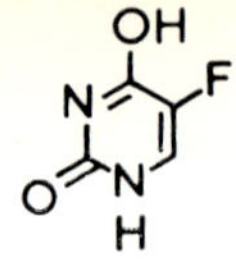

5-Fluorouracil

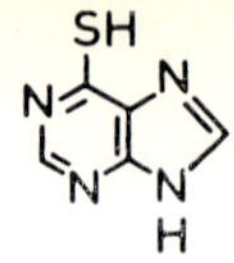

6-Mercaptopurine

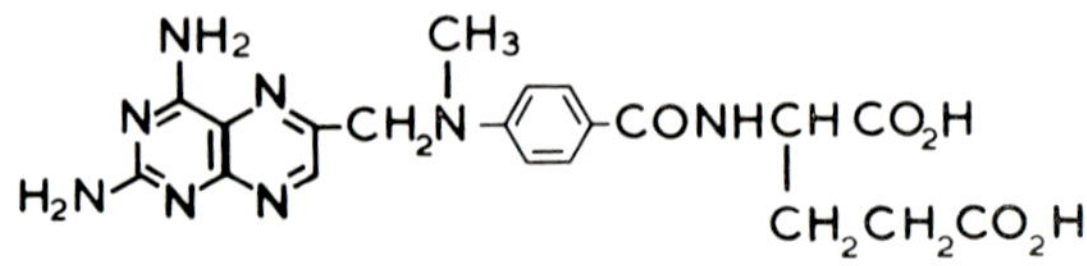

Methotrexate

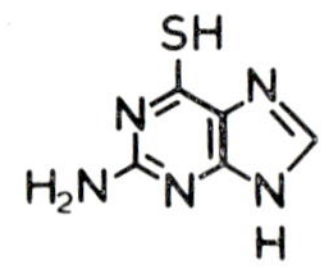

6-Thioguanine

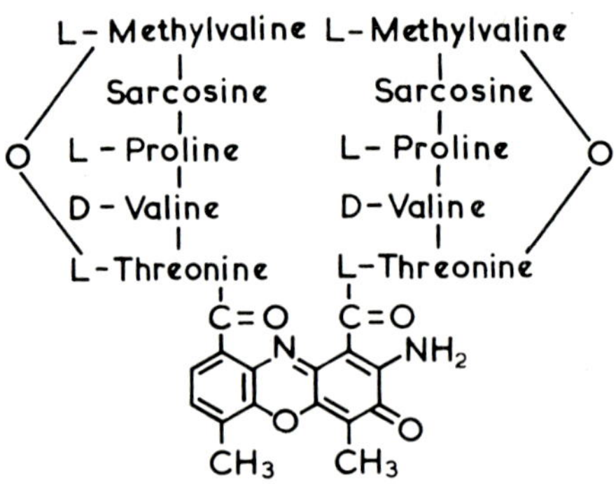

Actinomycin D

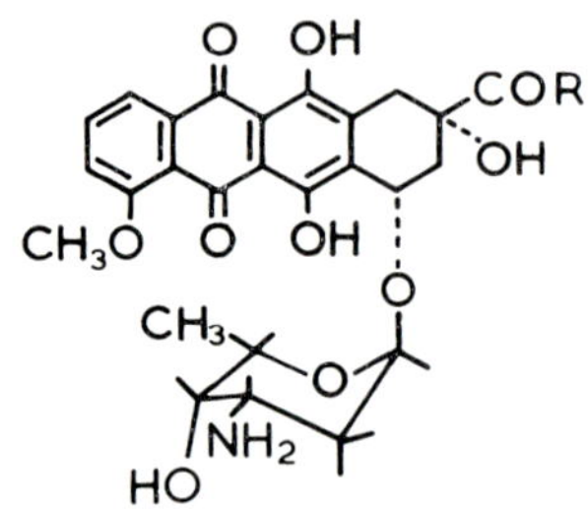

Adriamycin: R = CH_2OH

Daunorubicin: R = CH_3

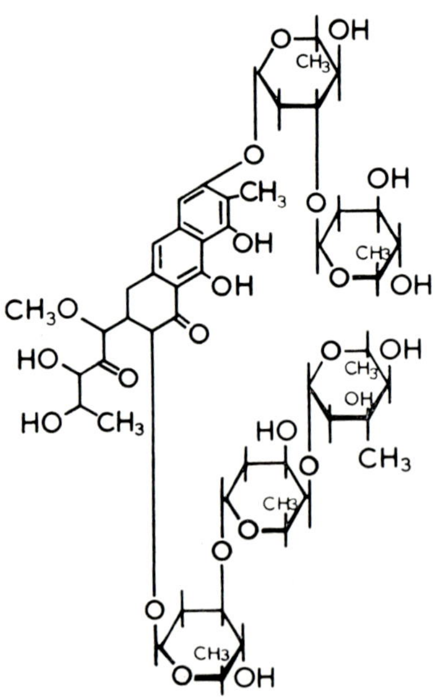

Mithramycin

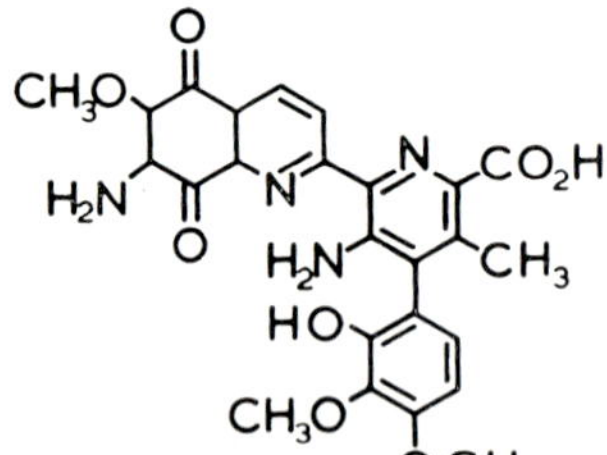

Streptonigrin

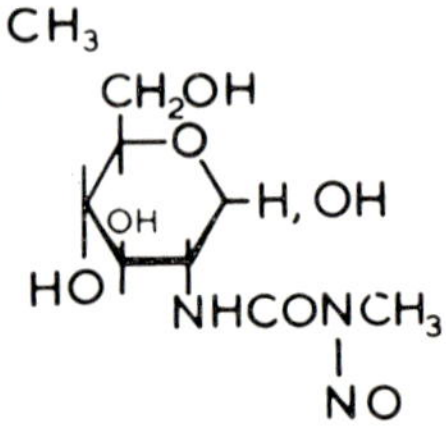

Streptozotocin

Fig. 13.5. Structures of antimetabolites and antibiotics.

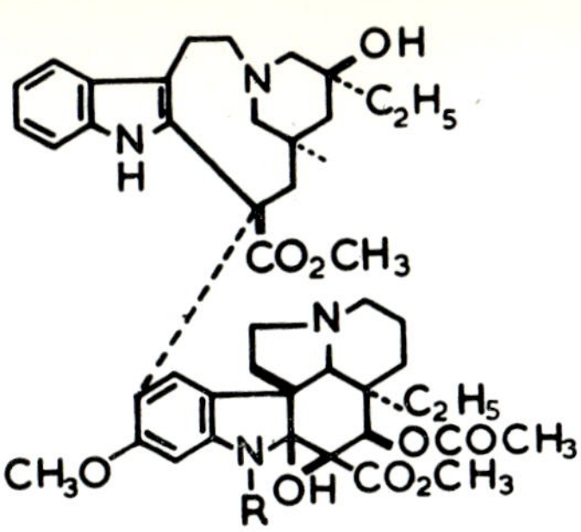

Vinblastine ; R = CH_3

Vincristine ; R = CHO

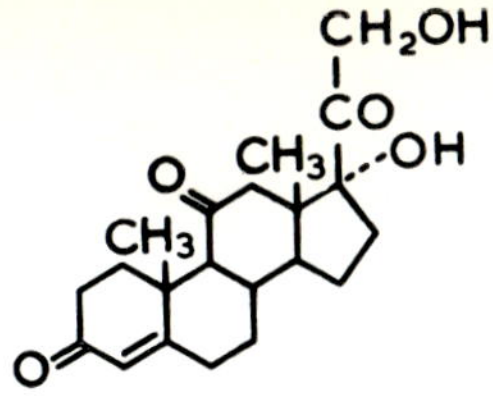

Cortisone

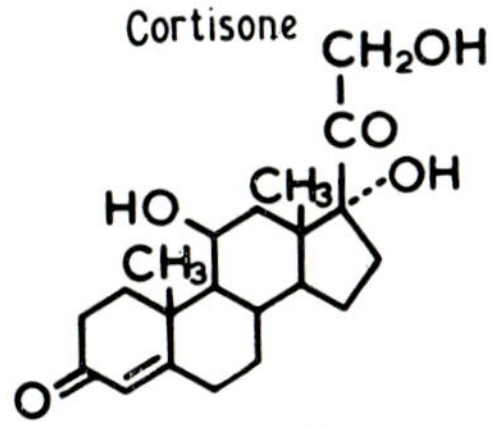

Hydrocortisone

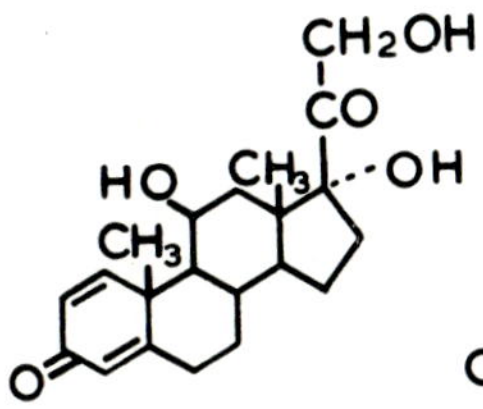

Prednisolone

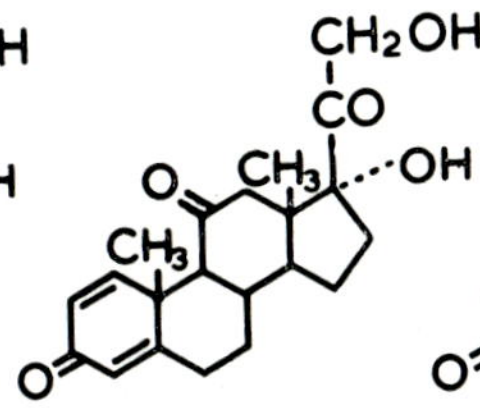

Prednisone

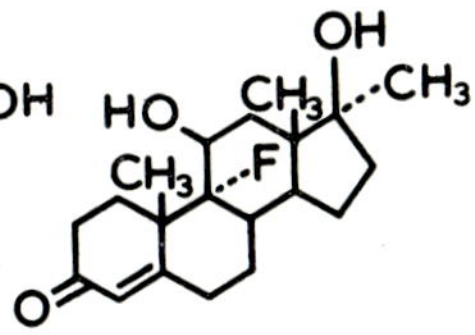

Fluoxymesterone

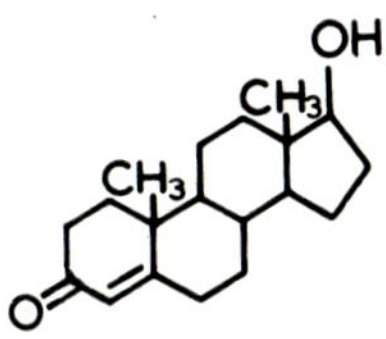

Testosterone

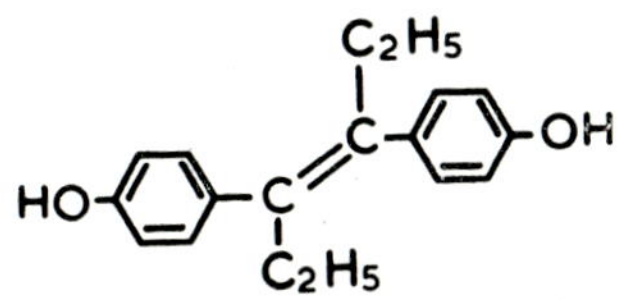

Diethylstilboestrol (stilboestrol)

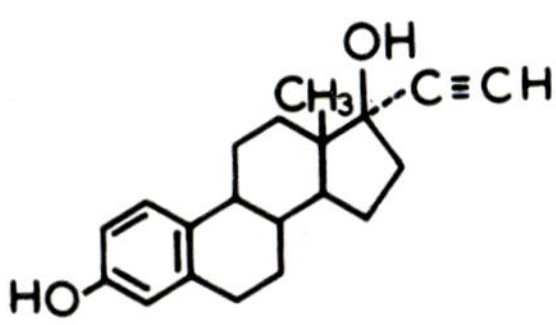

Ethinyl oestradiol

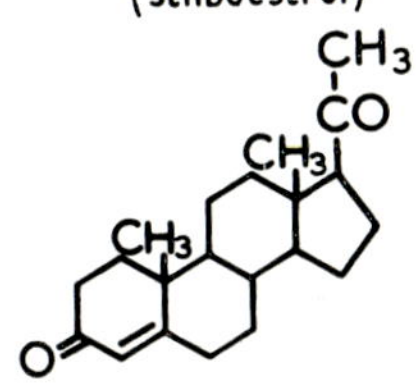

Progesterone

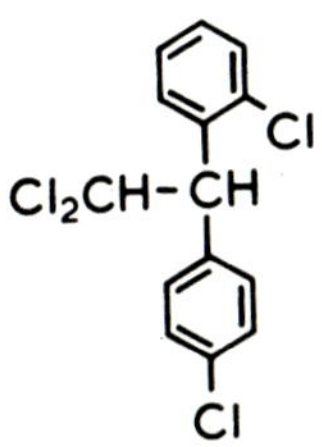

o,p′-DDD

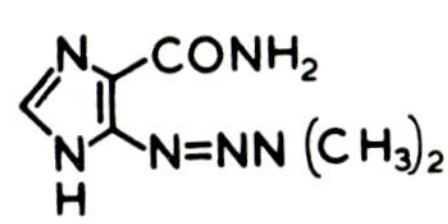

DIC

$H_2NCONHOH$

Hydroxyurea

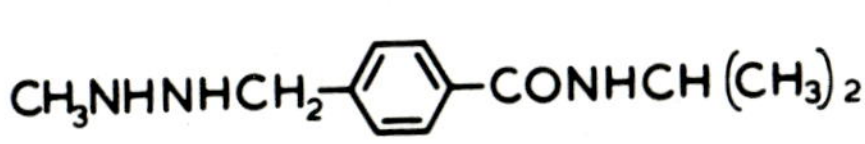

Procarbazine

Fig. 13.6. Structures of the *Vinca* alkaloids, hormones and some miscellaneous compounds

almost invariably necessary for antitumour activity, but there are a few exceptions (Stock, 1971[115]).

The alkylating agents are nucleophiles and are able to attack many kinds of cellular constituents (Ross, 1962[113]). The available evidence suggests that the biologically significant reactions of alkylating agents are those which cross-link nuclear DNA (see Chapter 10). This view is not, however, fully established yet because *in vivo* experiments have not provided a good correlation between the binding of an agent to cellular DNA and the sensitivity of that cell to the alkylating agent, even if repair processes are taken into consideration (Ball, 1969[14]; Connors, 1973[116]).

Whatever may be true for alkylating agents in general, it is likely that the activity of the bis-sulphonic ester, busulphan, results primarily from reaction with substrates other than DNA (Brookes and Lawley, 1965[117]).

Most alkylating agents begin to react immediately they are introduced into the organism, but some require activation. The best example is cyclophosphamide, currently the most widely used alkylating agent. This compound is converted in the liver by a microsomal oxidation process to the active form whose instability has so far obscured its structure (Connors *et al.*, 1972[118]).

Another example of current interest is the azo-bromo mustard (I), belonging to a type first investigated nearly 20 years ago (Ross *et al.*, 1955)[191]. Reduction of compound (I) by azo-reductase in liver or hepatoma cells would release locally a highly reactive derivative (II) of such short half-life that its effects would hopefully be confined to the liver and particularly to intrahepatic proliferating tumour cells; fortunately the mitotic index of normal liver parenchymal cells is extremely low (Bukhari *et al.*, 1973[120]). The compound is currently under investigation by Drs. E. H. Williams and G. P. Warwick in cases of primary liver cancer in Africa; preliminary results are encouraging.

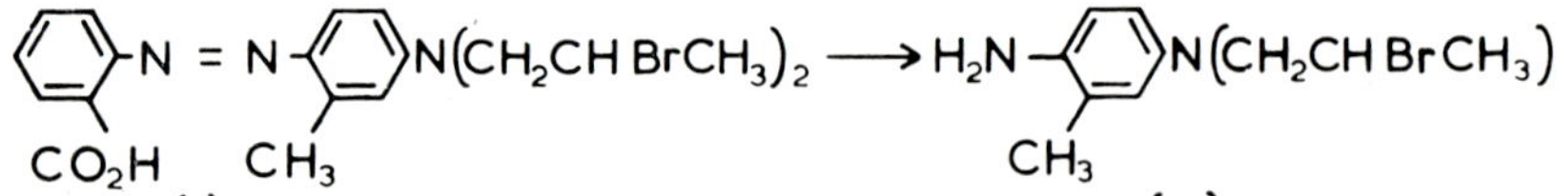

(I) (II)

Similarly, the biochemical involvement of both liver and tumour in an experimental system have suggested that the chemically simple aromatic *N*-mustard (III) may be of potential value in human tumours having a high glucuronidase activity (Connors and Whisson, 1966[121]).

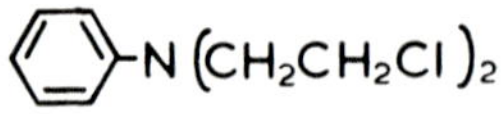

(III)

BCNU and CCNU are of special interest because of their value in the treatment of brain tumours. They are nominally *N*-mustard derivatives of nitrosoureas, but their mode of action is not known. They differ biologically from alkylating agents and it appears that their antitumour activity is due to products of chemical breakdown or metabolism (Montgomery *et al.*, 1967[122],

Livingston and Carter, 1970[76]; Oliverio *et al.*, 1970[123]; Hansen *et al.*, 1971[124] Carter *et al.*, 1972[125]).

The activity of dibromomannitol, used mainly in Hungary in the treatment of chronic granulocytic leukaemia, is thought to be largely due to its partial (non-enzymic) conversion to a bisepoxide (Livingston and Carter, 1970[76]; Elson *et al.*, 1968[126]).

The possible treatment of localized tumours by infusion of drugs into the supplying artery led to the design of the bromosulphur mustard (IV) (Davis and Ross, 1965[127]). The essential requirement in this approach was high chemical reactivity (short half-life) under physiological conditions, so that the drug is largely inactivated before it can reach sensitive normal tissues. Compound (IV) has been used clinically with some success, mainly in tumours of the head and neck (Meyza and Cobb, 1971[128]).

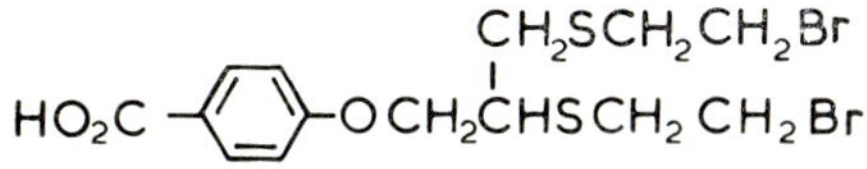

(IV)

Antimetabolites

All the commonly used antimetabolites (Table 13.1) other than the antifolates require an initial metabolic conversion to show activity.

Methotrexate remains the most important folate antagonist in cancer therapy, but much experimental work is still devoted to the general study of folate antagonism (Bertino, 1971[129]). Methotrexate and various analogues containing the 2, 4-diamino grouping strongly inhibit dihydrofolate reductase and thus prevent the conversion of the essential coenzyme, folic acid, into its active forms. A folate analogue, homofolate (V), is of interest because its reduced derivative, tetrahydrohomofolate (THHF; VI) prolonged the life of mice carrying methotrexate-resistant leukaemia. It was in fact less effective against methotrexate-sensitive lines. THHF strongly inhibited thymidylate synthetase from *E. coli*, and it was also reported that dihydrohomofolate was

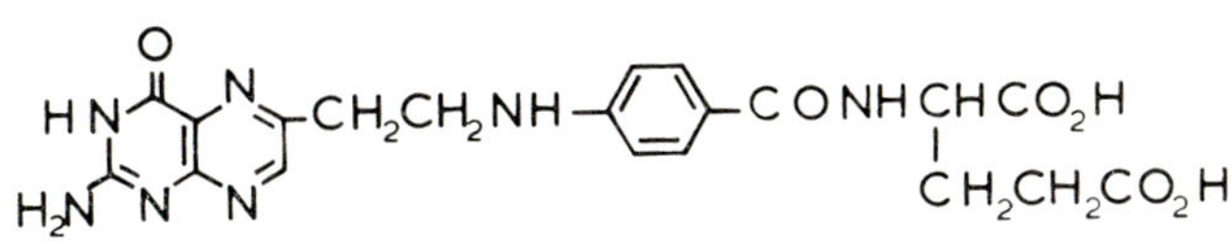

(V)

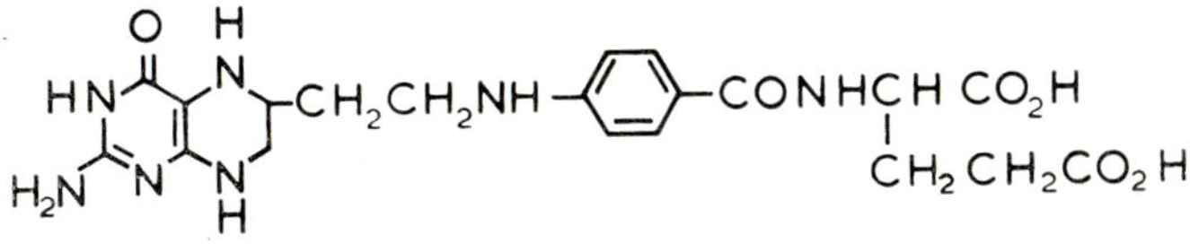

(VI)

reduced to the tetrahydro form by dihydrofolate reductase, present at high levels in methotrexate-resistant leukaemic cells. The consequent proposal that dihydrohomofolate would be the ideal drug in the therapy of methotrexate-resistant leukaemias seems, however, to have been premature: leukaemic cell reductase, unlike liver cell reductase, does *not* reduce dihydrofolate, and leukaemic-cell thymidylate synthetase is very much less sensitive than the bacterial enzyme to THHF. It appears at present that THHF may act by interfering with purine synthesis (Friedkin *et al.,* 1971[130]; Hakala, 1971[131]).

A group of 2, 4-diaminoquinazoline analogues are of special interest because of their high activity against L1210 leukaemia in mice. The aspartate series is more effective than the glutamate and one of the most effective members is methasquin (VII) (Hutchison, 1968, 1971[132,133]).

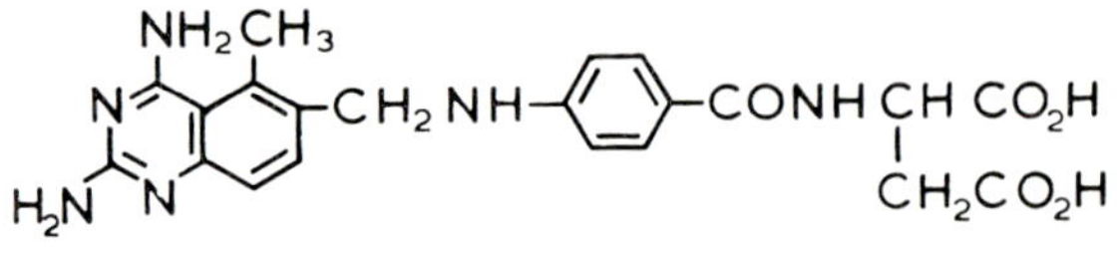

(VII)

6-Mercaptopurine (6MP) and 6-thioguanine (6TG) are the most important purine antagonists. The clinical value of the latter has become more fully recognized in recent years. Both compounds are converted by sensitive cells to their ribonucleotides, an essential step for cytotoxic activity (Montgomery, 1970[134]). Their modes of action are, however, different. 6MP appears to exert its effects by interfering directly, as its ribonucleotide or S-methylribonucleotide, with purine biosynthesis (Sartorelli and Creasey, 1969[135]; Bennett and Allan, 1971[136]). 6TG, unlike 6MP, is incorporated to a considerable extent into DNA in place of guanine; this is believed to cause subsequent faults either in DNA replication or RNA transcription or both (Le Page and Whitecar, 1971[137]; Beikirch *et al.* (1972)[138].

The most used of the pyrimidine antagonists at the present time is cytosine arabinoside. The agent appears to exert its major biological effects in the form of its triphosphate which inhibits DNA polymerase (Sartorelli and Creasey, 1969[179]; Muller *et al.,* 1972[139a]). The relationship of the compound with both cytidine and deoxycytidine has been studied (Roberts and Loehr, 1972[140]). The biochemistry of fluorouracils has been reviewed (Cheng, 1969[141]; Heidelberg, 1972[142]).

Antibiotics

The antibiotics listed in Table 13.1 are derived from various species of *Streptomyces.*

Studies of the way in which actinomycin D selectively inhibits DNA-dependent RNA synthesis have been reviewed by Goldberg and Friedman, (1971)[143] and Hash (1972)[144]. One model proposes that the antibiotic chromophore is bound by hydrogen bonding in the minor groove of helical DNA adjacent to a guanine residue. The cyclic peptides are packed into the minor groove, and form hydrogen bonds with the oxygen atoms of the DNA phosphate diester groups (Hamilton *et al.*, 1963[145]). A more recent suggestion is that the chromophore first intercalates between base pairs adjacent to a guanine-cytosine base pair, then the cyclic peptides undergo conformational changes that make dissociation of the complex very slow (Muller and Crothers, 1968[146]). The latter effect accounts for the high activity of actinomycin compared with simpler analogues. In any event, the bound antibiotic molecule appears to act by preventing the progression of RNA-polymerase along the DNA.

The inhibition of RNA synthesis by mithramycin can also be accounted for by the binding of the antibiotic to DNA (Goldberg and Friedman, 1971[143]).

Daunorubicin (daunomycin; rubidomycin) and adriamycin inhibit both DNA and RNA synthesis to varying degrees depending upon the test system (Bernard *et al.,* 1969[147]; Meriwether and Bachur, 1972[148]). Recently, an experimental therapeutic advantage was seen by administering daunorubicin as a complex with DNA to encourage pinocytototic ingestion by the tumour cells (Trouet *et al.,* 1972[149]).

Plant products

Vinblastine and vincristine are, like colchicine and its derivatives, metaphase poisons. They show many biological effects, among which is interference with microtubule formation and spindle assembly; but the antimitotic action is considered to be largely due to interference with nucleic acid synthesis (Sartorelli and Creasey, 1969[139]).

Enzymes

Recent reviews give detailed accounts of the biological and biochemical activity of L-asparaginase (Cooney and Handschumacher, 1970[150]; Grundmann and Oettgen, 1970[151]). Although early hopes concerning the therapeutic efficacy of the enzyme were not borne out, the agent plays a useful role in combination chemotherapy in certain malignant conditions. The asparaginase story is unique in that it revealed a qualitative difference—the ability or inability to synthesize asparagine—between normal and certain tumour cells.

The antitumour activity of a folate-cleaving bacterial enzyme, carboxypeptidase G_1, has been studied (Chabner *et al.,* 1972[152]). Daily doses of the enzyme increased the survival time of leukaemic (L1210) mice by up to nearly 90 per cent; inhibition of DNA synthesis in cells *in vitro* was characterized by a fall in the incorporation both of thymidine and uridine.

Hormone therapy

The use of the corticosteroids, (particularly prednisone and prednisolone) in the treatment of leukaemia has already been noted.

Tumours arising in tissues normally susceptible to changes in the hormonal environment tend to respond to treatment with hormones, especially in the earlier stages of the disease. In disseminated breast cancer in women, androgens (e.g., testosterone, as its propionate, or the synthetic fluoxymesterone) are commonly administered in the premenopausal patient; surgical ablation procedures, such as oophorectomy and adrenalectomy, are also often carried out to reduce the secretion of endogenous oestrogens. Sometimes, however, massive doses of oestrogen are of value in premenopausal women with metastatic breast cancer, probably because the formation of pituitary hormones is thereby suppressed. Treatment regimens for metastatic breast cancer may also employ corticosteroids and progestins. The basic rationale is not clear, but it is likely that steroid-induced remission is often a result of the interplay of a number of factors, including general metabolic effects, pituitary mediated action, and direct local action (Stoll, 1972[153]).

Oestrogen therapy is commonly used in the management of prostatic cancer. Its effects are thought to be due either to an anti-androgenic effect, or to suppression of gonadotrophin production or release. Stimulation of the immune mechanism of the host, or a direct effect on tumour DNA synthesis could conceivably also play a part (Fergusson, 1972[154]). Progestins are used in the management of metastatic endometrial carcinoma (Kistner, 1972[155]).

Miscellaneous agents

The mechanisms of action of hydroxyurea, procarbazine and some experimentally potent tumour-inhibitory thiosemicarbazones (Sartorelli and Creasey, 1969[139]), and of o, p′-DDD (Hart and Straw, 1971[156]) have been discussed.

The reason for the antitumour activity of various triazenes is not clear. The best known member of the group is DIC, of occasional value against melanoma (Cowan and Bergsagel, 1971[157]; Burke *et al.,* 1971[158]). The imidazole structure is not, however, essential for anti-tumour activity and can be replaced by an aryl group (Lin *et al.* (1972[159]; Audette *et al.,* 1973[160]). In both series, significant activity against the L1210 and TLX/5 tumours was shown only by compounds having at least one methyl group attached to the N^3 of the triazeno group; the 3, 3-bischloroethyl analogue of DIC is an exception to this rule. The mechanism of action of the triazenes is not known, but may depend upon carbonium ion formation and subsequent alkylation reactions (Shealy, 1970[161]). Of special interest is the fact that the cytotoxic effects of the triazenes against tumour cells *in vitro* is prevented by the addition of extracts of normal tissues but not those of tumour cells (Audette *et al.,* 1973[160]).

A series of bisdioxopiperazines were synthesized as potential latent chelating agents and some of the compounds were tumour inhibitory (Creighton *et al.,* 1969[162]). The most studied member, ICRF 159 (VIII), showed some encouraging results in a small clinical trial (Hellmann *et al.,* 1969[163]). Its experimental synergism with daunorubicin (Woodman *et al.,* 1972[99]) was referred to earlier. The compound is a potent inhibitor of DNA synthesis, an effect which could result from an acylation mechanism (Creighton and Birnie, 1970[164]). An interesting observation is the suppression of metastases from an experimental tumour, the Lewis lung carcinoma, probably resulting from the normalization of the tumour blood vessels (Le Serve and Hellman, 1972[165]). The non-ionic detergent, Triton WR 1339, can also affect the pattern of tumour growth. It inhibited the formation of metastases in one kind of *in vivo* system (Franchi *et al.,* 1971[166]) but enhanced tumour spread, as did some related surfactants, in another (Carter *et al.*, 1971[167]; Carter and Cotmore 1973[167a]; Cotmore and Carter 1973[167b]).

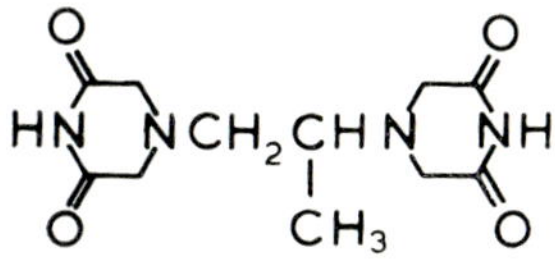

(VIII)

A number of platinum coordination compounds have been found to inhibit various experimental tumours. The active compounds are *cis*-diammino-dichloroplatinum-II (IX), *cis*-diammino-tetrachloroplatinum-IV (X), and corresponding structures in which the ammonia is replaced by organic bases. The *trans* analogues are not inhibitory (Rosenberg *et al.*, 1969[168];

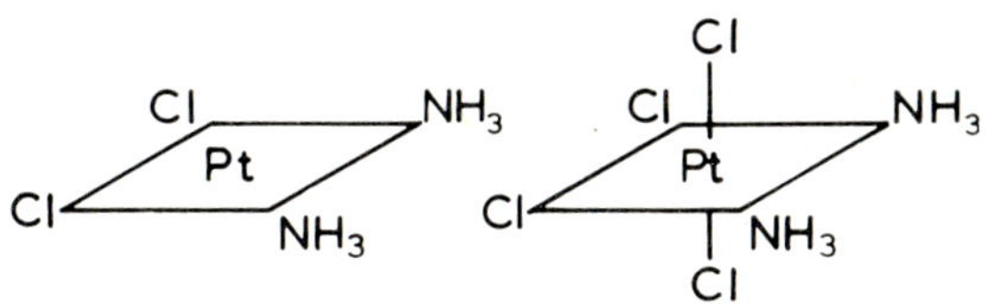

(IX) (X)

Rosenberg 1971[169]). Compound (IX) is being assessed clinically (Rosenberg, 1971[169]). The active compounds resemble the alkylating agents biologically. They inhibit DNA synthesis *in vitro* and compound (IX) cross-linked DNA in whole cells (Roberts and Pascoe, 1972[170]). Complexes containing cyclopentylamine and cyclohexylamine show a very much greater selectivity of action than the earlier compounds against an experimental plasma cell tumour[170a].

Rhodium acetate interfered with DNA replication and exhibited synergism with cytosine arabinoside against L1210 leukaemia in mice (Hughes *et al.*, 1972[171]). Gallium salts accumulated in certain human tumours and inhibited experimental solid tumours; they are currently in clinical trial (Arseneau *et al*, 1972[172]; Hart and Adamson, 1971[173]; Hart *et al.*, 1971[174]).

Interferon and interferon inducers are of potential value in the treatment of cancer. One inducer which has been extensively studied is polyinosinate-polycytidylate (Poly I: Poly C), an antiviral, anti-tumour synthetic twin-stranded polynucleotide (Levy, 1972[175]; Gresser, 1972[176]). It is not known whether, or to what extent, interferon produced by Poly I: Poly C contributes to the overall antitumour effect. It is also questionable whether the ability of Poly I: Poly C to enhance the immunological response of the host is a significant factor. It may be that the polynucleotide retards tumour growth by acting directly on tumour cells (Kreider and Benjamin, 1972[176a]).

Chalones are defined as endogenous mitotic inhibitors which control normal tissue proliferation. They are tissue specific rather than species specific. They were first studied by Bullough and his collaborators, and although they may have great potential, the practical problems of isolation and assay seem to mitigate their possible value at the present time (Iversen, 1970[177]; Maugh, 1972[178]).

Various derivatives of the antibiotic rifamycin, particularly rifampicin, originally of interest because of their antibacterial and antiviral activity, have been found to show a selective activity against reverse transcriptase (RNA-dependent DNA polymerase—see Gurgo *et al.,* 1972[179] and Yang *et al.,* 1972[180]). This enzyme is of interest because of its occurrence in animal tumour viruses and human leukaemic cells (Gallo *et al.,* 1970[181]), although its reported presence in normal cells Scolnick (1971[182]) suggests that it may not be specific to the oncogenic process. The extent of the specificity of its occurrence is not yet entirely clear. Toxicity for human leukaemic cells was greater and more selective (as compared with toxicity towards normal blood cells) when modified rifamycins were used which were potent inhibitors of viral reverse transcriptase. Some of these derivatives, however, are also active against DNA polymerase from normal cells, and it is not yet certain that their greater toxicity towards leukaemic cells can be related entirely to the sensitivity of reverse transcriptase (Smith *et al.,* 1972[183]).

Rifampicin inhibited the growth of virus-induced murine leukaemias *in vivo* (Gielkens *et al.,* 1972[184]), and also the Walker tumour (R. H. Adamson, 1971[185]).

Acknowledgement
I am indebted to Dr. C. D. R. Dunn for valuable discussions concerning the Bruce classification of anti-tumour chemotherapeutic agents.

References

1. Wood, H. B. *Cancer Chemother. Rep.*, Part 3, **2,** 9 (1971).
2. Burkitt, D. P. in *Burkitt's Lymphoma* (edited by D. P. Burkitt and D. H. Wright), pp. 45–51, Livingstone, Edinburgh and London (1970).
3. Clifford, P. in *Burkitt's Lymphoma* (edited by D. P. Burkitt and D. H. Wright), pp. 52–63, Livingstone, Edinburgh and London (1970).
4. Bagshawe, K. D. *Choriocarcinoma*, Arnold, London (1969).
5. Park, W. W. *Choriocarcinoma*, p.s, Heinemann Medical Books, London (1971).
6. Klein, G. in *Burkitt's Lymphoma* (edited by D. P. Burkitt and D. H. Wright), pp. 172–185, Livingstone, Edinburgh and London (1970).
7. Zubrod, C. G. *Proc. natn. Acad. Sci.* (*U.S.A.*), **69,** 1042 (1972).
8. Elderbout, P., Thomas, P. and Zwaveling, A. (editors), *Cancer Chemotherapy*, Leiden University Press, Leiden (1971).
9. Cobb., L. M. *Cancer Chemother. Rep.*, Part 1, **54,** 375 (1970).
10. Creech, O. and Krementz, E. T. *Adv. Cancer Res.*, **6,** 111 (1961).
11. Garai, O., Cooling, C. and Staunton, D. *Br. Med. J.*, **i,** 1231 (1962).
12. Gaudin, D. and Yielding, K. L. *Proc. Soc. exp. Biol. med.*, **131,** 1413 (1969).
13. Cohen, M. H. *J. natn. Cancer Inst.*, **48,** 927 (1972).
13a. Hutchison, D. J. *Adv. Cancer Res.*, **7,** 235 (1963).
14. Ball, C. R. in *Scientific Basis of Cancer Chemotherapy* (ed. by G. Mathé) (No. 21 of Recent Results in Cancer Research), pp. 26–40, Heinemann Medical Books, London (1969).
15. Wolpert, M. K. and Ruddon, R. W. *Cancer Res.*, **29,** 873 (1969).

16. Hill, B. T., Jarman, M. and Harrap, K. R. *J. med. Chem.*, **14,** 614 (1971).
17. Inaba, M., Moriwaki, A. and Sakurai, Y. *Int. J. Cancer*, **10,** 411 (1972).
18. Blakley, R. L. *Biochemistry of Folic Acid and Related Pteridines*, pp. 503–508, North Holland, Amsterdam and London (1969).
19. Paterson, A. R. P. and Hori, A. *Can. J. Biochem. Physiol.*, **40,** 181 (1962).
20. Kessel, D. and Bosmann, H. B. *Cancer Res.*, **30,** 2695 (1970).
21. Riehm, H. and Biedler, J. L. *Cancer Res.*, **31,** 409 (1971).
21a. Sköld, O. *Biochim. biophys. Acta,* **76,** 160 (1963).
22. Stock, J. A. in *Experimental Chemotherapy* (edited by R. J. Schnitzer and F. Hawking), Vol. **4,** pp. 79–237, Academic Press, London and New York (1966).
23. Sartorelli, A. C., LePage, G. A. and Moore, E. C. *Cancer Res.*, **18,** 1232 (1958).
24. Steuart, C. D. and Burke, P. J. *Nature New Biol., Lond.,* **233,** 109 (1971).
25. Harrap, K. R. and Hill, B. T. *Biochem. Pharmac.* **19,** 209 (1970).
26. Simard, R. and Cassingena, R. *Cancer Res.*, **29,** 1590 (1969).
27. Bieber, A. L. and Sartorelli, A. C. *Cancer Res.*, **24,** 1210 (1964).
28. Wolpert, M. K., Damle, S. P., Brown, J. E., Sznycer, E., Agrawal, K. C. and Sartorelli, A. C. *Cancer Res.*, **31,** 1620 (1971).
29. Haskell, C. M. and Canellos, G. P. in *Experimental and Clinical Effects of Asparaginase* (edited by E. Grundmann and H. F. Oettgen) (No. 33 of Recent Results in Cancer Research), pp. 188–193, Springer, Berlin, Heidelberg and New York (1970).
30. Calcutt, G. and Connors, T. A. *Biochem. Pharmac.*, **12,** 839 (1963).
31. Heidelberger, C., Kaldor, G., Mukherjee, K. L. and Danneberg, P. B. *Cancer Res.*, **20,** 903 (1960).
32. LePage, G. A. in *Oncology* (edited by R. L. Clark, R. W. Cumley, J. E. McKay and M. M. Copeland), Vol. **2,** pp. 275–278, Year Book Med. Publications, Chicago (1971).
33. Rosenau, W., Baxter, J. D., Rousseau, G. G. and Tomkins, G. M. *Nature New Biol., Lond.*, **237,** 20 (1972).
34. Willis, R. A. *Pathology of Tumours*, 4th edition, p. 133, Butterworth, London (1967).
35. Goldacre, R. J. and Sylvén, B. *Br. J. Cancer*, **16,** 306 (1962).
36. Griffiths, J. D. *Dis. Colon Rectum*, **8,** 114 (1965).
37. Connors, T. A. and Roe, F. J. C. in *Evaluation of Drug Activities: Pharmacometrics* (edited by D. R. Laurence and A. L. Bacharach), Vol. **2,** pp. 827–874, Academic Press, New York (1964).
38. Rosenoer, V. M. in *Experimental Chemotherapy* (edited by R. J. Schnitzer and F. Hawking), Vol. **4,** pp. 9–77, Academic Press, New York and London (1966).
39. Goldin, A., Sandberg, J. S., Henderson, E. S., Newman, J. W., Frei, E. and Holland, J. F. *Cancer Chemother. Rep.*, Part 1, **55,** 309 (1971).
40. E. O. R. T. C. Screening Group. *Europ. J. Cancer*, **8,** 185 (1972).
41. Larionov, L. F. *Cancer Chemother. Rep.*, Part 1, **54,** 71 (1970).
42. Cobb, L. M. *Br. J. Cancer*, **26,** 183 (1972).
43. Berenbaum, M. C. and Sheard, C. E. *Lancet*, **i,** 1116 (1972).
44. Annotation, *Lancet*, **i,** 827 (1972).
45. Foley, G. E. and Epstein, S. S. *Adv. Chemother.*, **1,** 175 (1964).
46. Thayer, P. S., Himmelfarb, P. and Watts, G. L. *Cancer Chemother. Rep.*, Part 2, **2,** 1 (1971).
47. Tanneberger, S. in *Aktuelle Probleme der Zellzüchtung* (edited by B. Mauersberger), p. 417, Stuttgart (1971).

48. Mitchell, J. S., Dendy, P. P., Dawson, M. P. and Wheeler, T. K. *Lancet*, **i,** 955 (1972).
49. Hudson, C. N. *Lancet*, **i,** 1116 (1972).
50. Dixon, R. L. *Cancer Chemother. Rep.* Part 3, **2,** 61 (1971).
51. Oliverio, V. T. *Cancer Chemother. Rep.* Part 3, **2,** 73 ;1971).
52. Skipper, H. E. *Cancer Res.*, **31,** 1173 (1971a).
53. Ball, C. R., Connors, T. A., Cooper, E. H. and Topping, N. E. *Neoplasma*, **14,** 253 (1967).
54. van Putten, L. M. in *The Design of Clinical Trials in Cancer Therapy* (Proceedings of a course in clinical pharmacology, Brussels, 1972 edited by M. Staquet), pp. 115–131, Editions Scientifiques Européenes, Brussels (1972).
55. Dunn, C. D. R. *Europ. J. Cancer*, **8.** 509 (1972a).
56. Dunn, C. D. R. *Europ. J. Cancer*, **8,** 517 (1972b).
56a. Blackett, N. M., and Adams, K. *Br. J. Haemat.*, **23,** 751 (1972).
56b. Ogawa, M., Bergsagel, D. E. and McCulloch, E. A. *Blood*, **41,** 7 (1973)
56c. Blackett, N. M. and Millard, R. E. *Nature*, **244,** 300 (1973).
57. Koss, L. G. *Ann. N.Y. Acad. Sci.*, **163,** 931 (1969).
58. Dunn, C. D. R. *J. natn. Cancer Inst.*, **48,** 639 (1972c).
59. Skipper, H. E., Schabel, F. M. and Wilcox, W. S. *Cancer Chemother. Rep.*, **35,** 1 (1964).
60. Goldin, A., Venditti, J. M., Humphreys, S. R. and Mantel, N. *J. natn. Cancer Inst.*, **17,** 203 (1956).
61. Lane, M. *Cancer Chemother. Rep.*, **3,** 1 (1959).
62. Skipper, H. E., Schabel, F. M. and Wilcox, W. S. *Cancer Chemother. Rep.*, **51,** 125 (1967).
63. Kline, I., Venditti, J. M., Tyrer, D. D. and Goldin, A. *Cancer Res.*, **26,** 853 (1966).
64. Skipper, H. E. in *The Cell Cycle and Cancer* (edited by R. Baserga), pp. 358–387, Dekkar, New York (1971b).
65. Straus, M. J., Mantel, N. and Goldin, A. *Cancer Res.*, **31,** 1429 (1971).
66. Venditti, J. M. *Cancer Chemother. Rep.*, Part 3, **2,** 35 (1971).
67. Schabel, F. M. *Cancer Res.*, **29,** 2384 (1969).
68. Bruce, W. R., Meeker, B. E. and Valeriote, F. A. *J. natn. Cancer Inst.*, **37,** 233 (1966).
69. van Putten, L. M. and Lelieveld, P. *Europ J. Cancer*, **7,** 11 (1971).
70. Valeriote, F. A. and Tolen, S. J. *Cancer Res.*, **32,** 470 (1972).
71. Dunn, C. D. R. Personal communication (1972d).
71a. Becker, A. J., McCulloch, E. A., Siminovitch, L. and Till, J. E. *Blood*, **26,** 296 (1965).
72. Valeriote, F. A. and Bruce, W. R. *J. natn. Cancer Inst.*, **38,** 393 (1967).
73. Bruce, W. R. and Meeker, B. E. *J. natn. Cancer Inst.*, **38,** 401 (1967).
74. Tannock, I. F. *Br. J. Cancer*, **22,** 258 (1968).
75. Steel, G. G. in *Natn. Cancer Inst. Monograph No.* 30 (Human Tumor Cell Kinetics), pp. 29–42 (1969).
76. Livingston, R. B. and Carter, S. K. *Single Agents in Cancer Chemotherapy*, IFI/Plenum, New York (1970).
77. Carter, S. K. *Cancer Chemother. Rep.* Part 3, **2,** 81 (1971).
78. Kellner, B., Nemeth, L. and Sellei, C. *Naturwissenschaften*, **42,** 528 (1955).
79. Larionov, L. F. *Cancer Chemotherapy*, Pergamon, Oxford (1965).
80. Gerhartz, H. in *Chemotherapy of Cancer* (edited by Pl. A. Plattner), pp. 62–72, Elsevier, Amsterdam (1964).
81. Hutter, A. M. and Kayhoe, D. E. *Am. J. Med.*, **41,** 581 (1966).

82. Holland, J. F. *J. Am. med. Ass.*, **209,** 1511 (1969).
83. Galton, D. A. G. and Spiers, A. S. D. *Progr. Haemeat.*, **7,** 343 (1971).
83a. Henderson, E. S. and Samaha, R. J. *Cancer Res.*, **29,** 2272 (1969).
84. Pinkel, D. *J. Am. med. Ass.*, **216,** 648 (1971).
85. Freireich, E. J., Bodey, G. P., Hart, J. S., Whitecar, J. P. and McCredie, K. B. in *Current Concepts in the Management of Lymphoma and Leukaemia* (edited by J. E. Ultmann, M. L. Griem, W. H. Kirsten and R. W. Wissler; No. 36 of Recent Results in Cancer Research), pp. 119–125, Heinemann Medical Books, London; and Springer, Berlin (1971).
86. Spiers, A. S. D. *Br. J. Haematol.*, **23,** 262 (1972).
87. Wiernick, P. H. and Serpick, A. A. *Cancer Res.*, **32,** 2023 (1972).
88. Powles, R. *Proceedings of Conference on B.C.G.,* October 1972, Washington, in press.
89. DeVita, V. T., Serpick, A. A. and Carbone, P. P. *Ann. intern. Med.*, **73,** 881 (1970).
90. Rubens, R. D., Wiltshaw, E., Boesen, E. and Galton, D. A. G. *Europ. J. Cancer*, **8,** 477 (1972).
91. Carter, S. K. in *The Design of Clinical Trials in Cancer Therapy* (Proceedings of a course in clinical pharmacology, Brussels, 1972; edited by M. Staquet), pp. 336–358, Editions Scientifique Européenes, Brussels (1972).
92. Mathé, G. (editor) *Aseptic Environments and Cancer Treatment* (No. 29 of Recent Results in Cancer Research), Springer, Berlin, Heidelberg and New York (1971).
93. Goldin, A., Venditti, J. M., Humphreys, S. R., Dennis, D. and Mantel, N. *Cancer Res.*, **15,** 742 (1955).
94. Djerassi, I. C. *Cancer Res.*, Part 1, **27,** 2561 (1967).
95. Mitchell, M. S., Wawro, N. W., DeConti, R. C., Kaplan, S. R., Papac, R. and Bertino, J. R. *Cancer Res.*, **28,** 1088 (1968).
96. Hryniuk, W. M. and Bertino, J. R. *J. clin. Invest.*, **48,** 2140 (1969).
97. Goldie, J., Price, L. A. and Harrap, K. R. *Europ. J. Cancer*, **8,** 409 (1972).
98. Kline, I., Gang, M. and Venditti, J. M. *Proc. Am. Ass. Cancer Res.*, **13,** 29 (1972).
99. Woodman, R. J., Kline, I. and Venditti, J. M. *Proc. Am. Ass. Cancer Res.*, **13,** 31 (1972).
100. Herman. E. H., Mhatre, R. M., Lee, I. P. and Waravdekar, V. S. *Proc. Soc. exp. Biol. Med.*, **140,** 234 (1972).
101. Capizzi, R. L., Summers, W. P. and Bertino, J. R. *Proc. Am. Ass. Cancer Res.*, **11,** 14 (1970).
102. Connors, T. A. and Jones, M. *Biochem. Pharmac.,* **19,** 2927 (1970).
103. Grindey, G. B. and Nichol, C. A. *Cancer Res.*, **32,** 527 (1972).
104. Tattersall, M. H. N., Connors, T. A. and Harrap, K. R. *Lancet*, **ii,** 1378 (1972).
105. Lieberman, M. W., Verlein, R. S., Landay, M., Liang, H., Farber, E., Lee, T.-N. and Starr, R. *Cancer Res.*, **30,** 942 (1970).
106. Borsa, J. and Whitmore, G. F. *Cancer Res.*, **29,** 737 (1969).
106a. Hryniuk, W. M., Fischer, G. A., and Bertino, J. R. *Molec. Pharmacol.*, **5,** 557 (1969).
106b. Borsa, J. *Ann. N.Y. Acad. Sci.*, **186,** 359 (1971).
107. Creighton, A. Personal communication (1972).
108. Currie, G. A. *Br. J. Cancer*, **26,** 141 (1972).
108a. Carter, R. L., Connors, T. A., Weston, B. J. and Davies, A. J. S. *Int. J. Cancer*, **11,** 345 (1973).
108b. Moore, M. and Withams, D. E., *Int. J. Cancer*, **11,** 358 (1973).

109. Currie, G. A. and Bagshawe, K. D. *Br. med. J.*, **i,** 541 (1970).
110. Mathé, G., Amiel, J. L., Schwarzenberg, L., Schneider, M., Cattan, A., Schlumberger, J. R., Hayat, M. and de Vassal, F. *Lancet*, **i,** 697 (1969).
111. M. R. C. Leukaemia Committee and Working Party on Leukaemia in Childhood *Br. med. J.*, **iv,** 189 (1971).
112. Ghose, T., Norvell, S. T., Guclu, A., Cameron, D., Bodurtha, A. and MacDonald, A. S. *Br. med. J.*, **iii,** 495 (1972).
113. Ross, W. C. J. *Biological Alkylating Agents*, Butterworths, London (1962).
114. Ochoa, M. and Hirschberg, E. in *Experimental Chemotherapy* (edited by R. J. Schnitzer and F. Hawking), Vol. **5,** pp. 1–132, Academic Press, New York and London (1967).
115. Stock, J. A. in *Drug Design* (edited by E. J. Ariens), Vol. **2,** pp. 531–571, Academic Press, New York and London (1971).
116. Connors, T. A. in *Antineoplastic and Immunosuppressive Agents* (edited by A. C. Sartorelli and D. G. Johns), in vol. 38 of *Handbook of Experimental Pharmacology* (edited by O. Eichler, A. Farah, H. Herken and A. D. Welch), in press, Springer, Berlin, Heidelberg and New York (1974).
117. Brookes, P. and Lawley, P. D. in *Isotopes in Experimental Pharmacology* (edited by L. J. Roth), pp. 403–414, University of Chicago Press, Chicago and London (1965).
118. Connors, T. A., Foster, A. B., Gilsenan, A. M., Jarman, M. and Tisdale, M. *Biochem. Pharmac.* **21,** 1373 (1972).
119. Ross, W. C. J., Warwick, G. P. and Roberts, J. J. *J. chem. Soc.*, 3110 (1955).
120. Bukhari, A., Connors, T. A., Gilsenan, A. M., Ross, W. C. J., Tisdale, M., Warwick, G. P. and Wilman, D. E. V. *J. natn., Cancer Inst.*, **50,** 245, (1973).
121. Connors, T. A. and Whisson, M. E. *Nature, Lond.*, **210,** 866 (1966).
122. Montgomery, J. A., James, R., McCaleb, G. S. and Johnston, T. P. *J. med. Chem.*, **10,** 668 (1967).
123. Oliverio, V. T., Vietzke, W. M., Williams, M. K. and Adamson, R. H. *Cancer Res.*, **30,** 1330 (1970).
124. Hansen, H. H., Selawry, O. S., Muggia, F. M. and Walker, M. D. *Cancer Res.*, **31,** 223 (1971).
125. Carter, S. K., Schabel, F. M., Broder, L. E. and Johnson, T. P. *Adv. Cancer Res.*, **16,** 273 (1972).
126. Elson, L. A., Jarman, M. and Ross, W. C. J. *Europ. J. Cancer*, **4,** 617 (1968).
127. Davis, W. and Ross, W. C. J. *J. med. Chem.*, **8,** 757 (1965).
128. Meyza, J. and Cobb, L. M. *Cancer*, **27,** 369 (1971).
129. Bertino, J. R. (editor) *Folate Antagonists as Chemotherapeutic Agents, Ann. N. Y. Acad. Sci.*, **186,** 1 (1971).
130. Friedkin, M., Crawford, E. J. and Plante, L. T. in *Folate Antagonists as Chemotherapeutic Agents* (edited by J. R. Bertino), *Ann. N.Y. Acad. Sci.*, **186,** 209 (1971).
131. Hakala, M. T. *Cancer Res.*, **31,** 813 (1971).
132. Hutchison, D. J. *Cancer Chemother. Rep.*, Part 1, **52.** 697 (1968).
133. Hutchison, D. J. in *Folate Antagonists as Chemotherapeutic Agents* (edited by J. R. Bertino), *Ann. N.Y. Acad. Sci.*, **186,** 496 (1971).
134. Montgomery, J. A. *Progr. med. Chem.*, **7,** 69 (1970).
135. Sartorelli, A. C. and Creasey, W. A. *Rev. Pharmac.*, **9,** 51 (1969).
136. Bennett, L. L. and Allan, P. W. *Cancer Res.*, **31,** 152 (1971).
137. LePage, G. A. and Whitecar, J. P. *Cancer Res.*, **31,** 1627 (1971).

138. Beikirch, H., Lentfer, D. and Lezius, A. *Z. physiol. Chem.*, **353,** 677 (1972).
139. Sartorelli, A. C. and Creasey, W. A. *A. Rev. Pharmac.*, **9,** 51 (1969).
139a. Muller, W. E. G., Yamazaki, Z. I., Sögtrop, H. H. and Zahn, R. K. *Europ. J. Cancer*, **8,** 421 (1972).
140. Roberts, D. W. and Loehr, E. V. *Cancer Res.*, **32,** 1160 (1972).
141. Cheng, C. C. *Progr. med. Chem.*, **6,** 67 (1969).
142. Heidelberger, C. in *Ciba Foundation Symposium on Carbon-Fluorine Compounds* (edited by K. Elliott and J. Birch), pp. 125–137, Elsevier-Excerpta Medica—North Holland, Amsterdam, London and New York (1972).
143. Goldberg, I. H. and Friedman, P. A. in *Drugs and Cell Regulation* (edited by E. Mihich), pp. 99–119 Academic Press, New York and London (1971).
144. Hash, J. H. *A. Rev. Pharmac.*, **12,** 35 (1972).
145. Hamilton, L., Fuller, W. and Reich, E. *Nature, Lond.*, **198,** 538 (1963).
146. Müller, W. and Crothers, D. M. *J. mol. Biol.*, **35,** 251 (1968).
147. Bernard, J., Paul, R., Boiron, M., Jacquillat, C. and Maral, R. (editors) *Rubidomycin* (No. 20 of Recent Results in Cancer Research), Springer, Berlin, Heidelberg and New York (1969).
148. Meriwether, W. D. and Bachur, N. R. *Cancer Res.*, **32,** 1137 (1972).
149. Trouet, A., de Campeneere, D. D. and de Duve, C. *Nature New Biol.*, **239,** 110 (1972).
150. Cooney, D. A. and Handschumacher, R. E. *A. Rev. Pharmac.*, **10,** 421 (1970).
151. Grundmann, E. and Oettgen, H. F. (editors) *Experimental and Clinical Effects of Asparaginase* (No. 33 of Recent Results in Cancer Research), Springer, Berlin, Heidelberg and New York (1970).
152. Chabner, B. A., Chello, P. L. and Bertino, J. R. *Cancer Res.*, **32,** 2114 (1972).
153. Stoll, B. A. in *Endocrine Therapy in Malignant Disease* (edited by B. A. Stoll), pp. 111–182, Saunders, London (1972).
154. Fergusson, J. D. in *Endocrine Therapy in Malignant Disease* (edited by B. A. Stoll), pp. 237–299, Saunders, London (1972).
155. Kistner, R. W. in *Endocrine Therapy in Malignant Disease* (edited by B. A. Stoll), pp. 323–327, Saunders, London (1972).
156. Hart, M. M. and Straw, J. J. *Biochem. Pharmac.*, **20,** 1679, 1689 (1971).
157. Cowan, D. H. and Bergsagel, D. E. *Cancer Chemother. Rep.*, Part 1, **55,** 175 (1971).
158. Burke, P. J., McCarthy, W. H. and Milton, G. W. *Cancer*, **27,** 744– (1971).
159. Lin, Y.-T., Loo, T. L., Vadlamudi, S. and Goldin, A. *J. med. Chem.*, **15** 201 (1972).
160. Audette, R. C. S., Connors, T. A., Mandel, H. G., Merai, K. and Ross, W. C. J. *Biochem, Pharmac.* **22,** 1855 (1973).
161. Shealy, Y. F. *J. pharm. Sci.* **59,** 1533 (1970).
162. Creighton, A. M., Hellman, K. and Whitecar, S. *Nature, Lond.*, **222,** 384 (1969).
163. Hellman, K., Newton, K. A., Whitmore, D. N., Hanham, I. W. F. and Bond, J. V. *Br. med. J.*, **i,** 822 (1969).
164. Creighton, A. M. and Birnie, G. D. *Int. J. Cancer*, **5,** 47 (1970).
165. Le Serve, A. W. and Hellmann, K. *Br. med. J.*, **i,** 597–601 (1972).
166. Franchi, G., Morasca, L., Reyers-Degli-Innocenti, I. and Garattini, S. *Europ. J. Cancer*, **7,** 533 (1971).
167. Carter, R. L., Birbeck, M. S. C. and Stock, J. A. *Int. J. Cancer*, **7,** 34 (1971).
167a. Carter, R. L., and Cotmore, S. In *Chemotherapy of Cancer Dissemination*

and Metastasis. Eds. S. Garattini and G. Franchi. Raven Press, New York. (1973).
167b. Cotmore, S. and Carter, R. L. *Int. J. Cancer*, **11,** 725 (1973).
168. Rosenberg, B., VanCamp, L., Trosko, J. E. and Mansour, V. H. *Nature, Lond.*, **222,** 385 (1969).
169. Rosenberg, B. *Platinium Metals Rev.*, **15,** 42 (1971).
170. Roberts, J. J. and Pascoe, J. M. *Nature, Lond.*, **235,** 282 (1972).
170a. Connors, T. A., Jones, M., Ross, W. C. J., Braddock, P. D., Khokhar, A. R. and Tobe, M. L. *Chem.-Biol. Interactions*, **5,** 415 (1972).
171. Hughes, R. G., Bear, J. L. and Kimball, A. P. *Proc. Am. Ass. Cancer Res.*, **13,** 120 (1972).
172. Arseneau, J., Adamson, R. H., Hart, M. M., Larson, S., Aamodt, R., Johnson, G. and Cannelos, G. P. *Proc. Am. Ass. Cancer Res.*, **13,** 40 (1972).
173. Hart, M. M. and Adamson, R. H. *Proc. natn. Acad. Sci.* (*U.S.A.*), **68,** 1623 (1971).
174. Hart, M. M., Smith, C. F., Yancey, S. T. and Adamson, R. H. *J. natn. Cancer Inst.*, **47,** 1121 (1971).
175. Levy, H. B. in *Cancer Chemotherapy* (edited by I. Brodsky and S. B. Kahn), Vol. **2,** pp. 53–61, Grune and Stratton, New York (1972).
176. Gresser, I. *Adv. Cancer Res.*, **16,** 97–140 (1972).
176a. Kreider, J. W. and Benjamin, S. A. *J. natn. Cancer Inst.*, **49,** 1303 (1972).
177. Iversen, O. H. *Cancer Res.*, **30,** 1481 (1970).
178. Maugh, T. H. *Science*, **176,** 1407 (1972).
179. Gurgo, C., Ray, P. and Green, M. *J. natn. Cancer Inst.*, **49,** 61 (1972).
180. Yang, S. S., Herrera, F. M., Smith, R. G., Reitz, M. J., Lancini, G., Ting, R. C. and Gallo, R. C. *J. natn. Cancer Inst.*, **49,** 7 (1972).
181. Gallo, R. C., Yang, S. S. and Ting, R. C. *Nature, Lond.*, **228,** 927 (1970).
182. Scolnick, E. M., Aaronson, S. A., Todaro, G. J. and Parks, W. P. *Nature, Lond.*, **229,** 318 (1971).
183. Smith, R. G., Whang-Peng, J., Gallo, R. C., Levine, P. and Ting, R. C. *Nature new Biol. Lond.*, **236,** 166 (1972).
184. Gielkens, A. L. J., Burghouts, J. T. M. and Bloemendal, H. *Int. J. Cancer*, **9,** 595 (1972).
185. Adamson, R. H. *Lancet*, **i,** 398 (1971).

ADDENDUM

A few comments and references to work published since this manuscript was prepared are given under headings used above.

Introduction

Several reviews on cancer chemotherapy have recently become available (Brodsky *et al.*, 1972[186]; Holland and Frei, 1973[187]; Brule *et al.*, 1973[188]; Raven, 1973[189]; Ansfield, 1973[190]).

The chemotherapy of human tumours including combination chemotherapy

More details of the treatment of AGL by chemotherapy combined with immunotherapy have been given (Powles *et al.*, 1973[191]; Freeman *et al.*, 1973[192]). The use of combinations of drugs in the treatment of breast cancer has been reviewed (Kelley, 1973[193]). Further to the report[112] that the action of chlorambucil was augmented by complexing it with tumour-specific antibodies, it has now been shown that a comparable degree of enhancement is achieved by giving the specific antibodies separately from the drug (Davies and O'Neill, 1973[194]; Rubens and Dulbecco, 1974[195]).

Notes on chemotherapeutic agents and their mechanisms of action

It now seems clear that the metabolite mainly responsible for the biological activity of cyclophosphamide is N,N-di(2-chloroethyl)phosphorodiamidic acid (Connors *et al.*, 1974[196]: Colvin *et al.*, 1973[197]). A new model of the binding of actinomycin D to DNA has been proposed and combines features of earlier[145, 146] suggestions (Sobell, 1973[198]). The properties of L-asparaginase have been reviewed (Wriston and Yellin 1973[199]). Bleomycin, a complex polypeptide antibiotic, is active against squamous cell carcinomas, lymphomas and testicular carcinomas. Toxic effects are seen in skin and lung, but the substance is exceptional in that it does not depress the marrow. The drug seems unlikely to be of great value used alone, but may prove a useful component of drug combinations (Blum *et al.*, 1973[200]). The mode of action of ICRF 159 is not known. It is active at concentrations below those which inhibit DNA synthesis, and blocks the cell cycle at the end of G2 or the beginning of mitosis (Hallowes *et al.*, 1974[201]). Chalones have been extensively reviewed (Forscher and Houck, 1973[202]). It is now established that reverse transcriptase is not a specific marker for malignancy. Studies on the enzyme may, however, be relevant to the possible viral aetiology of some forms of human cancer (*Lancet* annotation, 1973[203], Gallo and Spiegelman, 1974[204]).

References

186. Brodsky, I., Kahn, S. B. and Mayer, J. H. (editors), *Cancer Chemotherapy II* Grune and Stratton, New York and London (1972).
187. Holland, J. F. and Frei, E. (editors), *Cancer Medicine*, Lea and Febiger, Philadelphia (1973).
188. Brule, G., Eckhardt, S. J., Hall, T. C. and Winkler, A. *Drug Therapy of Cancer*, World Health Organization, Geneva (1973).
189. Raven, R. W. (editor), *Modern Trends in Oncology*—**1**, Parts I and II, Butterworths, London (1973).
190. Ansfield, F. J. *Chemotherapy of Malignant Neoplasms*, 2nd edition, Thomas, Springfield (1973).
191. Powles, R. L., Crowther, D., Bateman, C. J. T., Beard, M. E. J., McElwain, T. J., Russell, J., Lister, T. A., Whitehouse, J. M. A., Wrigley, P. F. M., Pike, M., Alexander, P. and Hamilton Fairley, G. *Br. J. Cancer*, **28**, 365 (1973).
192. Freeman, C. B., Harris, R., Geary, C. G., Leyland, M. J., MaCiver, J. E. and Delamore, I. W. *Br. med. J.*, iv, 571 (1973).
193. Kelley, R. M. in *Breast Cancer: a Challenging Problem* (edited by M. L. Griem, E. V. Jensen, J. E. Ultmann and R. W. Wissler; No. 42 of Recent Results in Cancer Research), Heinemann Medical Books, London; and Springer, Berlin (1973).
194. Davies, D. A. L. and O'Neill, G. J. *Br. J. Cancer*, **28**, Suppl. I, 285 (1973).
195. Rubens, R. D. and Dulbecco, R. *Nature, Lond.*, **248**, 81 (1974).

196. Connors, T. A., Cox, P. J., Farmer, P. B., Foster, A. B. and Jarman, M. *Biochem. Pharmac.*, **23,** 115 (1974).
197. Colvin, M., Padgett, C. A. and Fenselau, C. *Cancer Res.*, **33,** 915 (1973).
198. Sobell, H. M. *Progr. Nucleic Acid Res. mol. Biol.*, **13,** 153 (1973).
199. Wriston, J. C. and Yellin, T. O. *A. Enzymol.*, **39,** 185 (1973).
200. Blum, R. H., Carter, S. K. and Agre, K. *Cancer*, **31,** 903 (1973).
201. Hallowes, R. C., West, D. G. and Hellmann, K. *Nature, Lond.*, **247,** 487 (1964).
202. Forscher, B. K. and Houck, J. C. *Natn. Cancer Inst. Monograph No.* **38** (Chalones: Concepts and Current Researches) (1973).
203. Annotation, *Lancet*, **ii,** 542 (1973).
204. Gallo, R. C. and Spiegelman, S. *Lancet*, **i,** 1117 (1974).

INDEX